Techniques in Large Animal Surgery

Third Edition

Techniques in Large Animal Surgery

Third Edition

By

Dean A. Hendrickson
DVM, MS

Diplomate, American College of Veterinary Surgeons
Professor of Surgery, Department of Clinical Sciences
College of Veterinary Medicine and Biomedical Sciences
Colorado State University, Fort Collins, Colorado

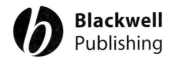

Blackwell
Publishing

Dean A. Hendrickson, DVM, MS, DACVS, is a professor of large animal surgery at Colorado State
University College of Veterinary Medicine, Fort Collins, Colorado.

Blackwell Publishing Professional
2121 State Avenue, Ames, Iowa 50014, USA

Orders: 1-800-862-6657
Office: 1-515-292-0140
Fax: 1-515-292-3348
Web site: www.blackwellprofessional.com

Blackwell Publishing Ltd
9600 Garsington Road, Oxford OX4 2DQ, UK
Tel.: +44 (0)1865 776868

Blackwell Publishing Asia
550 Swanston Street, Carlton, Victoria 3053, Australia
Tel.: +61 (0)3 8359 1011

First and Second editions, © Lea & Febiger
Third edition, © Blackwell Publishing

Library of Congress Cataloging-in-Publication Data

Hendrickson, Dean A.
    Techniques in large animal surgery. – 3rd ed. / by Dean A. Hendrickson.
        p.   ;   cm.
    Rev. ed. of: Techniques in large animal surgery / A. Simon Turner, C. Wayne McIlwraith. 2nd ed. 1989.
    Includes bibliographical references and index.
    ISBN 978-0-7817-8255-5 (alk. paper)
    1. Veterinary surgery.   2. Horses–Surgery.   3. Cattle–Surgery.   I. Turner, A. Simon (Anthony
Simon) Techniques in large animal surgery.   II. Title.
    [DNLM: 1. Surgery, Veterinary–methods.   2. Goats–surgery.   3. Horses–surgery.   4. Surgical
Procedures, Operative–veterinary.   5. Swine–surgery. SF 911 H498t 2007]

SF911.T87 2007
636.089'7–dc22
                                                    2007019840

The last digit is the print number: 9 8 7 6   2012

TABLE OF CONTENTS

PREFACE TO THE FIRST EDITION

The purpose of this book is to present some fundamental techniques in large animal surgery to both veterinary students and large animal practitioners. It is designed to be brief, discussing only the major steps in a particular operation, and each discussion is accompanied by appropriate illustrations. Most of the techniques presented in this book can be performed without the advantages of a fully equipped large animal hospital or teaching institution.

The book assumes a basic understanding of anatomy and physiology. Those who wish to know more about a particular technique are encouraged to consult the bibliography.

We and our colleagues at the Colorado State University Veterinary Teaching Hospital consider the procedures discussed in this book to be time honored. Some practitioners may perform certain techniques in slightly different ways. We would be happy to receive input about modifications of these techniques for future editions of this book.

All of the drawings in the book are original and based on rough sketches and photographs taken at various points during actual surgery. Occasionally, dissections were performed on cadavers.

The surgical procedures described in this text represent not only our thoughts, but suggestions from many of our colleagues as well. Their help was an important contribution to the production of this book. We are indebted to Dr. Wilbur Aanes, Professor of Surgery, Colorado State University, who unselfishly shared 30 years of his personal experience in large animal surgery with us. We are proud to be able to present in Chapter 10 of this book "Aanes' Method of Repair of Third-Degree Perineal Laceration" in the mare, a technique that he pioneered over 15 years ago. We also wish to give credit to the following faculty members at Colorado State University Veterinary Teaching Hospital who willingly gave us advice on the diagrams and manuscript of various techniques discussed in this book: Dr. Leslie Ball, Dr. Bill Bennett, Dr. Bruce Heath, Dr. Tony Knight, Dr. LaRue Johnson, Dr. Gary Rupp, Dr. Ted Stashak, Dr. Gayle Trotter, Dr. James Voss, and Dr. Mollie Wright. We also wish to

express appreciation to Dr. John Baker, Purdue University, and Dr. Charles Wallace, University of Georgia, for their comments on some questions we had. Dr. McIlwraith is also grateful to Dr. John Fessler, Professor of Surgery, Purdue University, for his inspiration and training.

We are particularly grateful to Dr. Robert Kainer, Professor of Anatomy, Colorado State University, for checking the manuscript and the illustrations and advising us on nomenclature. His input impressed upon us the importance of the relationship between the dissection room and the surgery room.

The terrific amount of time and effort involved with the illustrations will be clear to the reader who cares only to leaf through the book. For these illustrations, we are indebted to Mr. Tom McCracken, Director, Office of Biomedical Media, Colorado State University. We are thankful for his expertise, as well as his cooperation and understanding. The diagrams for "Aanes' Method of Repair of Third-Degree Perineal Laceration" were done by Mr. John Daughtery, Medical Illustrator, Colorado State University. We must also thank Kathleen Jee, who assisted with various aspects of the artwork. We would also like to thank Messrs. Al Kilminster and Charles Kerlee for taking photographs during the various surgical procedures that were used to assist with the artwork of this text.

The manuscript was typed by Mrs. Helen Mawhiney, Ms. Teresa Repphun, and Mrs. Jan Schmidt. We thank them for their patience and understanding during the many changes we made during the generation of the final manuscript.

We are grateful to the following instrument companies for allowing us to use some of the diagrams from their sales catalogs for inclusion in Chapter 3, "Surgical Instruments": Schroer Manufacturing Co., Kansas City, MO; Intermountain Veterinary Supply, Denver, CO; Miltex Instrument Co., Lake Success, NY; J. Skyler Manufacturing Co., Inc., Long Island, NY.

The idea for this book was conceived in 1978 when one of us (AST) was approached by Mr. George Mundroff,

Executive Editor, Lea & Febiger. We would like to thank him for his encouragement and guidance. We are also grateful to Mr. Kit Spahr, Jr., Veterinary Editor; Diane Ramanauskas, Copy Editor; Tom Colaiezzi, Production Manager; and Samuel A. Rondinelli, Assistant Production Manager, Lea & Febiger, for their assistance, as well as to others at the Publisher who assisted in the production of this book.

A. Simon Turner
C. Wayne McIlwraith
Fort Collins, Colorado

PREFACE TO THE SECOND EDITION

The second edition of *Techniques in Large Animal Surgery* is in response to the acceptance of the first edition and the continued need for such a book for both veterinary students and large animal practitioners. In many instances, the techniques are time honored and require no change from 5 years ago. In other instances, however, refinements in technique as well as improved perception of indications, limitations, and complications have made changes appropriate.

A significant change is the addition of Dr. R. Bruce Hull, Professor of Veterinary Clinical Sciences, The Ohio State University, as a contributor. He has carefully analyzed the entire bovine section, and his suggested changes and additions have been incorporated into the text. In addition, two procedures, "teaser bull preparations by penile fixation" and "treatment of vaginal prolapse by fixation to the prepubic tendon," have been added. We are most grateful in having Dr. Hull's help and expertise. Among the introductory chapters, the section on anesthesia required the most updating, and we are grateful to our colleague Dr. David Hodgson at Colorado State University for his review and advice. Two new procedures, "superior check ligament desmotomy" and "deep digital flexor tenotomy," were considered appropriate additions to this edition. We are grateful to Dr. Larry Bramlage, Ohio State University, for his comments and help with the first of these procedures. Many of the other changes in this edition are in response to the book reviews and comments on the first edition returned to Lea & Febiger. To these people, we appreciate your feedback.

A chapter on llama tooth removal was added because of the increased popularity of this species, especially in our own part of the country. Although we only discuss this one technique, it should not be inferred that other operations are unheard of in llamas. We have corrected angular limb deformities, repaired fractures, and performed gastrointestinal surgery, among other procedures, but tooth removal is the most common. Descriptions of these other procedures in llamas are beyond the scope of this book at this stage.

The need for more sophisticated equine techniques prompted us to produce the textbook *Equine Surgery: Advanced Techniques* in 1987. It is envisioned that the book will be used as a companion to this second edition, to provide a full spectrum of equine procedures, with the well-accepted format of concise text and clear illustrations.

Again, we are thankful to Mr. Tom McCracken, Assistant Professor, Department of Anatomy and Neurobiology, Colorado State University, for his talent in capturing the techniques described in his line drawings. We are also indebted to Helen Acvedo for typing our additions and to Holly Lukens for copyediting. Finally, our thanks again to the excellent staff at Lea & Febiger for the production of this edition.

A. Simon Turner
C. Wayne McIlwraith
Fort Collins, Colorado

PREFACE TO THE THIRD EDITION

The first two editions of *Techniques in Large Animal Surgery* have been well accepted, much to the credit of Drs. Turner and McIlwraith. They have been excellent texts for the veterinary student and the large animal practitioner. I was fortunate to be able to take on the task when it came time to update the information for a third edition. I am deeply appreciative of the opportunity to take such an excellent text and update it with new information and techniques.

The third edition of *Techniques in Large Animal Surgery* has been updated in response to the continued need for such a book for both veterinary students and large animal practitioners. There are some techniques that are time tested and continue to be included. There are other techniques that have been refined or replaced, and these are included in the new text.

New information has been included in essentially every chapter. We have made extensive use of tables to simplify the information. The anesthesia section includes new and updated information on sedation and anesthetic agents. The instrument section has been evaluated, adding new instruments where applicable and removing outdated or unavailable instruments. The section on suture materials has been updated to include new materials. There are new illustrations in the suture pattern section to better aid the practitioner with surgical techniques. The sections on wound management and reconstructive surgery have been increased to provide up-to-date information on wound care. Tables of required instrumentation have been added to all sections of the remaining surgical chapters to aid in surgical planning and preparation.

I am very grateful for our new illustrator Anne Rains; she has done an excellent job and has made my life very easy. I am indebted to Joanna Virgin who has done the lion's share of the research to make sure this text was as up-to-date and accurate as possible. I could not have done this work without her. Thanks to the folks at Blackwell for their help and assistance in the production of this edition.

Dean A. Hendrickson
Fort Collins, Colorado

Techniques in Large Animal Surgery

Third Edition

Chapter 1

PRESURGICAL CONSIDERATIONS

Objectives

1. Discuss some of the presurgical considerations that can affect the success of a procedure, including the physiological state and condition of the patient; predisposing factors for infection; and the limitations of the surgeon, facilities, and equipment.
2. Describe the methods of asepsis and antisepsis.
3. Describe the classification of different procedures with regard to risk of infection and degree of contamination.
4. Discuss the judicious use of antibiotics and their applications prophylaxis and postoperative infection.
5. Describe proper techniques for surgical site preparation.

Preoperative Evaluation of the Patient

Before a surgical procedure, a physical examination is generally indicated. This applies to both emergency and elective surgery. The following are laboratory tests that are generally indicated for horses based upon animal age and systemic status at our clinic:

- For horses younger than 4 years old and healthy:
  - Packed cell volume (PCV)
  - Total protein
- Appropriate for horses greater than 4 years old or those that are systemically ill:
  - Complete blood count (CBC)
  - Chemistry

Exactly where to draw the line on laboratory tests is largely a matter of judgment on the part of the surgeon.

Obviously, if the surgery consists of castration of several litters of piglets, then for purely economic reasons laboratory tests prior to surgery will not be performed. In many cases, however, additional tests will be necessary. The following are examples of other optional tests and their indications:

- Electrolyte measurement for right-sided abomasal diseases of dairy cow
- Urinalysis in the dairy cow to evaluate presence of ketosis
- Measurement of blood urea nitrogen (BUN) and creatinine if urinary problems are suspected
- Analysis of peritoneal fluid prior to laparotomy for horses with colic
- Full chemistry panels when there are age or systemic considerations

If any laboratory parameters are abnormal, the underlying causes should be investigated and efforts made to correct them. In "elective" surgery this is possible, but it may not be possible in an emergency. The owner should be made aware of any problems prior to subjecting the animal to surgery. Risks are always present in normal elective surgery, and these should be explained to the owner.

Fluid replacement should be performed if necessary. In the elective case, the surgical procedure should be postponed if the animal's physical condition or laboratory parameters are abnormal. In some animals, internal and external parasitism may have to be rectified to achieve this goal.

Medical records should be kept at all times. Obviously this can be difficult in such cases as castration of several litters of piglets, but record keeping should become an essential part of the procedure for horses and cattle in a hospital and herd records should be kept in all other situations. Finally, if the animal is insured, the insurance company must be notified of any surgical procedure; otherwise, the policy may be void.

Surgical Judgment

Surgical judgment cannot be learned overnight by reading a surgery textbook, nor is it necessarily attained by years of experience. The surgeon who continually makes the same mistake will probably never possess good surgical judgment. Not only should the surgeon learn from his own mistakes; he also should learn from the mistakes of others, including those documented in the surgical literature. As part of surgical judgment, the surgeon must ask the following questions:

Is the surgery necessary?
What would happen if the surgery were not performed?
Is the procedure within the capabilities of the surgeon, the facilities, and the technical help?
What is the economical and/or sentimental value of the animal; does it outweigh or reinforce the cost of the surgery?

If the surgeon finds that the procedure is too advanced for his or her capabilities and/or facilities, the surgery should be referred. Some veterinarians have a fear that this will mean loss of the client's business in the future, but this is rarely the case. If the surgeon explains why the case should be referred elsewhere, most clients will be grateful for such frankness and honesty. It is inexcusable to operate on a patient and then have complications arise due to inadequate training and facilities, when the surgery could easily have been referred to a well-equipped, well-staffed hospital with specially qualified personnel. Clearly, this rule has exceptions—mainly the emergency patient, which may fare better by undergoing immediate surgery than being subjected to a long trailer ride to another facility.

Many of the procedures described in this book can be done "on the farm." Some, such as arthrotomy for removal of chip fractures of the carpal and sesamoid bones in horses, should be done in a dust-free operating theater. If clients want these latter procedures to be done "in the field," they should understand the disastrous consequences of postsurgical infection. The surgeon must be the final judge of whether his facilities or experience are suitable.

Principles of Asepsis and Antisepsis

There are three determinants of an infection in a surgical site: host defense, physiologic derangement, and bacterial contamination risk at surgery.[2] Control methods include aseptic surgical practices as well as identification of the high-risk patient, correction of systemic imbalances prior to surgery, and the proper use of prophylactic antibiotics.[3]

We are sometimes reminded by fellow veterinarians in the field that we must teach undergraduates how to do surgery in the real world. By this they mean that we must ignore aseptic draping and gloving and lower the standard to a "practical" level. This is fallacious in our opinion. Although we recognize that the ideal may be unattainable in private practice, one should always strive for the highest possible standard; otherwise, the final standard of prac-

Table 1-1. Surgical classifications.

Classification	Description	Examples
Clean	Gastrointestinal, urinary, or respiratory tract is not entered.	Arthrotomy for removal of a chip fracture of a carpal bone of a horse
Clean-contaminated	Gastrointestinal, respiratory, or urinary tract is entered. There is no spillage of contaminated contents.	Abomasopexy for displaced abomasums in the dairy cow
Contaminated-dirty	Gross spillage of contaminated body contents or acute inflammation occurs.	Wounds Abscesses Devitalized bowel

tice may be so low that the well-being of the patient is at risk, not to mention the reputation of the veterinarian as a surgeon. For this reason, we believe that it behooves us as instructors of the undergraduate to teach the *best possible methods with regard to asepsis as well as technique.*

The extent to which the practice of asepsis or even antisepsis is carried out depends on the classification of the operation, as shown in Table 1.1. This classification may also help the veterinarian decide whether antibiotics are indicated or whether postoperative infection can be anticipated.

Surgical Classifications

Once the surgeon has categorized the surgical procedure, appropriate precautions to avoid postoperative infection can be determined. In all cases, however, the surgical site is prepared properly, including clipping and aseptic scrubbing.

Whatever category of surgery is performed, clean clothing should be worn. The wearing of surgical gloves is good policy even if to protect the operator from infectious organisms that may be present at the surgical site. Surgical gowns, gloves, and caps are recommended for clean surgical procedures, although such attire has obvious practical limitations for the large animal surgeon operating in the field. The purpose of this book is to present guidelines rather than to lay down hard-and-fast rules. For example, the decision between wearing caps, gowns, and gloves and wearing just gloves can be made only by the surgeon. Good surgical judgment is required. In general, it is better to be more careful than what may appear necessary in order to be better prepared when problems arise.

Role of Antibiotics

Antibiotics should never be used to cover flaws in surgical technique. The young surgeon is often tempted, sometimes under pressure from the client, to use antibiotics prophylactically. However, the disadvantages of antimicrobial therapy often outweigh its benefits. Extended periods of antimicrobial therapy can select for resistant organisms and adversely affect the gastrointestinal tract by eliminating many of the normal enteric organisms and allowing outgrowths of pathogenic bacteria, such as *Clostridia* spp., which can result in colitis and diarrhea.[4] When selecting an antibiotic regimen, the surgeon should consider the following aspects:

Does the diagnosis warrant antibiotics?
Which organisms are most likely to be involved and what is their in vitro antimicrobial susceptibility?
What is the location or likely location of the infection?
How accessible is the location of the infection to the drug?
What possible adverse reactions and toxicities to the drug could occur?
What dosage and duration of treatment are necessary to obtain sufficient concentrations of the drug?

Again, some judgment is required, but suffice to say, antibiotics should never be a substitute for "surgical conscience." *Surgical conscience* consists of the following: dissection along tissue planes, gentleness in handling tissues, adequate hemostasis, selection of the best surgical approach, correct choice of suture material (both size and type), closure of dead space, and short operating time.

If the surgeon decides that antibiotics are indicated, special attention should be given to selecting the type of antimicrobial drug, dosage, and duration of use. Ample scientific literature indicates that for maximum benefit, antimicrobials should be administered prophylactically prior to surgery and, at the latest, during surgery. Beyond 4 hours postsurgically, the administration of prophylactic antibiotics has little to no effect on the incidence of postoperative infection.[1] The duration of treatment should not exceed 24 hours because most research indicates that antimicrobial use after this period of time does not confer further benefits. If longer duration of antimicrobial coverage is necessary, the full duration of the specific antimicrobial drug selected should be given. This varies depending on the drug; however, in most cases the duration is at least 3 to 5 days. If the surgeon is operating on a food animal, there are regulations for withdrawal times from different antimicrobial drugs prior to slaughter that must be taken into account.

If topical antibiotics are used during surgery, they should be nonirritating to the tissues; otherwise, tissue necrosis from cellular damage will outweigh any advantageous effects of the antibiotics. It is also beneficial when using topical antibiotics to use antibiotics that are not generally used systemically.

All equine surgical patients should have tetanus prophylaxis. If the immunization program is doubtful, the horse can receive 1500 to 3000 units tetanus antitoxin. Horses on a permanent immunization program that have not had tetanus toxoid within the previous 6 months should receive a booster injection.

Tetanus prophylaxis is generally not provided for food animals, but an immunization program may be considered, especially if a specific predisposition is thought to exist.

Preoperative Planning

The surgeon should be thoroughly familiar with the regional anatomy. In this book we illustrate what we consider to be the important structures in each technique. If more detail is required, a suitable anatomy text should be consulted. Not only should the procedure be planned prior to the surgery, but the surgeon also should visit the dissection room and review local anatomy on cadavers prior to attempting surgery on a client's animal. We are fortunate in veterinary surgery to have greater access to cadavers than our counterparts in human surgery.

Preparation of the Surgical Site

For the large animal surgeon, preparation of the surgical site can present major problems, especially in the winter and spring when farms can be muddy. Preparation for surgery may have to begin with removal of dirt and manure. Some animals that have been recumbent in mud and filth for various reasons may have to be hosed off. Hair should then be removed, not just from the surgical site, but from an adequate area surrounding the surgical site.

The clipping should be done in a neat square or rectangular shape with straight edges. Surprisingly, this, along with the neatness of the final suture pattern in the skin, is how the client judges the skill of the surgeon. Clipping may be done initially with a no. 10 clipper blade, and then the finer no. 40 blade may be used. The incision site can be shaved with a straight razor in horses and cattle, but debate exists regarding the benefit or problems associated with this procedure. In sheep and goats, in which the skin is supple and pliable, it is difficult to shave the edges.

Preparation of the surgical site, such as the ventral midline of a horse about to undergo an exploratory laparotomy, may have to be performed when the animal is anesthetized. If surgery is to be done with the animal standing, an initial surgical scrub, followed by the appropriate local anesthetic technique and a final scrub, is standard procedure.

For cattle or pigs, the skin of the surgical site can be prepared for surgery with the aid of a stiff brush. For the horse, gauze sponges are recommended. Sheep may require defatting of the skin with ether prior to the actual skin scrub. The antiseptic scrub solution used is generally a matter of personal preference. Either povidone-iodine scrub (Betadine Scrub) alternated with a 70% alcohol rinse, or Chlorhexidine alternated with water, can be used. Finally, the skin can be sprayed with povidone-iodine solution (Betadine Solution) and allowed to dry.

Scrubbing of the proposed surgical site is done immediately prior to the operation. Scrubbing should commence at the proposed site of the incision and progress toward the periphery; one must be sure not to come back onto a previously scrubbed area. Some equine surgeons clip and shave the surgical site the night before the surgery, perform an aseptic preparation as previously described, and wrap the limb in a sterile bandage until the next day. A shaving nick made the day before surgery may be a pustule on the day of surgery, however, and this is generally not recommended for anything proximal to the pastern region.

When aseptic surgery is to be performed, an efficient draping system is mandatory. Generally, time taken to drape the animal properly is well spent. The draping of cattle in the standing position can be difficult, especially if the animal decides to move or becomes restless. It can be difficult to secure drapes with towel clamps in the conscious animal because only the operative site is anesthetized. If draping is not done, the surgeon must minimize contact with parts of the animal that have not been scrubbed. The tail must be tied to prevent it from flicking into the surgical field.

Several operations described in this book require the strictest of aseptic technique, and sterile, antimicrobial, adhesive, incise drapes are indicated. Characteristics of sterile plastic adhesive drapes include their ability to adhere, their antimicrobial activity, and their clarity when applied to the skin. Probably the most desirable feature is the one first mentioned. With excessive traction or manipulation, some brands of drapes quickly separate from the skin surfaces, and this separation instantly defeats their purpose.

Rubberized drapes are helpful when large amounts of fluids (such as peritoneal and amniotic fluid) are encountered during the procedure. Rubberized drapes are also useful to isolate the bowel or any other organ that is potentially contaminated, to prevent contamination of drapes. Newer fluid-impermeable paper drapes that are disposable make the surgeon's job even easier.

Postoperative Infection

Prevention of postoperative infection should be the goal of the surgeon, but infection may occur despite all measures taken to prevent it. If infection occurs, the surgeon must decide whether antibiotic treatment is indicated, or whether the animal is strong enough to fight it using its own defense mechanisms. Some surgical wounds require drainage at their most ventral part, whereas others require more aggressive treatment. If, in the judgment of the surgeon, the infection appears to be serious, a Gram stain, culture, and sensitivity testing of the offending microorganism(s) will be indicated. A Gram stain may give the surgeon a better idea of what type of organism is involved and may in turn narrow the selection of antibiotics. Sometimes in vitro sensitivities have to be ignored because the antibiotic of choice would be prohibitively expensive. This is especially true for adult cattle and horses. A broad-spectrum antibiotic should be given, if possible, as soon as practical.

References

1. Burke, J.F.: Preventing bacterial infection by coordinating antibiotic and host activity. *In* Symposium on prophylactic use of antibiotics. South Med. J., *70:*24, 1977.
2. Cristou, N.V., Nohr, C.W., and Meakins, J.L.: Assessing operative site infection in surgical patients. Arch. Surg., *122:*165, 1987.
3. Nelson, C.L.: Prevention of sepsis. Clin. Orthop., *222:*66, 1987.
4. Papich, M.G.: Antimicrobial therapy for gastrointestinal disease. Vet. Clin. Eq., *19:*645–663, 2003.

Chapter 2

ANESTHESIA AND FLUID THERAPY

Objectives

1. Describe routine local and regional anesthetic techniques in large animals.
2. Discuss some of the species differences in reference to anesthetic techniques.
3. Describe the indications for, advantages of, and disadvantages of general anesthesia in large animal species.
4. Provide a basic discussion of the fundamentals of fluid therapy, including methods for ascertaining fluid deficits, acid-base imbalances, and electrolyte abnormalities.
5. Discuss specific fluid therapies in patients undergoing elective surgery and compromised patients, either with or without preliminary data.

Anesthesia

The purpose of this section is not to present an in-depth discussion of anesthesia. Details on the principles of anesthesia, recognition of stages of anesthesia, monitoring, and the pharmacology and physiology associated with anesthesia are well documented in other texts.[34,58,77] In this section, anesthetic techniques used routinely by us are presented. Many alternatives are available and personal preferences differ, but we consider these to be suitable for the individual surgical techniques presented in this textbook.

Local and Regional Anesthesia (Analgesia)

Local or *infiltration anesthesia* is the injection of a surgical site directly with analgesic agent. *Regional anesthesia* is desensitization by blocking the major nerve(s) to a given region. Both techniques permit the desensitization of the surgical site. Because they are purely analgesic techniques, the term *analgesia* is preferred to the term anesthesia. The two analgesic agents most commonly used are 2% lidocaine hydrochloride (Lidocaine Hydrochloride Injection 2%) and 2% mepivacaine hydrochloride (Carbocaine). Although lidocaine has essentially replaced procaine hydrochloride as the standard local analgesic agent, mepivicaine is also widely used because of its rapid onset, longer duration, and less associated tissue reaction.[7]

In the ox in particular, surgical procedures are commonly performed under local or regional analgesia. In many instances, surgery is performed on the standing animal, and no sedation is used. In other instances, a combination of sedation and casting is used in conjunction with a local analgesic regimen. Local and regional analgesic techniques that are used routinely in individual species follow.

Infiltration Analgesia

The principles of infiltration analgesia are simple and are similar for all species. The limits of the region to be infiltrated may be well defined by making a subcutaneous wheal. A small amount of analgesic agent is injected at an initial site with a small needle and then, if a long region of analgesia is required, a longer needle is inserted through the initial region of desensitization. Needles should always be reinserted through a region that has already been infiltrated. The skin and subcutis should be infiltrated first and then the deeper layers, such as muscle and peritoneum. Avoid the injection of significant amounts of analgesic solution into the peritoneal cavity; rapid absorption can take place, with the possibility of resultant toxicity. Infiltrating injections should be made in straight lines, and "fanning" should be avoided as much as possible because of the tissue trauma it causes.

Infiltration analgesia is commonly used for suturing wounds and for removing cutaneous lesions in all large animal species. It may also be used in the form of a *line block* for laparotomy, in which case the analgesic agent is infiltrated along the line of incision. Although convenient, the infiltration of analgesic agent into the incision line causes edema in the tissues and may affect wound healing. In this respect, regional analgesic techniques are generally considered preferable.

Techniques of Regional Analgesia

Inverted L Block

Inverted L block is the simplest technique of regional analgesia for laparotomy and laparoscopy approaches in large animal species. It may be used for either flank or paramedian laparotomies, laparoscopic procedures such as cryptorchidectomies and ovariectomies, and urogenital surgery. The principles of the technique are illustrated in the ox in Figure 2-1. It is a nonspecific technique in which local analgesic agent is deposited in the form of an inverted L to create a wall of analgesia enclosing the surgical field. All nerves entering the operative field are blocked. The procedure is facilitated by the use of an 8- to 10-cm, 16- to 18-gauge needle. Up to 100 ml of local analgesic agent may be used in an adult-sized horse or cow; however, the author recommends using no more than 60 ml. The vertical line of the L passes caudal to the last rib, and the horizontal line is just ventral to the transverse processes of the lumbar vertebrae. Ten to fifteen minutes should be allowed for the analgesic agent to take effect.

Special consideration should be given to regional and local analgesia in sheep and goats. Systemic toxicity is a potential complication with these species, and dosage limits should be considered. Experiments in sheep have shown that convulsions occur in adult sheep at a dose of lidocaine hydrochloride of 5.8 ± 1.8 mg/kg intravenously.[59] Subconvulsive doses of lidocaine hydrochloride often produce drowsiness, however. Above convulsive doses, hypotension occurs at 31.2 ± 2.6 mg/kg, respiratory arrest at 32.4 ± 2.8 mg/kg, and circulatory collapse at 36.7 ± 3.3 mg/kg. An initial dose of 6 mg/kg is within a reasonable margin to avoid serious complications. If convulsions do occur, they can be controlled with an intravenous dose of 0.5 mg/kg of diazepam (Valium). Diluted solutions of lidocaine in local blocks of sheep and goats are advantageous in these species.[27,34]

Paravertebral Block

The *paravertebral block* is not commonly used in equine species, but is frequently performed in cattle, sheep, and goats.[10,27] In ruminants, the thirteenth thoracic nerve (T13), the first and second lumbar nerves (L1 and L2), and the dorsolateral branch of the third lumbar nerve (L3) supply sensory and motor innervation to the skin, fascia, muscles, and peritoneum of the flank. Regional analgesia

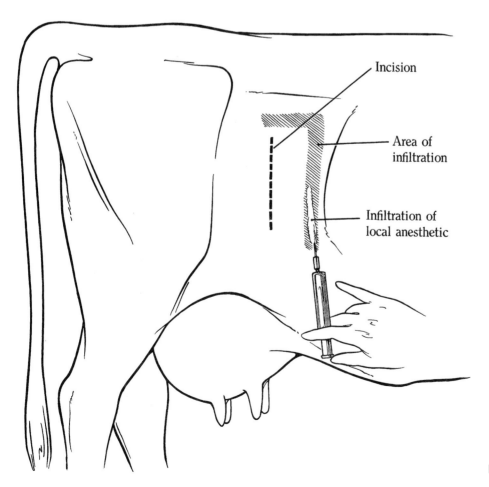

Incision

Area of infiltration

Infiltration of local anesthetic

Fig. 2-1. Inverted L block.

of these nerves is the basis of the paravertebral block. For practical purposes with flank laparotomy, blocking of the dorsolateral branch of L3 is not generally considered necessary and may be contraindicated because if one has miscounted the vertebrae, one may actually block L4, which has nerve fibers running to the back legs.

Various techniques for paravertebral block have been described. Walking the needle off the caudal edge of the transverse process, as illustrated in Figure 2-2, is most satisfactory. Anatomically, the nerve is most localized at its intervertebral foramen. By walking the needle off the caudal edge of the transverse process, one can deposit the analgesic solution close to the foramen; therefore, one has to block only a single site rather than the dorsal and ventral branches individually. The transverse processes are used as landmarks. Remembering that the transverse processes slope forward, the transverse process of L1 is used as a landmark to block T13, and the transverse processes of L2 and L3 are similarly used to locate nerves L1 and L2, respectively. When the transverse process has been located, a line is drawn from its cranial edge to the dorsal midline. The site for injection is 3 to 4 cm from the midline (Figure 2-2). The transverse process of L1 is difficult to locate in fat animals, in which case the site is estimated relative to the distance between the processes of L2 and L3. Local blebs are placed, and a 1-in, 16-gauge needle is inserted to act as a trocar in placing a 10-cm, 20-gauge needle. This second needle is inserted perpendicularly until the transverse process is encountered. The needle is then walked off the caudal border of the transverse process and advanced 0.75 cm; 10 ml of local analgesic solution are placed at each site. The incision site should be tested with a needle, and if the block has been properly placed, it will be effective almost immediately. In testing the block, one must remember that the distribution of the nerves is such that T13 innervates the ventral flank area, whereas L2 innervates the area close to the transverse processes.

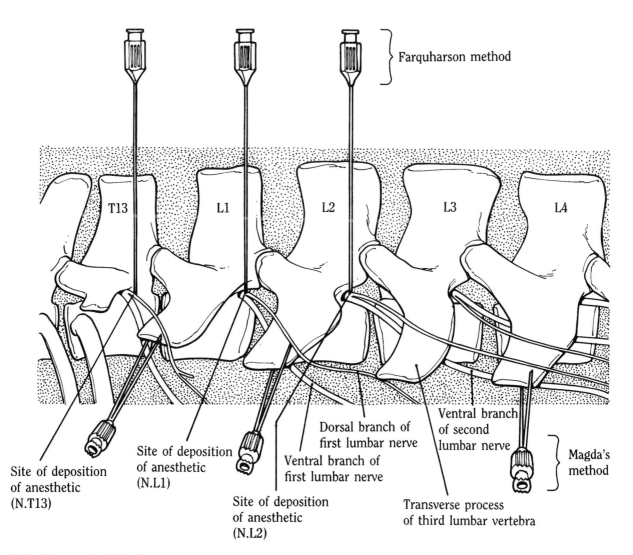

Fig. 2-2. Paravertebral block.

A temporary lateral deviation of the spine due to muscle paralysis is observed in association with paravertebral analgesia.

Another technique favored by some surgeons is that developed by Magda and modified by Cakala.[12] It uses a lateral approach to the nerves and would be more accurately described as a *paralumbar* rather than a paravertebral technique. The branches of T13, L1, and L2 are blocked close to the ends of the first, second, and fourth transverse processes, respectively, as illustrated in Figure 2-2. The skin is clipped and prepared at the ends of the first, second, and fourth lumbar transverse processes. An 18-gauge needle is inserted under each transverse process toward the midline, and 10 ml of solution are injected. The needle is then withdrawn a short distance and is redirected craniad and caudad while more solution is injected. In this fashion, a diffuse region ventral to the transverse process is infiltrated to block the ventral branch of the nerve. The needle is then redirected slightly dorsal and caudal to the transverse process to block the dorsolateral branches of the nerves. About 25 ml of solution are used for each site. Because the Cakala paralumbar technique does not paralyze the lumbar muscles, lateral deviation of the spine does not occur.

The technique for paravertebral nerve block is the same in sheep and goats as it is in cattle. Up to 5 ml of 1 or 2% lidocaine is recommended for each of the injection sites.[34] The total dose should not exceed 6 mg/kg, and onset may occur in as little as 5 minutes. Lidocaine with epinephrine may be used to increase the duration of analgesia to an hour or longer.[34]

Epidural Analgesia

Epidural analgesia is used frequently in large animal surgery for standing procedures in cattle and horses, cesarean sections in swine, urogenital surgery in goats, and postoperative analgesia. Sheep can be easily handled and may require only local analgesia and physical restraint for some procedures. On the other hand, goats have a low pain threshold and require analgesia and sedation. The technique for epidural injection is basically the same among small ruminants, cattle, and horses. Swine are more easily injected in the lumbrosacral space, however, than other species.

This technique consists of the deposition of local analgesic solution between the dura mater and periosteum of the spinal canal (epidural space), which in turn desensitizes the caudal nerve roots after they emerge from the dura. The degree of paralysis that is achieved depends chiefly on the volume of solution injected and on the concentration and diffusibility of the analgesic agent. The rate of absorption of local analgesic agent from the epidural space may contribute to the analgesic effect.

Epidural analgesia can be classified into *cranial (high)* or *caudal (low)*, according to the area of spread of the analgesic solution and the extent of the area in which sensory and motor paralysis develops. Caudal epidural anesthesia implies that motor control of the hindlegs is not affected. Sensory innervation is lost from the anus, vulva, perineum, and caudal aspects of the thighs. The anal sphincter relaxes, and the posterior part of the rectum balloons. Tenesmus is relieved and obstetric straining is prevented. Caudal epidural anesthesia is inexpensive and routinely used in ruminants and horses.

The injection site for caudal epidural analgesia is the same among ruminants and horses. The injection of the analgesic agent may be made between the first and second coccygeal vertebrae or in the sacrococcygeal space, although the former site is preferable because it is a larger space and is more easily detected, especially in fat animals. This site is 1 to 2 inches cranial to the long tail hairs in the horse. To locate the space, the tail is grasped and is moved up and down; the first obvious articulation caudal to the sacrum is the first intercoccygeal space. After clipping and skin preparation, a skin bleb is made with 2% lidocaine using a 2.5-cm, 25-gauge needle, to facilitate needle placement. An 18-gauge, 3- to 5-cm needle (or a spinal needle) is introduced through the center of the space on the midline at a 45° angle in the ox until its point hits the floor of the spinal canal (Figure 2-3). In the horse, this needle may be inserted at an angle of 30° from a perpendicular line through the vertebrae, or at an angle of 60° (as illustrated later in Figure 2-4). The needle is then retracted slightly to ensure that the end is not embedded in the intervertebral disc. If the needle is correctly placed in the epidural space, there should be no resistance to injection. In addition, one should make sure that the bevel of the needle is pointed forward, rather than to one side, to obtain even anesthesia.

In cattle and small ruminants, 2% lidocaine may be used for epidural anesthesia (doses shown in Table 2-1). Injections of 2 ml of 2% lidocaine can be used in the sacrococcygeal space of sheep and goats to provide caudal epidural analgesia for obstetric procedures.[34,78] To achieve epidural analgesia for perineal and hindlimb surgical procedures in small ruminants, a lower dose of lidocaine is used (1 ml/7 kg). The total volume of lidocaine should not exceed 3 ml in sheep and goats and 10 ml in cattle to avoid hindlimb uncoordination and recumbency.[78] Xylazine and 2% lidocaine are now more frequently used in cattle to achieve a longer duration of analgesia and quick onset.[31]

Local anesthetics are not as frequently used alone for caudal epidural anesthesia in horses; their onset of analgesia (about 20 minutes) is much slower than in cattle and the duration is relatively short (87.2 ± 7.5 min).[32,34] For this reason, α_2 agonists such as detomidine, xylazine, and medetomidine, are commonly used in combination with local anesthetics to increase the duration of analgesia and decrease ataxia.[7,71] It is recommended that regardless of the drug used, the dose should not exceed 10 ml in horses to avoid hindlimb ataxia. Alternative anesthetic combinations are shown in Table 2-2.

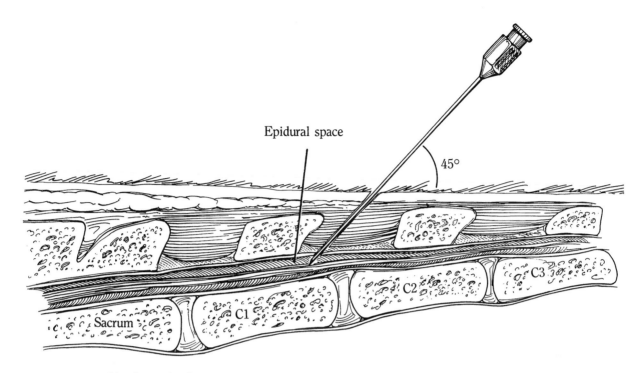

Epidural space

45°

Sacrum C1 C2 C3

Fig. 2-3. Bovine epidural anesthesia.

Cranial epidural injection is considered contraindicated in horses but has some uses in other species. For example, this technique may be used to provide 2 to 4 hours of analgesia in cattle for laparotomy, pelvic limb surgery, or udder amputation. A higher dose of local anesthetic [1 ml/10 lb (3.73 kg) body weight] is used; the animal will go down and should be maintained in sternal recumbency for 10 to 15 minutes to ensure the even distribution of the analgesic solution. When inducing cranial epidural analgesia in cattle, the possible development of hypotension must be considered. No signs of hypotension have been observed using volumes of 100 to 150 ml of 2% lidocaine, but they have been recorded with volumes of 150 to 200 ml.[33±]

Continuous caudal epidural anesthesia using a commercial epidural catheter kit (Continuous Epidural Tray, American Hospital Supply, McGraw Park, IL.) is also used in horses and in some instances, food animals, for repeated epidural delivery of analgesics and postoperative pain relief.[28,55,71] The kit contains a Huber-point directional needle with stylet (Tuohy spinal needle) inserted through a pilot hole at 45° to the horizontal until one encounters an abrupt reduction in resistance. The catheter is then inserted through the needle, it is advanced 2.5 to 4 cm beyond the end of the needle, and the needle is withdrawn. Combinations of either a local anesthetic or alpha-2 adrenergic agonist and morphine administered in the caudal epidural space have been shown to have useful clinical applications for postoperative and long-term pain relief in both humans and animals. Preoperative epidural administration of detomidine (30 μg/kg) and morphine

(0.2 mg/kg) provides effective, long-lasting pain relief and decreases postoperative lameness in horses that undergo bilateral stifle arthroscopy.[23]

Epidural analgesia has been used in both young and adult pigs and, in particular, for cesarean section in the sow. In this instance, cranial (high) epidural analgesia has been used to effect both immobilization and analgesia without fetal depression. Cranial, rather than caudal, epidural analgesia is commonly performed.

The injection site for epidural analgesia in the pig is the lumbosacral space; this space is located at the intersection of the spine with a line drawn through the cranial borders of the ilium. An 18-gauge needle is inserted 1 to 2 cm caudal to this line in small pigs and 2.5 to 5 cm caudal to the line in larger animals. The needle is then directed ventrad and slightly caudad until it is felt to pass through the dorsal ligament of the vertebrae and into the epidural space. The needle size varies with the size of the pig: 8 cm is used for the pig weighing up to 75 kg, and 15 cm is used for pigs heavier than 75 kg. The dose is about 1 ml/5–10 kg of 2% lidocaine for pelvic limb block; the higher dose rate is used in small pigs, and the smaller dose rate is used in large pigs. Other drug combinations used for epidural anesthesia in swine are listed in Table 2-3.

Although epidural analgesia may have advantages based on a requirement for minimal depression of the central nervous system and decreased expense, its use in swine practice has been limited by the time required to perform the technique and the temperament of the animal. Food and Drug Administration (FDA) regulations must also be considered in animals destined for

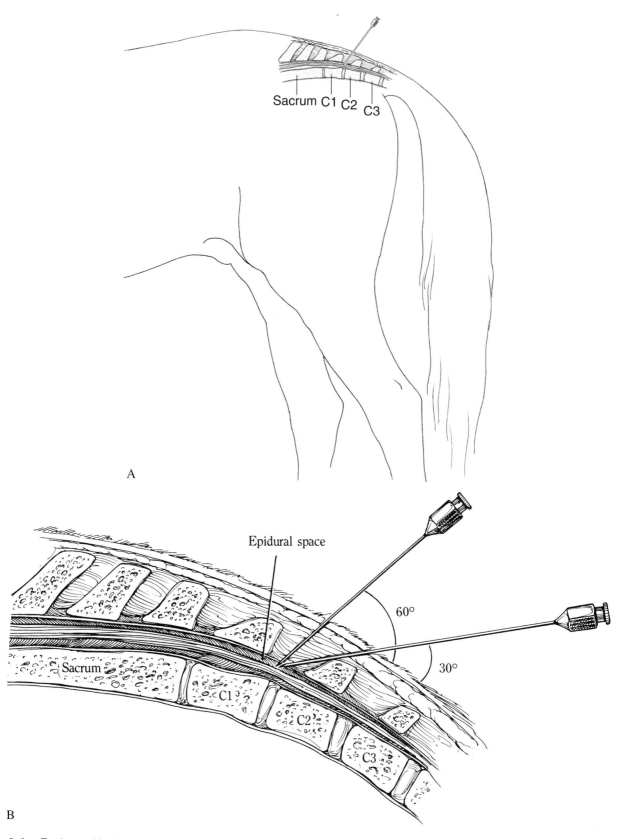

Fig. 2-4. Equine epidural anesthesia. A, Overall view of hindquarters. B, Close-up of caudal vertebra.

Table 2-1. Epidural analgesia in the ox and small ruminants.

Drug	Indications	Dosage	Comments
2% Lidocaine	Cranial and caudal epidural anesthesia Caudal epidural anesthesia in sheep and goats	Cattle: 1 ml /10 lb or 0.5 to 1 ml/100 lb Sheep/goats: 2 to 3 ml	Short onset and duration (20–180 minutes). Commonly used in the ox. Doses greater than 10 ml in cattle and 3 ml in sheep and goats can cause hindlimb uncoordination and recumbency.[77,78]
2% Lidocaine/ xylazine	Caudal epidural anesthesia in cattle	0.22 mg/kg lidocaine, 0.05 mg/kg xylazine Total volume: 5.7 ml/kg[31,86]	The addition of xylazine lengthens the duration of analgesia (303 ± 11 minutes) compared to either drug alone.[31] The onset is also quicker than lidocaine alone. Xylazine should be avoided in pregnant cows.
Medetomidine	Caudal epidural anesthesia in cattle Lumbrosacral epidural anesthesia in goats	Cattle: 15 μg/kg diluted to 5 ml with 0.9% saline[52] Sheep/goats: 20 μg/kg diluted to 5 ml in sterile water[60]	Greatest duration of analgesia (412 ± 156 minutes) and comparable onset time to lidocaine/xylazine in cattle.[52]
Medetomidine/ Mepivacaine	Caudal epidural anesthesia in cattle	Medetomidine: 15 μg/kg mepivicaine: 0.5 to 1 ml/100 lb	
Morphine	Epidural anesthesia and postoperative pain relief in goats and sheep	15 mg/ml morphine diluted to 0.15 to 0.20 ml/kg in 0.9% saline[38]	Provides analgesia without paralysis in goats and provides postoperative analgesia.[38]

Table 2-2. Caudal epidural analgesic agents in the horse.

Drug	Indications	Dosage	Comments
Detomidine	Sedation, some analgesic effects	40–60 μg/kg Total volume: 10–15 ml	Detomidine is more potent in horses than xylazine. Associated with moderate ataxia, mild cardiopulmonary depression, and renal diuresis. Detomidine may be combined with morphine to provide longer-lasting analgesia and provide postoperative pain relief.[23]
Detomidine/ morphine	Sedation/analgesia	Detomidine: 30–40 μg/kg Morphine: 0.1–0.2 mg/kg diluted to total volume of 10–15 ml with 0.9% saline	
Xylazine/2% lidocaine	Sedation/analgesia	0.22 mg/kg lidocaine, 0.17 mg/kg xylazine	Local anesthetics alone are not ideal for caudal epidural analgesia due to their undesirable level of hindlimb ataxia and weakness in horses. Usually, they are combined with an α-2 agonist.[32,34]
2% Mepivacaine	Sedation/analgesia	4–4.5 ml or 2% solution (80–90 mg)[7]	Rapid onset (5–10 minutes) and medium duration (70–210 minutes). Reported to cause less tissue irritation than lidocaine.[7]

market. Few analgesics are approved for use in swine, and withdrawal and food residue values are not available for most of these drugs.

Regional Analgesia of the Eye

The main indication for analgesia of the eye in cattle is for orbital exenteration. For this purpose, the technique of local infiltration using the *retrobulbar* (four-point) block is convenient and satisfactory. The technique is described and illustrated under eye enucleation in Chapter 15, "Miscellaneous Bovine Surgical Techniques."

An alternate technique for regional analgesia to the eye is the *Peterson block*. For this technique, an 11-cm, 18-gauge needle bent to a curvature of a 10-in circle is required. A skin bleb is made at the point where the supraorbital process meets the zygomatic arch, and a

Table 2-3. Epidural analgesic agents in swine.

Drug	Indication	Dosage	Comments
Detomidine	Lumbosacral epidural anesthesia in swine	0.5 mg/kg in 5 ml 0.9% saline	Onset of 10 minutes, duration of 30 minutes. Minimal analgesia caudal to umbilicus.[77,78]
2% Lidocaine	Lumbosacral epidural anesthesia in swine	0.5–1 ml/5 kg, depending on the size of the pig.	2% lidocaine has been used successfully for castration of boars and cesarean section in sows.[77,78]
Xylazine	Lumbosacral epidural anesthesia in swine	2 mg/kg diluted in 5 ml of 0.9% saline	Xylazine produces bilateral analgesia from the anus to the umbilicus within 5 to 10 minutes and lasting for at least 120 minutes.[49] Addition of lidocaine may increase duration to 5 to 8 hours. Typically used for cesarean sections.
10% Xylazine and 2% lidocaine		Xylazine (10%): 1 mg/kg Lidocaine (2%): 10 ml	

puncture wound is made in this bleb with a short 14-gauge needle. The 11-cm needle is then directed mediad, with the concavity of the needle directed caudad. In this fashion, the point of the needle will pass around the cranial border of the coronoid process of the mandible, and the needle is then directed further mediad until it hits the pterygoid crest. The needle is then moved slightly rostrad and down to the pterygopalatine fossa at the foramen orbitorotundum, and 15 to 20 ml of local analgesic solution are injected. The needle is withdrawn and is directed caudad just beneath the skin, to infiltrate the subcutaneous tissues along the zygomatic arch. A small region just dorsal to the medial canthus should also be infiltrated.

Although the Peterson block is preferred by some practitioners for eye analgesia, it is unpredictable, and the injection of 15 ml of local anesthetic inadvertently into the internal maxillary artery can have fatal results. The latter problem can be avoided by injecting 5 ml in one place, repositioning the needle slightly, aspirating and injecting another 5 ml, and then repeating this procedure. Placing a subcutaneous line block across (perpendicular) to the medial canthus of the eye (probably blocking a branch of the infratrochlear nerve) is also a useful adjunct in achieving complete desensitization of the eye. The retrobulbar (four-point) block has been convenient and satisfactory.

Regional Analgesia of the Horn
The *cornual block* is a simple technique that provides analgesia for dehorning cattle and goats. An imaginary line is drawn from the lateral canthus of the eye to the base of the horn along the crest dorsal to the temporal fossa; on this line, an 18-gauge, 2.5-cm needle is inserted halfway from the lateral canthus to the horn, and an injection is made under the skin and through the frontalis muscle at the lateral border of the crest. Generally, 5 ml of 2% lidocaine are sufficient, but up to 10 ml may be used in a larger animal.

Unlike cattle, goats have two cornual branches, one arising from the lacrimal nerve and one from the infratrochlear nerve. The locations of these branches and the technique for blocking is described in Chapter 17, "Miscellaneous Surgical Techniques." Some exotic breeds of cattle, especially the Simmental, also require additional blockade of the infratrochlear nerve, which innervates the medial aspect of the horn.[6] This can be achieved by using a line block subcutaneously from the midline of the head to the facial crest across the forehead dorsal to the eye.

Intravenous Limb Anesthesia of Ruminants
For local analgesia of the distal limb, the technique of *intravenous local analgesia* is considered superior to previously used techniques of specific nerve blocks or ring blocks. The technique involves intravenous injection of local analgesic solution distal to a previously applied tourniquet.[95] The animal is cast and restrained, and the tourniquet of rubber tubing is applied distal to the carpus or hock (Figure 2-5). A protective pad may be placed under the tourniquet. A superficial vein is detected, either the dorsal common digital vein III in the metacarpus or the cranial branch of the lateral saphenous vein in the metatarsus. For cattle, an intravenous injection of 10 to 20 ml of 2% lidocaine or mepivacaine is given after the area has been clipped and prepared. For sheep and particularly goats, a lower dose of 2–3 ml should be used initially. It is important to avoid the use of lidocaine with epinephrine because the combination may cause vasoconstriction sufficient to prevent desensitization. Increased amounts of lidocaine may be necessary to achieve adequate analgesia of the interdigital area. The needle is withdrawn, and the injection site is massaged briefly to prevent hematoma formation. Anesthesia of the distal limb is complete in 5 minutes and persists 1 to 2 hours if the tourniquet remains in place. At the end of the operation, the tourniquet is released slowly over a period of 10 seconds, and the limb will regain normal sensation and motor function in about 5 minutes. Toxicity related to the entrance of the local anesthetic into the circulation has not been observed.[95]

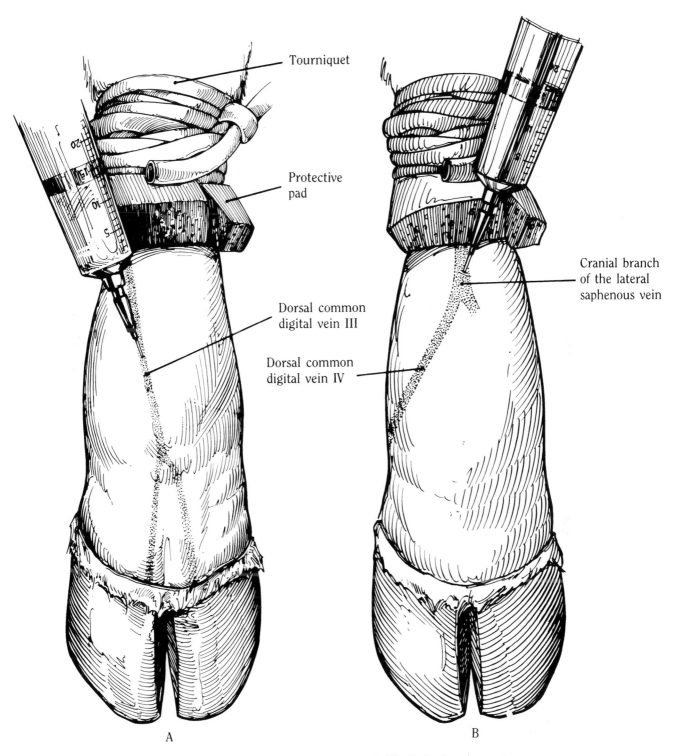

Fig. 2-5. Intravenous limb anesthesia. A, Forelimb, dorsal aspect; B, Hindlimb, dorsal aspect.

Tourniquet

Protective pad

Dorsal common digital vein III

Dorsal common digital vein IV

Cranial branch of the lateral saphenous vein

A

B

Other Nerve Blocks

Nerve blocks and ring blocks are usually performed in the limb for lameness diagnosis and wound repair. Local nerve blocks of the limbs and intraarticular analgesic techniques have an important place in the diagnosis of lameness and are well described elsewhere.[1] These techniques are not repeated in this text.

Tranquilization and Sedation

There are three general purposes for the tranquilization or sedation of large animals: (1) sedation of intractable animals for routine diagnostic and therapeutic procedures, (2) sedation for minor surgical procedures in conjunction with local anesthesia, and (3) preanesthetic medication. The terms *tranquilization* and *sedation* with the horse implies that the animal is standing, whereas with the bovine patient, it generally implies that the animal will be placed in recumbency and secured with ropes or restrained on a tilt table. Selected drugs with commonly used dosages are found in Table 2-4. The two primary phenothiazine tranquilizers used in the horse are promazine hydrochloride (Promazine Hydrochloride Injection) and acetylpromazine maleate (Acepromazine Maleate Injectable). Hypotension, tachycardia, and persistent penile paralysis are potential side effects of the phenothiazine tranquilizers.[46] Alpha-2 adrenoceptor agonists, such as xylazine hydrochloride, detomidine, medetomidine, and romifidine, have become popular. In general, alpha-2 agonists are associated with a transient period of hypertension followed by hypotension and decreased heart rate, respiratory rate, and cardiac output. Opioids and alpha-2 agonists are both commonly used to produce sedation in cattle.[29] Note that xylazine is not approved for use in cattle. Phenothiazine tranquilizers are rarely used in cattle. Tables 2-4 and 2-5 depict a few of the commonly used drugs for sedation in cattle and horses, respectively.

Sedation in swine can be achieved with azaperone, a safe, inexpensive drug used by herdsmen to control fighting and aggression. Droperidol also produces a similar quality of sedation in pigs. Acepromazine, diazepam, or xylazine may be used for sedation in goats and sheep. Goats are more sensitive to xylazine than sheep and require a dose of only 0.04 to 0.05 mg/kg intravenously. Dosages are listed in Tables 2-6 and 2-7.

General Anesthesia

General anesthesia should be used whenever it is considered the optimal technique. Many surgical procedures have been either cancelled or performed under compromised circumstances because of reluctance to anesthetize the patient. General anesthesia offers the ultimate in restraint and, therefore, the ideal situation for aseptic surgery, proper handling of tissues, and hemostasis. General anesthesia should never be done casually, however, and the operator should be experienced in performing general anesthesia before electing to use the technique.

Many procedures in the equine are performed under general anesthesia. Most surgical procedures in cattle can be performed either standing or in dorsal recumbency with physical or chemical restraint and local anesthesia. General anesthesia in ruminants presents many challenges due to the animals' physiological characteristics. Prolonged recumbence in cattle may cause the abdominal contents to interfere with normal diaphragm movement and result in hypoventilation, hypoxia, hypercarbia, and respiratory acidosis.[14,29] Regurgitation and postoperative bloat are also a concern in ruminants under general anesthesia. General anesthesia in these animals requires a

Table 2-4. Tranquilizers and sedatives used in cattle.

Drug	Indications	Dosage	Comments
Detomidine	Standing sedation in cattle	0.03–0.06 mg/kg i.v.	No associations with drug residues in milk after dosing in dairy cows or increased risk of abortion.[29,73]
Medetomidine	Deep sedation and recumbency at high doses in cattle	0.005–0.01 mg/kg i.v	The lower dose results in deep sedation whereas the higher produces recumbency.
Xylazine	Casting agent or standing sedation in cattle Standing sedation/analgesia	0.11–0.22 mg/kg i.m. 0.055–0.11 mg/kg i.v. Xylazine: 0.02 mg/kg i.v.	Profound effects in cattle, causes recumbency at the higher intramuscular dose and standing sedation with the lower intravenous dose. Gastrointestinal side effects in large bulls have been noted
Xylazine/butorphanol	Standing sedation	Butorphanol: 0.05–0.07 mg/kg i.v.[14]	with xylazine.[50] Increased risk of spontaneous abortion during the third trimester in pregnant cows.[29]

Table 2-5. Tranquilizers and sedatives used in horses.

Drug	Indications	Dosage	Comments
Acepromazine/ meperdine hydrochloride (Demerol)	Sedation	Ace: 0.06 mg/kg Meperdine: 0.5 mg/kg	Acepromazine at a dose of 0.05 mg/kg i.v. or i.m. can be used for mild sedation that lasts approximately 90 minutes and begins within 15 to 20 minutes.[58] Acepromazine should not be used after recent treatment with organophosphate antihelmintics. Due to its alpha-adrenergic blocking effect, this drug should not be used in cases of hypovolemic shock, except when volume replacement has been adequate and peripheral vasodilation to increase perfusion is desired.
Detomidine Detomidine/ butorphanol tartate (Torbugesic)	Sedation	4–20 µg/kg i.v. Detomidine: 10–20 µg/kg Butorphanol: 0.02–0.05 mg/ kg i.v.	Cardiovascular effects are more profound than with xylazine or medetomidine. Duration of 60–120 minutes.[7] Detomidine can be administered with a loading dose of 7.5 µg/kg i.v. followed by constant rate infusion to effect.
Medetomidine	Sedation	5 µg/kg i.v.	Longer duration than xylazine.[7] Similar to detomidine, may be infused intravenously to effect to achieve desired length of sedation.
Medetomidine	Sedation	5 µg/kg i.v.	Longer duration than xylazine.[7] Similar to detomidine, may be infused intravenously to effect to achieve desired length of sedation.
Romifidine	Sedation	40–120 µg/kg i.v.	Produces sedation of a longer duration than detomidine or xylazine.[7]
Xylazine	Sedation or preanesthetic	1.1 mg/kg i.v.[42] 0.33–0.66 mg/kg i.v. for preanesthetic	Bradycardia and transient cardiac arrhythmias (usually partial atrioventricular block) occur when xylazine is given intravenously, but may be prevented by prior administration of atropine.[47] At maximum doses, significant ataxia may complicate standing procedures. Animal behavior under heavy sedation may be unpredictable. Good for short procedures.
Xylazine/acepromazine	Sedation	Xylazine: 0.5 mg/kg Ace: 0.05 mg/kg i.v.	Addition of acepromazine, butorphanol, or morphine results in longer duration of sedation, quicker onset, and increased analgesia than xylazine alone.
Xylazine/butorphanol tartate Xylazine/morphine		Xylazine: 1.1 mg/kg Butorphanol: 0.1 mg/kg i.v.[70] Xylazine: 0.66 mg/kg Morphine: 0.66 mg/kg i.v.[48,65]	

cuffed endotracheal tube to prevent aspiration, and fasting prior to surgery is crucial. Sedation and local analgesia are frequently used in goats instead of general anesthesia because there is less risk of regurgitation and depression of the cardiovascular and respiratory systems.[34]

A thorough preanesthetic evaluation of the patient should be made, followed by appropriate preoperative preparation. The preanesthetic patient evaluation should include a history, clinical examination, and a complete blood count (CBC) or at least a packed cell volume (PCV)/total protein determination. Complete serum chemistry profiles are indicated in certain situations. The patient should be carefully monitored during the procedure and throughout postoperative recovery.

Table 2-6. Tranquilizers and sedatives used in swine.

Drug	Indications	Dosage	Comments
Azaperone	Sedation in swine	1 to 8 mg/kg	Not recommended for use in boars at doses greater than 1 mg/kg due to the risk of penile protrusion and subsequent injury.[34] Onset is approximately 20 minutes.
Droperidol	Sedation in swine	0.1 to 0.4 mg/kg	Produces sedation similar to azaperone.
Ketamine/diazepam	Sedation in swine	10–15 mg/kg ketamine, 0.5–2.0 mg/kg diazepam i.m.	Longer duration than previous drugs (1 to 2 hours).
Ketamine/midazolam		10–20 mg/kg ketamine, 0.1 to 0.5 mg/kg midazolam i.m.	

Table 2-7. Tranquilizers and sedatives used in small ruminants.

Drug	Indications	Dosage	Comments
Acepromazine	Mild sedation	0.05–0.1 mg/kg i.m.	May be used for restraint prior to induction.
Detomidine	Sedation	0.03 mg/kg i.v.	Detomidine and butorphanol may be used as preanesthetics. Detomidine produces dose- and route-dependent sedation in goats; doses of 0.02 mg/kg i.v. result in sedation and moderate analgesia and a dose of 0.04 mg/kg i.v. or i.m. causes sternal recumbency and severe ataxia.[76] Butorphanol provides effective preemptive and postoperative analgesia in goats.[14]
Detomidine/butorphanol	Sedation	Detomidine: 0.01 mg/kg Butorphanol: 0.1 mg/kg i.v.	
Xylazine	Sedation	0.1–0.4 mg/kg i.v in sheep 0.05–0.1 mg/kg i.v. in goats	Goats are more sensitive to xylazine than sheep and thus require lower doses.

Premedication

Feed should be withheld from all patients before general anesthesia unless the urgency of the problem precludes it. This is especially crucial in ruminants, where bloat, regurgitation, and aspiration of ingesta are concerns. Adult cattle should be kept off roughage and feed for 48 hours prior to surgery, grain concentrates for 24 hours, and water for 12 hours. Regurgitation is less of a problem in younger cattle, and feed needs to be withheld for only 12 to 24 hours and water withheld overnight prior to surgery.[2] Feed should be withheld from sheep and goats 24 hours prior to surgery and from pigs 6 to 8 hours prior to surgery. Water should be withheld 12 hours prior to surgery in sheep and goats and 2 hours prior to surgery for pigs. Feed should be withheld from horses for 12 hours prior to surgery; water can be available free choice.

Sedation or tranquilization of the equine patient is almost always indicated prior to inducing general anesthesia, but seldom in cattle or small ruminants. Most tranquilizers and sedatives are not approved for use in ruminants by the Food and Drug Administration and the surgeon must assume responsibility when using these drugs. Compromised horses, such as a patient with an acute abdominal disorder, may preclude the need for sedation prior to induction. If pain in a colic patient makes induction of anesthesia impossible, it is preferable to administer an analgesic agent rather than a phenothiazine tranquilizer. Preanesthetic tranquilizers are not generally administered to foals because of inadequate development of the microsomal enzyme system in the liver and the consequent slow metabolism of these drugs. Pigs are commonly sedated with intramuscular azaperone prior to surgery.[34]

The alpha-2 agonists are commonly used as preinduction agents in horses and cattle when appropriate (refer to Table 2-5). Acepromazine is not considered a good preanesthetic tranquilizer in cattle because it is associated with an increased risk of regurgitation during intubation and may cause penile prolapse.

Anticholinergic drugs, such as atropine, are also not used frequently as preanesthetic agents. The advantages do not outweigh the disadvantages, which include postoperative ileus, increased myocardial oxygen consumption, tachycardia, and ocular effects in sheep and goats.[19,46,34] In high doses, atropine will reduce salivation in the small ruminants and render it more viscous to facilitate intubation. However, tachycardia and other side effects occur at these doses. Atropine or glycopyrrolate (0.2–2.0 mg/kg) is useful in pigs to control excessive salivation during general anesthesia.[34]

Induction of Anesthesia

There are many alternate regimens for the intravenous induction of anesthesia in horses and ruminants. The methods discussed here currently receive the most use. Common induction agents and doses are included in Tables 2-8 and 2-9.

Traditionally, thiobarbiturates were used to induce recumbency in sedated horses, but have been largely replaced by dissociative drugs such as ketamine and tiletamine. Thiamylal sodium (Surital) is no longer commercially available in the United States, but thiopental sodium (Pentothal) is still used although it is seldom practical in field situations due to its unpredictability in

many horses. Guaifenesin, used alone as a casting agent[74] or in combination with thiobarbiturates or ketamine, has become a common adjunct to induction agents.[21,46] It is now used generally in combination with a short-acting thiobarbiturate or ketamine. The drug is a muscle relaxant that acts at the level of the internuncial neurons and provides a calm state similar to sleep, but it is not an anesthetic. Because it is centrally acting, guaifenesin provides some analgesia. It has minimal depressant effects on the respiratory and cardiac systems, and induction is smooth, without involuntary movements of the forelimbs (dog paddling). The drug is administered as a 5% solution in 5% dextrose or as a 10% solution in sterile distilled water.[22,24]

The safest and most satisfactory way of inducing anesthesia in foals is by "masking down" with halothane. The mask is applied, and initially, oxygen alone (6 to 7 L/min) is administered. The vaporizer is then set at 0.5 to 1% to introduce the foal to the smell of halothane, and the

Table 2-8. Anesthetic induction regimens in the equine patient.

Drug	Dosage	Comments
Guaifenesin/ketamine	5–10% solution of guaifenesin i.v. followed by bolus of ketamine (1.8–2.2 mg/kg)	Excellent for debilitated patients. Provides relatively nonexcitable induction of anesthesia with little cardiopulmonary depression.[22] The solution is mixed immediately prior to use. 600 to 800 ml of a 5% solution are required to induce anesthesia in a 450-kg horse.[44] A wide-bore needle (10 to 12 gauge) or catheter facilitates rapid administration. A second method of administration is to give the guaifenesin solution intravenously until the horse becomes slightly ataxic and then give a 2-g dose of thiobarbiturate intravenously as a bolus.[22] Recovery from guaifenesin/thiopental combinations is smooth.
Guaifenesin/thiopental	4–6 mg/kg thiopental per liter of guaifenesin solution	
5–10% Thiopental	5–6 mg/kg rapid i.v.	Practicality in the field is limited due to its unpredictability in many horses. Rapid induction is convenient for the single-handed practitioner, but it can produce some profound physiological effects, including marked drops in perfusion pressure and cardiac output, a period of initial apnea, and cardiac arrhythmias. As a sole anesthetic agent, thiopental is useful only for short procedures. Halothane used in conjunction to maintain anesthesia may exacerbate hypotension caused by the barbiturate. The dose must be decreased in acidotic patients.
Tiletamine/zolazepam (Telazol®)	0.7–1.0 mg/kg i.v.	Considered to have superior induction quality and produce greater muscle relaxation than other agents, but it is also associated with a prolonged ataxia during recovery.[54]
Xylazine/ketamine	1.1 mg/kg xylazine i.v. followed 2 to 3 minutes later by 2.2 mg/kg ketamine i.v.	This regimen provides anesthesia for a short duration (12 to 15 minutes) and eliminates the need for large-volume administration through a catheter or needle. Induction is smooth when xylazine takes effect before ketamine is administered. Disadvantages include increased cost and the inability to control the duration of anesthesia by repeat injections. Repeat injections of ketamine can result in convulsions, muscle tremors, and spasms. Active palpebral, cornual, and swallowing reflexes are maintained, and passing an endotracheal tube can be difficult. Diazepam (0.22 mg/kg) administered a few minutes prior to xylazine may improve induction.[11]

Table 2-9. Anesthetic induction regimens in cattle and small ruminants.

Drug	Dosage	Comments
Guaifenesin	6–12 mg/kg i.v. in cattle Use to effect in small ruminants	Administered the same as in horses. Guaifenesin is not approved for use in food animals.[68]
Guaifenesin/thiopental	2–3 g thiopental per liter of 5% guaifenesin solution i.v. at 2 ml/kg (max dose rate) in cattle. Use to effect in small ruminants.	
Guaifenesin/ketamine/ xylazine	Solution prepared as 1 g ketamine and 25–50 mg xylazine added to 1 liter 5% guaifenesin. Administered i.v. initially at 0.5–1.1 ml/kg to effect. May be maintained at 2.2 ml/kg/hr.[87]	Xylazine (0.1–0.2 mg/kg i.m.) may be used as premedication for guaifenesin- thiopental combinations. This combination has been found to be safe in cattle, sheep, and goats. Addition of xylazine is optional.
Ketamine	2 mg/kg i.v. bolus of ketamine following premedication with atropine and xylazine in cattle.[89]	Jaw relaxation is not as effective as with guaifenesin and thiobarbiturates, but endotracheal intubation can be performed.[89]
Ketamine/diazepam	5–7.5 mg/kg i.v. ketamine/0.2–0.3 mg/kg i.v. diazepam in sheep and goats 50:50 mixtures of ketamine and diazepam (Ket-Val) may be administered i.v. at 1 ml/15 kg in small cattle, sheep, goats, and calves.	Butorphanol (0.1 mg/kg) may be administered just prior to injection to improve muscle relaxation. Onset is approximately 5 minutes and duration is 30 to 40 minutes. If anesthesia is maintained with halothane or isoflurane, may result in low arterial blood pressure.[34]
Tiletamine/zolazepam (Telazol®)	6–12 mg/kg i.v. in cattle	To avoid overdosage in sheep and goats, it is recommended to administer an initial bolus dose of 5–7 mg/kg of 2.5% thiopental followed by smaller boluses. Duration of anesthesia is short (5 to 10 minutes) and recovery is smooth in sheep and goats.[34]
Thiopental sodium	7–20 mg/kg i.v. in sheep and goats	

concentration is gradually increased to 4% until anesthesia is induced. The foal is then intubated and placed on a maintenance plane of anesthesia.

Similar to the horse, combinations of guafenesin are frequently used in cattle to induce and maintain anesthesia. A "triple drip" solution of 5% guaifenesin solution, 1 mg/ml of ketamine, and 0.1 mg/ml of xylazine has been found to be safe and effective for general anesthesia in cattle, sheep, and goats. Initially 0.55 mg/kg of the solution is given rapidly, and then a 2.2-ml/kg/hr maintenance level is used.

Intravenous agents, such as chloral hydrate, may be used as well but it is preferred as a sedative rather than an induction agent. Table 2.9 lists some of the frequently used induction agents in cattle, sheep, and goats.

On induction of anesthesia, a mouth speculum is immediately inserted, and an endotracheal tube is introduced. To avoid the aspiration of regurgitated rumen contents, intubation should be performed even if anesthesia is to be maintained by an intravenous agent. Endotracheal intubation in cattle can be accomplished digitally by direct visualization of the larynx or by blind passage of the tube into the pharynx coupled with external manipulation of the larynx.[45] In adult cattle, digital intubation can be performed by placing a speculum to hold the patient's mouth open and by directing the tube into the larynx with one's hand cupped over the end of the tube. Blind intubation can also be performed by extending the animal's head, elevating the larynx by external manipulation, and passing the tube into the trachea. In calves and smaller cattle, the use of a laryngoscope is beneficial.

Although intubation can be performed after sedation with xylazine, the incidence of regurgitation is lower if surgical anesthesia is induced before endotracheal intubation is performed.[93] Regurgitation while an endotracheal tube is in place is of minor concern, provided the pharynx is cleared and drained and the nasal cavity is flushed before extubation.[93]

Induction of anesthesia in young animals may be performed with a combination of halothane and oxygen.

Solutions of guaifenesin, ketamine, and xylazine (GKX) may be used to induce and maintain anesthesia in mature swine.[55] It is administered through the central ear vein using a 16- to 18-gauge catheter.

Halothane, administered by face mask, may also be used to induce anesthesia in pigs.[68] Other induction agents and their doses commonly used in swine are depicted in Table 2-10. Ketamine hydrochloride used alone should be

Table 2-10. Anesthetic induction regimens in swine.

Drug	Dosage	Comments
Guaifenesin/ketamine/ xylazine	5% guaifenesin solution in 5% dextrose, 1 mg/ml ketamine, and 1 mg/ml of xylazine i.v. at dose rate of 0.5–1.0 mg/kg[89]	May be used to induce and maintain anesthesia in swine. It is administered through the central ear vein using a 16- to 18-gauge catheter. This combination of drugs is initially given rapidly at a dose of 0.5 to 1.0 mg/kg to induce anesthesia. This infusion may be continued at a rate of 2 ml/kg/hr to maintain anesthesia for up to 2.5 hours.[89] Recovery is rapid once the infusion is discontinued.
Ketamine	11 mg/kg i.m	The patient is given atropine (0.4 mg/kg) and droperidol-fentanyl (1 ml/14.6 kg) intramuscularly. With the onset of sedation (10 to 15 minutes), ketamine is administered intramuscularly and surgical anesthesia is induced in 5 to 10 minutes. The duration of anesthesia is 30 to 45 minutes, but it may be prolonged with supplemental ketamine given intramuscularly at the rate of 2.2 to 6.6 mg/kg or intravenously to effect. Pentobarbital sodium is effective for controlling reactions that may occur during recovery.
Pentobarbital sodium	30 mg/kg i.v. in unsedated pigs	Administered by slow i.v. injection into an ear vein until the desired degree of anesthesia is achieved.[34]
Thiopental sodium	5–10 mg/kg i.v. of 2.5% solution	The quantity necessary to induce anesthesia is dependent upon the rate of injection. Azaperone is recommended for premedication.[34]
Tiletamine/zolazepam (Telazol®)/ketamine/ xylazine (TKX)	Add 4 ml ketamine (100 mg/ml) and 1 ml xylazine (100 mg/ml) to 5 ml Telazol® Administer 0.5–1 ml/20 kg i.m.	Duration of anesthesia of 10 to 30 minutes.

supplemented with thiobarbiturates or inhalational agents to prevent excitement during the recovery period.[91] Ketamine in combination with droperidol-fentanyl has been successfully used for various surgical procedures in pigs weighing less than 45 kg.[5]

Endotracheal intubation can be difficult in swine. The larynx in the pig is long and mobile, and there is a middle ventricle in the floor of the larynx near the base of the epiglottis. The arch of the cricoid cartilage is on an oblique angle with the trachea. Laryngeal spasm is easily induced. A laryngoscope is used for intubation of swine, and a malleable metal-rod stylet is placed inside the lumen of the endotracheal tube with the tip slightly curved to facilitate the maneuvers necessary to place the tube in the trachea. A topical anesthetic should be sprayed on the larynx to prevent laryngospasm. A technique for nasal intubation has also been described.[68] Nasal intubation works well, but one disadvantage is the lack of protection against regurgitation and aspiration because the trachea is not intubated. Anesthesia in pigs may be maintained by mask, but this technique uses excess halothane if leaks are present between the mask and the animal's snout and is not in the best interest of the operators' health.

Maintaining Anesthesia
Inhalation anesthesia is the preferred method of maintaining general anesthesia in ruminants and horses, especially when procedures involve a total anesthetic time of longer than an hour. However, because most procedures performed on swine on the farm are of relatively short duration, they lend themselves to the use of injectable agents, and the indications for inhalation anesthesia in swine are few. The physical features and temperament of swine make induction of any form of general anesthesia difficult. Accessible superficial veins are few, intubation is generally more difficult than in other species, and swine are prone to malignant hyperthermia.[3,34] For the purpose of this text, details on inhalation anesthetic machines, equipment, techniques, and monitoring will not be described here but are available elsewhere.[33,53,68,79,80]

The combination most commonly used in cattle and horses is that of halothane and oxygen because the depth of anesthesia is easily controlled, recovery time and induction are rapid, and muscle relaxation is adequate. Halothane is considered to cause cardiopulmonary depression in a dose-dependent manner in cattle. It has been shown, however, that a guaifenesin and thiobarbiturate induction and a halothane maintenance regimen would cause bulls to be hypertensive, despite a decrease in cardiac output.[75]

Halothane and methoxyflurane both work satisfactorily for sheep, goats, and swine. The longer recovery time with methoxyflurane is not as critical in these species as it is in the equine and bovine species. Nitrous oxide is commonly added to halothane and methoxyflurane in swine (Table 2-11). Halothane is one of several anesthetic agents capable of triggering hyperthermia in certain breeds of pigs. Pigs should be carefully monitored for body temperature. A rapid rise in temperature to 41°C (106°F) or above accompanied by tachypnea, hyperventilation, muscular rigidity, blotchy cyanosis, and tachycardia is an indication for cessation of anesthesia.[3]

Other primary anesthetic agents include isoflurane, sevoflurane, and desflurane. Isoflurane and sevoflurane have been evaluated in ruminants and horses,[4,30,81,83,88] and their effectiveness has been established. The advantages of sevoflurane and isoflurane are a smooth, rapid recovery and quick induction. Cost and anesthetic potency have been limiting factors for the widespread use of sevoflurane and desflurane, however.[4,30,44] The intravenous

Table 2-11. Anesthetic maintenance in large animals.

Drug	Species	Dosage	Comments
Guaifenesin/ ketamine/ detomidine	Horses	10% Guaifenesin Ketamine: 2 mg/ml Detomidine: 0.02 mg/ml Infusion rate: 1–3 ml/kg/hr[61]	Generally administered to effect. 10% solutions of guaifenesin are combined with detomidine, medetomidine, and romifidine. A 5% solution is used for GKX solutions. Triple drips can be used as an adjunct to inhalational anesthesia to reduce the concentration of inhalant required and improve the quality of transition made to inhalation anesthesia or used to maintain anesthesia (total intravenous anesthesia).[97]
Guaifenesin/ ketamine/ medetomidine	Horses	10% Guaifenesin Ketamine: 2 mg/ml Medetomidine: 0.02 mg/ml Infusion rate: 1–3 ml/kg/hr	
Guaifenesin/ ketamine/ romifidine	Horses	10% Guaifenesin Ketamine: 2 mg/ml Romifidine: 0.06 mg/ml Infusion rate: 1–3 ml/kg/hr[61]	
Guaifenesin/ ketamine/ xylazine (GKX)	Cattle	5% Guaifenesin: 500 ml Ketamine: 1 g/ml Xylazine: 50 mg/ml Infusion rate: 0.5–2.2 ml/kg[14,29]	
	Sheep and goats	10% Guaifenesin Ketamine: 2 mg/ml Xylazine: 1 mg/ml Infusion rate: 1–3 ml/kg/hr	
	Horses	5% Guafenesin: 500 ml Ketamine: 500 mg Xylazine: 250 mg Infusion rate: 2.75 ml/kg or to effect	
Halothane/oxygen	Cattle	4–5 L/min oxygen flow and 1–3% halothane for adult cattle (1–1.5% halothane in calves[42])	Rapid induction and recovery, adequate muscle relaxation, and easy monitoring of anesthetic depth. Intravenous constant infusion of butorphanol (0.05 mg/kg) and acepromazine (0.05 mg/kg) will decrease the minimum alveolar concentration of halothane by 38% in horses.[17]
	Sheep and goats Horses	11 ml/kg/min oxygen and 1–2% halothane	
	Swine	1.5–3% halothane 1 to 2% halothane and 25–40% nitrous oxide[68]	
Isoflurane	Goats and sheep Horses	1.5–1.6% MAC 1.5–2.5% MAC[62,82]	Smoother, more rapid recovery and quicker induction than halothane 4, 50, 52, 54.[30,44] Greater respiratory depression and less cardiac output than halothane. Xylazine (0.5–1.0 mg/kg i.v.) or a triple drip of guaifenesin, ketamine, and medetomidine may be infused at a constant rate to decrease the minimum alveolar concentration of isoflurane.[97]
Methoxyflurane	Sheep and goats Swine	0.24–0.28% 25–40% nitrous oxide administered with 1 to 1.5% methoxyflurane[68]	

constant infusion of some drugs, such as GKX triple drip, xylazine, acepromazine, and butorphanol, has been proven to be a useful adjunct to inhalation maintained anesthesia (Table 2-11).

Although the maintenance of anesthesia with intravenous agents is not ideal, it may be the only method available to the practitioner in the field. Intravenously maintained anesthesia has the advantages of minimal equipment requirements, economy, and less postoperative stress; however, lengthy maintenance on any of the injectable regimens is associated with a prolonged, and sometimes stormy, recovery. Because excretion of the anesthetic agent is slower than with an inhalation agent, the plane of anesthesia cannot be reduced quickly, particularly in debilitated or young animals. In general, any period of intravenously maintained anesthesia should last no longer than an hour.

Intravenous maintenance of anesthesia in horses and ruminants is usually accomplished by a "triple drip" combination of guaifenesin, ketamine, and an alpha-2 antagonist (Table 2-11).[62] Guafenesin-ketamine and guafenesin-ketamine-xylazine (GKX) solutions may also be used for maintenance using either constant intravenous infusion or repeat boluses.[29] GKX solutions will maintain anesthesia in cattle for up to 2.5 hours at a dose rate of 2.2 ml/kg (5% guaifenesin, ketamine 1 mg/L, and xylazine 0.1 mg/ml).[14] The use of an intramuscularly administered regimen of xylazine (0.1–0.2 mg/kg) and ketamine (6 mg/kg) provides satisfactory anesthesia for short surgical procedures in calves and small ruminants.[29] The xylazine and ketamine can be mixed and given in the same syringe, or they can be given separately. About 30 to 40 minutes of anesthesia can be expected from this combination. If anesthesia becomes too light, the ketamine can be repeated at a half-dose (0.5 mg/kg).[69] Other injectable anesthetic regimens for small ruminants are shown in Table 2-10. Their effects in these animals seem more satisfactory than in equine and bovine species. Other combinations are shown in Table 2-11. Large doses of thiobarbiturates are generally avoided to maintain anesthesia because recovery will be prolonged.

Careful clinical monitoring of the patient during anesthesia is important, including measurement of reflexes and physical monitoring of the cardiovascular system.[46] More definitive monitoring of the cardiovascular system is accomplished by direct or indirect blood pressure measurements and electrocardiograms (ECG). For performance of short procedures in the field, monitoring equipment is minimal. For longer procedures in a hospital situation, however, the measurement of arterial blood pressure (using arterial catheterization and a pressure transducer or indirect measurement with the Doppler system over the coccygeal artery), in addition to the normal monitoring of vital signs, is desirable. ECG monitoring is also useful.

Patients in hypotensive states that do not respond to intravenous fluids require the use of vasoactive agents. Dopamine, dobutamine, and ephedrine are practical and effective drugs used to increase blood pressure.[46,63,84] Clinical experience in anesthetized horses indicates that dopamine or dobutamine is superior to ephedrine in time-to-peak response, improvement of blood pressure, and increases in cardiac output. Atrial and ventricular arrhythmias occur at higher doses (75 mg/kg/min) of dopamine and dobutamine, but they are easily controlled by reducing the rate of administration. Cardiac arrhythmias are mainly observed after ephedrine administration.[63]

Positioning of the patient is important when procedures of over 30 minutes are performed in a hospital situation. Faulty positioning of the hindlimbs can lead to peroneal or femoral nerve paresis.[37] In addition, failure to support the upper pelvic limb when the horse is in lateral recumbency can lead to venous occlusion and subsequent rhabdomyolysis. The recumbent thoracic limb should be pulled craniad to relieve pressure between the rib cage, brachial plexus, and vessels along the humerus; otherwise, rhabdomyolysis or nerve paresis may result. The routine use of a waterbed, air mattress, or deep foam pad is recommended when placing anesthetized animals on an operating table for periods of longer than 30 minutes. Hypotension during anesthesia is a significant contributor to postanesthetic myopathy in horses anesthetized with halothane.[25]

Ventilatory compromise is of concern in anesthetized, recumbent horses. The causes include pharmacologic depression of the respiratory control center, decreased lung volume, inadequate thoracic expansion or diaphragmatic excursions, and mismatched distribution of ventilation and perfusion in recumbency.[35,43,56,57,79,83] Hypercarbia and hypoxemia develop unless ventilation is assisted. Controlled ventilation is the most effective means of maintaining normal blood gas levels, but it has detrimental cardiovascular effects. Assisted ventilation reduces arterial carbon dioxide levels and raises oxygen levels, when compared to spontaneous ventilation, with less cardiovascular depression than during controlled ventilation.[40] Hypoxemia is another potential problem in the recovery period.[57] Only oxygen supplementation through a demand valve seems sufficient to maintain arterial blood gas tensions similar to those in awake horses.[57]

Clinical monitoring during bovine anesthesia with halothane includes careful attention to the cardiovascular and respiratory parameters and to the eyes.[45] Rotation of the eyeball is a reliable means of monitoring anesthetic depth, as well as progression of recovery from halothane anesthesia.[89,92] As the anesthesia deepens, the eyeball rotates ventrad and mediad. As depth of anesthesia further increases, the cornea is completely hidden by the lower eyelid (this is plane 2 to 3 of surgical anesthesia). A further increase in the depth of anesthesia causes the eye to rotate dorsad to a central position between the palpebral folds. This point denotes deep surgical anesthesia. Palpebral reflexes dull progressively, but the corneal reflex should remain strong. During recovery, eyeball rotation occurs in reverse order to that observed during induction of anesthesia. Cardiovascular monitoring is performed as with the horse. The recovery of cattle from general anesthesia is usually smooth. As the animal recovers, it should be supported in sternal recumbency to reduce the chances of inhaling rumenal contents or developing bloat.

In sheep and goats, jaw tone should be used cautiously because some exists at deep levels of anesthesia. Swallowing movements signify lightening of anesthesia. Eye rotation is not a useful method of assessing anesthetic depth as it is in cattle.[27] Pupillary dilation is evident during light anesthetic planes and may also be evident during deep anesthesia.

Ocular reflexes are usually of no value in monitoring anesthesia in pigs. The lack of superficial arteries makes it difficult to monitor anesthesia on the basis of pulse strength. Heart rate should range from 80 to 150/min in normal swine under anesthesia, and the respiratory rate should be 10 to 25/min. The depth of anesthesia can also be judged by the degree of muscle relaxation and muscle fasciculations in response to the surgical stimulus.[68]

References

1. Adams, O.R.: Lameness in Horses, 3rd Ed. Philadelphia, Lea & Febiger, 1974.
2. Ames, K.N., and Reibold, T.W.: Anesthesia in cattle. *In* Proceedings of the 11th Annual Convention of the American Association of Bovine Practitioners in 1978: 1979, p. 75.
3. Anderson, I.: Anaesthesia in the pig. Aust. Vet. J., *49*:474, 1973.
4. Auer, J.A., et al.: Recovery from anaesthesia in ponies: a comparative study of the effects of isoflurane, enflurane, methoxyflurane and halothane. Equine Vet. J., *10*:18, 1978.
5. Benson, G.J., and Thurmon, J.C.: Anesthesia of swine under field conditions. J. Am. Vet. Med. Assoc., *174*:594, 1979.
6. Benson, G.J., and Thurmon, J.C.: Regional analgesia of food animals. *In* Current Veterinary Therapy: Food Animal Practice. Vol. 2. Edited by J.L. Howard. Philadelphia, W.B. Saunders, 1986, p. 71.
7. Bertone, J., and Horspool, L.J.I.: Equine Clinical Pharmacology. Philadelphia, W.B. Saunders, 2004.
8. Bettschart-Wolfensberger, R., Jaggin-Schmucker, N., Lendl, C., Bettschart, R.W., and Clarke, K.W.: Minimal alveolar concentration of desflurane in combination with an infusion of medetomidine for the anaesthesia of ponies. Vet. Rec., *148*:264–267, 2001.
9. Bettschart-Wolfensberger, R., Clarke, K.W., Vainio, O., Aliabadi, F., and Demuth, D.: Pharmacokinetics of medetomidine in ponies and elaboration of a medetomidine infusion regime which provides a constant level of sedation. Res. Vet. Sci., *67*:41–46, 1999.
10. Brock, K.A., and Heard, D.J.: Field anesthesia techniques in small ruminants. Part 1. Local analgesia. Compend. Contin. Educ., *7*:S407, 1985.
11. Butera, T.S., et al.: Diazepam/xylazine/ketamine combination for short-term anesthesia. VM/SAC, *74*:490, 1978.
12. Cakala, S.: A technique for the paravertebral lumbar block in cattle. Cornell Vet., *51*:64, 1961.
13. Cantor, G.H., Brunson, D.B., and Reibold, T.W.: A comparison of four short-acting anesthetic combinations for swine. VM/SAC, *76*:716, 1981.
14. Carroll, G.L., and Hartsfield, S.M.: General anesthetic techniques in ruminants. Vet. Clin. Food Anim. Prac., *12*:627–661, 1996.
15. Chevalier, H.M., Provost, P.J., and Karas, A.Z.: Effect of caudal epidural xylazine on intraoperative distress and post operative pain in Holstein heifers. Vet. Anesth. Analg., *31*:1–10, 2004.
16. Copland, M.D.: Anaesthesia for caesarean section in the ewe: a comparison of local and general anesthesia and the relationship between maternal and foetal values. N. Z. Vet. J., *24*:233, 1976.
17. Doherty, T.J., Geiser, D.R., and Rohrbach, B.W.: Effect of acepromazine and butorphanol on halothane minimum alveolar concentration in ponies. Eq. Vet. J., *29*:374–376, 1997.
18. England, G.C., Clarke, K.W., and Goossens, L.: A comparison of the sedative effects of three alpha 2-adrenoceptor agonists (romifidine, detomidine, and xylazine) in the horse. J. Vet. Pharmacol. Ther., *15*:194–201, 1992.
19. Ducharme, N.G., and Fubini, S.L.: Gastrointestinal complications associated with use of atropine in horses. J. Am. Vet. Med. Assoc., *182*:229, 1983.
20. Freeman, S.L., and England, G.C.: Comparison of sedative effects of Romifidine following intravenous, intramuscular, and sublingual administration to horses. Am. J. Vet. Res., *60*:954–959, 1999.
21. Funk, K.A.: Glyceryl guaiacolate: some effects and indications in horses. Eq. Vet. J., *5*:15, 1973.
22. Geiser, D.R.: Practical equine injectable anesthesia. J. Am. Vet. Med. Assoc., *182*:574, 1983.
23. Goodrich, L.R., Nixon, L.R., Fubini, S.L., Ducharme, N.G., et al.: Epidural morphine and detomidine decreases postoperative hindlimb lameness in horses after bilateral stifle arthroscopy. Vet. Surg., *31*:232–239, 2002.
24. Grandy, J.L., and McDonell, W.N.: Evaluation of concentrated solutions of guaifenesin for equine anesthesia. J. Am. Vet. Med. Assoc., *176*:619, 1980.
25. Grandy, J.L., et al.: Arterial hypotension and the development of postanesthetic myopathy in halothane-anesthetized horses. Am. J. Vet. Res., *48*:192, 1987.
26. Gray, P.R., and McDonell, W.: Anesthesia in goats and sheep. Part II. General anesthesia. Compend. Contin. Educ., *8*:S127, 1986.
27. Gray, P.R., and McDonell, W.N.: Anesthesia in goats and sheep. Part I. Local analgesia. Compend. Contin. Educ., *8*:S33, 1986.
28. Green, E.M., and Cooper, R.C.: Continuous caudal epidural anesthesia in the horse. J. Am. Vet. Med. Assoc., *184*:971–974, 1984.
29. Greene, S.A.: Protocols for anesthesia of cattle. Vet. Clin. Food. Anim., *19*:679–693, 2003.
30. Grosenbaugh, D.A., and Muir, W.W.: Cardiorespiratory effects of sevoflurane, isoflurane, and halothane anesthesia in horses. Am. J. Vet. Res., *59*:101–106, 1998.
31. Grubb, T.L., Riebold, T.W., Crismann, R.O., and Lamb, L.D.: Comparison of lidocaine, xylazine, and lidocaine-xylazine for caudal epidural analgesia in cattle. Vet. Anaesth Analges., *29*:64–68, 2002.

32. Grubb, T.L., Riebold, T.W., and Huber, M.J.: Comparison of lidocaine, xylazine, and xylazine/lidocaine for caudal epidural analgesia in horses. J. Am. Vet. Med. Assoc., 201:1187–1190, 1992.

33. Hall, L.W.: Wright's Veterinary Anaesthesia and Analgesia, 7th Ed. Philadelphia, Lea & Febiger, 1971.

34. Hall, L.W., Clarke, K.W., and Trim, C.M.: Veterinary Anesthesia. Philadelphia, W.B. Saunders, New York, 2001.

35. Hall, L.W., Gillespie, J.R., and Tyler, W.S.: Alveolar-arterial oxygen tension differences in anesthetized horses. Br. J. Anaesth., 40:560, 1968.

36. Heath, R.B.: Inhalation anesthesia. In Proceedings of the American Association of Equine Practitioners in 1976:1977, p. 335.

37. Heath, R.B., et al.: Protecting and positioning the equine surgical patient. VM/SAC, 68:1241, 1972.

38. Hendrickson, D.A., Kruse-Elliott, K.T., and Broadstone, R.V.: A comparison of epidural saline, morphine, and bupivacaine for pain relief after abdominal surgery in goats. Vet. Surg., 25:83–87, 1996.

39. Henny, D.P.: Anaesthesia of boars by intratesticular injection. Aust. Vet. J., 44:418, 1968.

40. Hodgson, D.S., et al.: Effects of spontaneous, assisted and controlled ventilatory modes in halothane-anesthetized geldings. Am. J. Vet. Res., 47:992, 1986.

41. Hodgson, D.S., Dunlop, C.I., Chapman, P.L., and Smith, J.A.: Cardiopulmonary effects of xylazine and acepromazine in pregnant cows in late gestation. Am. J. Vet. Res., 63:1695–1699, 2002.

42. Hoffman, P.E.: Clinical evaluation of xylazine as a chemical restraint agent, sedative and analgesic in horses. J. Am. Vet. Med. Assoc., 164:42, 1974.

43. Hornof, W.J., et al.: Effects of lateral recumbency on regional lung function in anesthetized horses. Am. J. Vet. Res., 47:277, 1986.

44. Hubbell, J.A.E.: Anesthesia of the equine athlete. In Veterinary Management of the Performance Horse. Philadelphia, W.B. Saunders, 2004.

45. Hubbell, J.A.E., Hull, B.L., and Muir, W.W.: Perianesthetic considerations in cattle. Compend. Contin. Educ., 8:F92, 1986.

46. Hubbell, J.A.E., et al.: Perianesthetic considerations in the horse. Compend. Contin. Educ., 6:S401, 1984.

47. Kerr, D.D., et al.: Sedative and other effects of xylazine given intravenously to horses. Am. J. Vet. Res., 33:526, 1972.

48. Klein, L.V., and Baetjar, C.: Preliminary report: xylazine and morphine sedation in horses. Vet. Anesth., 2:2-C, 1974.

49. Ko, J.C.H., Thurmon, J.C., Benson, J.G., et al.: Evaluation of analgesia induced by epidural injection of detomidine or xylazine in swine. J. Vet. Anaesth., 19:56–60, 1992.

50. Knight, A.P.: Xylazine. J. Am. Vet. Med. Assoc., 176:454, 1980.

51. Kumar, A., Thurmon, J.C., and Hardenbrook, J.H.: Clinical studies of ketamine HCl and xylazine HCl in domestic goats. VM/SAC, 72:1707, 1976.

52. Lin, H.C., Trachte, E.A., DeGraves, F.J., Rodgerson, D.H., Steiss, J.E., and Carson, R.L.: Evaluation of analgesia induced by epidural administration of medetomidine to cows. Am. J. Vet. Res., 59:162–167, 1998.

53. Lumb, W.V., and Jones, E.W.: Veterinary Anesthesia, 2nd Ed. Philadelphia, Lea & Febiger, 1984.

54. Mama, K.R.: Traditional and non-traditional uses of anesthetic drugs—an update. Vet. Clin. Eq., 18:169–179, 2002.

55. Martin, C.A., Kerr, C.L., Pearce, S.G., Lansdowne, J.L., and Boure, L.P.: Outcome of epidural catheterization for delivery of analgesics in horses: 43 cases (1998–2001). J. Am. Vet. Med. Assoc., 222:1394–1398, 2003.

56. McDonell, W.N., Hall, L.W., and Jeffcott, L.B.: Radiographic evidence of impaired pulmonary function in laterally recumbent anesthetized horses. Equine Vet. J., 11:24, 1979.

57. Mason, D.E., Muir, W.W., and Wade, A.: Arterial blood gas tensions in the horse during recovery from anesthesia. J. Am. Vet. Med. Assoc., 190:989, 1987.

58. McGrath, C., Richey, M.: Large animal anesthesia. In Veterinary Anesthesia and Analgesia. Edited by D. McKelvey, K.W. Hollingshead. Mosby, 2003, pp. 387–412.

59. Morishima, O.H., et al.: Toxicity of lidocaine in adult, newborn and fetal sheep. Anesthes., 55:7, 1981.

60. Mpanduji, D.G., Bittegeko, S.B., Mgasa, M.N., and Batamuzi, E.K.: Analgesic, behavioural, and cardiopulmonary effects of epidurally injected medetomidine (Domitor) in goats. J. Vet. Med. A. Physiol. Pathol. Clin. Med., 47:65–72, 2000.

61. Muir, W.W.: Total IV anesthesia in horses. In: 10th ACVA Vet. Symp., Sept, 2000, p. 109.

62. Muir, W.W.: Inhalant anesthesia in horses. In: 10th ACVA Vet. Symp., Sept, 2000, p. 109.

63. Muir, W.W., and Bednarski, R.M.: Equine cardiopulmonary resuscitation. Part II. Compend. Contin. Educ., 5:S287, 1983.

64. Muir, W.W., Skarda, R.T., and Milne, D.W.: Evaluation of xylazine and ketamine hydrochloride for anesthesia in horses. Am. J. Vet. Res., 38:195, 1977.

65. Muir, W.W., Skarda, R.T., and Sheehan, W.C.: Hemodynamic and respiratory effects of xylazine-morphine sulfate in horses. Am. J. Vet. Res., 40:1417, 1979.

66. Prado, M.E., Streeter, R.N., Mandsager, R.E., Shawley, R.V., and Claypool, P.L.: Pharmacologic effects of epidural versus intramuscular administration of detomidine in cattle. Am. J. Vet. Res., 60:1242–1247, 1999.

67. Ragan, H.A., and Gillis, M.F.: Restraint, venipuncture, endotracheal intubation and anesthesia of miniature swine. Lab. Anim. Sci., 25:409, 1975.

68. Reibold, T.W., Goble, D.O., and Geiser, D.R.: Principles and Techniques of Large Animal Anesthesia. East Lansing, Mich. State Univ. Press, 1978.

69. Rings, D.M., and Muir, W.W.: Cardiopulmonary effects of intramuscular xylazine-ketamine in calves. Can. J. Comp. Med., 467:386, 1982.

70. Robertson, J.T., and Muir, W.W.: A new analgesic drug combination in the horse. Am. J. Vet. Res., 44:1667, 1983.

71. Robinson, E.P., and Natalini, C.C.: Epidural anesthesia and analgesia in horses. Vet. Clin. North Am. Eq. Pract., 18:61–82, 2002.

72. Runnels, L.J.: Practical anesthesia and analgesia for porcine surgery. In Proceedings of the American Association of Swine Practitioners in 1976:1976, p. 80.

73. Salonen, J.S., Vaha-Vahe, T., Vainio, O., and Vakkuri, O.: Single-dose pharmacokinetics of detomidine in the horse and cow. J. Vet. Pharmacol. Ther., 12:65–72, 1989.

74. Schatzmann, U., et al.: An investigation of the action and haemolytic effect of glyceryl guaicolate in the horse. Equine Vet. J., 10:224, 1978.

75. Sembrad, S.D., Trim, C.M., and Hardee, G.E.: Hypertension in bulls and steers anesthetized with guaifenesin-theobarbiturate-halothane combination. Am. J. Vet. Res., 47:1577, 1986.

76. Singh, A.P., Peshin, P.K., Singh, J., et al.: Evaluation of detomidine as a sedative in goats. Acta. Vet. Hung., 39:109–114, 1991.

77. Skarda, R.T.: Local and regional anesthetic and analgesic techniques in ruminants and swine. In Lumb and Jones' Veterinary Anesthesia. 3rd Ed. Edited by J.C. Thurmon, W.J. Tranquili, G.J. Benson. Baltimore: Williams and Wilkins; 1996, pp. 479–514.

78. Skarda, R.T.: Local and regional anesthesia in ruminants and swine. Vet. Clin. Food. Anim. Pract., 12:579–626, 1996.

79. Soma, L.R.: Equine anesthesia: causes of reduced oxygen and increased carbon dioxide tensions. Compend. Contin. Educ., 2:S57, 1980.

80. Soma, L.R.: Textbook of Veterinary Anesthesia. Baltimore, Williams & Wilkins, 1971.

81. Steffey, E.P.: Enflurane and isoflurane anesthesia: a summary of laboratory and clinical investigations in horses. J. Am. Vet. Med. Assoc., 172:367, 1978.

82. Steffey, E.P.: Recent advances in inhalation anesthesia. Vet. Clin. Eq. Pract., 18:159–169, 2002.

83. Steffey, E.P., et al.: Body position and mode of ventilation influences arterial pH, oxygen and carbon dioxide tensions in halothane-anesthetized horses. Am. J. Vet. Res., 38:379, 1977.

84. Steffey, E.P., et al.: Enflurane, halothane and isoflurane potency in horses. Am. J. Vet. Res., 38:1037, 1977.

85. Steffey, E.P., Pascoe, P.J., Woliner, M.J., and Berryman, E.R.: Effects of xylazine hydrochloride during isoflurane-induced anesthesia in horses. Am. J. Vet. Res., 61:1255–1231, 2000.

86. St. Jean, G., Skarda, R.T., Muir, W.W., and Hoffsis, G.F.: Caudal epidural analgesia induced by xylazine administration in cows. Am. J. Vet. Res., 51:1232–1236, 1990.

87. Tadmor, A., Marcus, S., and Eting, E.: The use of ketamine hydrochloride for endotracheal intubation in cattle. Aust. Vet. J., 55:537, 1979.

88. Taylor, P.M., and Hall, L.W.: Clinical anaesthesia in the horse: comparison of enflurane and isoflurane. Equine Vet. J., 17:51, 1985.

89. Thurmon, J.C., and Benson, G.J.: Anesthesia in ruminants and swine. In Current Veterinary Therapy: Food Animal Practice. Vol. 2. Edited by J.L. Howard. Philadelphia, W.B. Saunders, 1986, p. 51.

90. Thurmon, J.C., Kumar, A., and Link, R.P.: Evaluation of ketamine hydrochloride as an anesthetic in sheep. J. Am. Vet. Med. Assoc., 162:293, 1973.

91. Thurmon, J.C., Nelson, D.R., and Christy, D.J.: Ketamine anesthesia in swine. J. Am. Vet. Med. Assoc., 160:1325, 1972.

92. Thurmon, J.C., Romack, F.E., and Garner, H.E.: Excursion of the bovine eyeball during gaseous anesthesia. VM/SAC, 63:967, 1968.

93. Trim, C.M.: Sedation and general anesthesia in ruminants. Calif. Vet., 4:29, 1981.

94. Trim, C.M., Moore, J.N., and White, N.A.: Cardiopulmonary effects of dopamine hydrochloride in anaesthetized horses. Eq. Vet. J., 17:41, 1985.

95. Weaver, A.D.: Intravenous local anesthesia of the lower limbs in cattle. J. Am. Vet. Med. Assoc., 160:55, 1972.

96. Yamashita, K., Muir, W.W. III, Tsubakishita, S., Abrahamsen, E., Lerch, P., et al.: Infusion of guaifenesin, ketamine, and medetomidine in combination with inhalation of sevoflurane versus inhalation of sevoflurane alone for anesthesia in horses. J. Am. Vet. Med. Assoc., 221:1150–1155, 2002.

97. Yamashita, K., Tsubakishita, S., Futaoka, S., Ueda, I., et al.: Cardiovascular effects of medetomidine, detomidine, and xylazine in horses. J. Vet. Med. Sci., 62:1025–1032, 2000.

Fluid Therapy

The need for fluid therapy in the physiologically compromised patient is well recognized. The horse undergoing exploratory laparotomy for acute abdominal crisis is often in a state of impending or fulminant shock. Similarly, the bovine patient with abomasal torsion often has major fluid volume and electrolyte deficits.

In the majority of the procedures in this textbook, the patients are systemically healthy and do not have fluid imbalances prior to surgery; however, such animals do need attention with respect to intravenous fluid therapy while they are under anesthesia. The purposes of fluid therapy for normal animals during anesthesia are to maintain adequate renal perfusion, to provide fluids for the patient's maintenance requirements, to maintain normal acid-base balance, and to maintain an intravenous route for emergency medication if needed.[17]

Two basic approaches are available in fluid management of the surgical patient: The first approach is to adopt a standard protocol devised to meet likely or anticipated deficits; the second approach is to acquire clinical and laboratory data on an individual patient and to administer the appropriate fluids to meet the patient's specific requirements. The first approach is simple and particularly convenient for the practitioner in the field, where it is not possible to obtain laboratory data instantly. In addition, this approach is satisfactory for fluid administration during routine elective surgery. For the patient with a systemic illness, however, such as an acute abdominal crisis in the horse or ox, it is desirable to obtain as accurate an assessment of the patient's fluid volume, acid-base balance, and electrolyte status as possible.

Diagnosis of Fluid Volume Deficits

The degree of dehydration or fluid volume deficit may be estimated by knowing the duration of the problem and evaluating various clinical signs, including skin elasticity, pulse rate and character, character of the mucous membranes, temperature of the extremities, and nature and position of the eyes (these parameters are defined in Table 2-12). Skin elasticity is estimated by picking up skin on the side of the neck and pinching it: If the skin flattens out in 1 to 2 seconds, it has normal elasticity; if the skin takes longer than 6 to 8 seconds to flatten, severe dehydration is present. In dehydration, the mucous membranes

Table 2-12. Assessment of degrees of clinical dehydration.

	Mild	Moderate	Severe*
Skin	Elasticity	Decreased elasticity	No elasticity
Eyes	Slightly sunken, bright	Slightly sunken, duller than normal	Deeply sunken, dry cornea
Mouth	Moist, warm	Sticky or dry	Dry, cold, cyanotic
Body weight decrease estimated (%)	4 to 6%	8%	10%
Fluid deficit (450-kg animal)	18 to 27 L	36 L	45 L

*Will see more dramatic clinical signs in acute hypovolemic shock.

change from moist and warm to sticky and dry, and then to cold and cyanotic. Volume deficits also increase the capillary refill time from its normal 1 to 3 seconds.

A severe hypovolemic situation, such as fulminant endotoxic shock, presents a sequence of obvious clinical signs. These include a weak, irregular pulse and color changes in the mucous membranes (brick red in the vasodilatory phase of septic shock, progressing through the cyanotic "muddy" appearance in the vasoconstricted phase). Capillary refill time is greater than 3 seconds, and the extremities are cold. Although these signs do not give a quantitative estimate of the volume deficit, they do indicate an urgent need for rapid infusion of intravenous fluids. The quantity of fluids given is based on the patient's response to therapy, rather than on any previous calculations.

It is possible to estimate the approximate fluid volume deficit by using clinical signs (Table 2-12). Under a state of mild dehydration, the fluid deficit is considered to be 4 to 6% of body weight. If signs of severe dehydration are observed, one generally considers that a fluid deficit is at least 10% of the body weight. This means that, in a 450-kg cow, a fluid volume deficit of 45 L exists.

A simple laboratory estimate of the degree of hypovolemia may be obtained by simultaneous measurement of the PCV and total plasma protein (TPP). The use of PCV has been criticized because of its wide normal range (in the horse, the normal range is 32 to 52%) and its tendency to undergo changes associated with splenic contraction or hemorrhage, thus confusing attempts to estimate intravascular volume. When the PCV is considered in conjunction with the TPP, however, it is a valuable tool. The range of normal TPP values is more limited. Under certain conditions, such as peritonitis, protein loss can occur, and again, both PCV and TPP need to be evaluated simultaneously and serially.

The use of PCV and TPP estimations is particularly valuable as a monitoring aid during volume replacement. If TPP remains at a normal level while PCV decreases, or if TPP and PCV concurrently decrease, this generally signifies that volume replacement is proceeding satisfactorily. A continued increase in PCV and TPP despite intensive fluid therapy is a poor sign, signifying a continued decrease in intravascular volume, associated with persistent pooling of fluid peripherally. A decreasing TPP accompanied by an increasing PCV usually signifies that the intravascular volume is not increasing and that protein is being lost from the vascular system.

Admittedly, the foregoing parameters actually provide an estimate of intravascular hydration, and acute loss from the interstitial or intracellular compartments may not be recognized initially. Equilibration between compartments takes place, however, and with sequential monitoring, most disadvantages in the use of PCV and TPP are eliminated.

Other laboratory tests thought to have advantages in the evaluation of fluid deficits include the estimation of serum sodium, plasma osmolarity, and serum creatinine.[12,18,20] Serum sodium estimation helps characterize the nature of the fluid loss, but in most clinical situations, the clinician can decide whether the fluid loss is hypotonic, isotonic, or hypertonic based on the clinical problem. In addition, serum sodium estimation generally is not immediately available to the clinician. An accurate method of assessing volume deficits is through estimation of plasma osmolality.[14] Unfortunately, this test is not routinely available in clinical institutions, let alone in practice. Serum creatinine and urea concentrations are highly elevated in patients with acute dehydration and may be used to assess the degree of fluid replacement that is needed.

The practical methods available for assessing volume deficits in the surgical patient include the surgeon's clinical assessments and knowledge of the pathophysiology of the disease; estimation of the PCV and TPP; and probably most important, serial evaluation of the response to replacement therapy by both clinical examination and PCV and TPP estimation.

Diagnosis of Acid-Base Imbalance

Acid-base physiology is complex, and consequently, discussions on the cause, diagnosis, and treatment of acid-base imbalance are frequently confusing. The following is a simplified (and one hopes practical) summary of the identification of acid-base imbalance. Although some accuracy may be compromised because of simplification, it is of little significance to the animal.

Abnormalities of acid-base can be ascertained based upon clinical signs, serum biochemical profiles, or blood gas analyses. The advent of relatively inexpensive and portable blood gas analyzers has increased their practicality in the field and allows for quick and easy measurements of pH, P_{CO_2} and P_{O_2}. An alternative method is to measure total carbon dioxide with a Harleco CO_2 appartus.[12]

The pH represents the net effect of the influences of respiratory and metabolic mechanisms. The magnitude of the respiratory component is identified by the P_{CO_2}. A P_{CO_2} greater than 45 mm Hg generally indicates respiratory acidosis, whereas a P_{CO_2} less than 35 mm Hg indicates respiratory alkalosis. The magnitude of the metabolic component is identified by either the bicarbonate concentration (HCO_3^-) or the base deficit/excess.[15]

The bicarbonate concentration can be misleading as a quantitative estimate of the metabolic component, because a primary change in carbon dioxide concentration directly causes a change in bicarbonate concentration that is not due to any change in the metabolic component. In addition, because of the presence of other buffer systems, the bicarbonate system is not responsible for buffering all of a given acid or base load. Base deficit/excess is a more accurate measure of quantitative changes in the metabolic component. Base deficit/excess is defined as the titratable acid or base, respectively, when titrating to a pH of 7.4 under standard conditions of P_{CO_2} (40 mm Hg), temperature (38°C), and complete hemoglobin saturation.[18] The base deficit/excess is estimated by aligning the measured values of pH and P_{CO_2} on a nomogram or is computed directly by the blood-gas machine. A base deficit less than −4 mEq/L indicates metabolic acidosis, whereas a base excess greater than +4 mEq/L indicates metabolic alkalosis.[15]

Despite the theoretic deficiencies in using bicarbonate levels as the measure of the metabolic component, the difference is negligible in most practical clinical situations. When P_{CO_2} is within normal range, the bicarbonate deficit (actual HCO_3^- − normal HCO_3^-) approximates the base deficit. It is commonly assumed in clinical practice

that these two values are the same. If this approximation is accepted, the bicarbonate may be read off a nomogram in the same fashion as the base deficit.

To identify a respiratory-derived acid-base imbalance, arterial blood samples are necessary. In most presurgical and postsurgical patients, any acid-base problems have a primary metabolic component, and it is not usually necessary to obtain arterial samples. In large animals, most acid-base imbalances with a primary respiratory origin occur during anesthesia, when arterial blood samples may be conveniently obtained. Treatment of respiratory acidosis involves proper ventilation. Respiratory alkalosis is generally iatrogenic or compensatory.

In evaluating metabolically derived acid-base imbalance, venous blood samples are satisfactory. Normal values for venous blood gases are listed in Table 2-13. Severe metabolic acidosis is treated with an infusion of sodium bicarbonate. The following is an example of a calculation of the amount of bicarbonate needed using the blood-gas data from a patient with severe metabolic acidosis.

pH	7.113
P_{CO_2}	43.8 mm Hg
HCO_3^-	11.9 mEq/L
TCO_2	12.9 mEq/L
Base deficit	13.6 mEq/L

Using the base deficit, the patient's bicarbonate deficit is calculated by the following equation:

$$\frac{\text{Base deficit} \times \text{body weight(kg)} \times .3}{\text{Equivalent weight of } HCO_3^-}$$
$$= \frac{13.6 \times 405 \times .3}{12}$$
$$= 153 \text{ g bicarbonate}$$

The bicarbonate deficit may also be calculated from the bicarbonate level using this formula:

Table 2-13. Normal values used in the evaluation of fluid balance in large animals.

	Horse	Ox	Sheep	Swine
PCV (%)	32–52	24–46	24–50	32–50
Total protein (g/dl)	6–8	6–8	6–7.5	6–7
Electrolytes				
Sodium (mEq/L)	128–140	130–147	139–150	135–150
Potassium (mEq/L)	2.8–4.3	4.3–5.0	3.9–5.4	4.4–6.7
Chloride (mEq/L)	99–109	97–111	95–103	94–106
Blood gases (venous)				
pH	7.32–7.44	7.31–7.53	7.32–7.53	
P_{CO_2} (mm Hg)	38–46	35–44	36–40	
HCO_3 (mEq/L)	24–27	25–35	20–25	18–27
TCO_2 (mM/L)	24–32	21.2–32.2	21–28	

$$\dfrac{\left(\begin{array}{l}\text{Measured} \quad \text{normal} \\ \text{bicarbonate} - \text{bicarbonate} \\ \text{level} \qquad \text{level}\end{array}\right) \times BW \times .3}{12}$$

$$= \dfrac{(11.9 - 25) \times 450 \times .3}{12}$$

$$= \dfrac{13.1 \times 450 \times .3}{12}$$

$$= 147\,g\ \text{bicarbonate}$$

This example demonstrates the general approximation between using base deficit and bicarbonate levels.

The factor 0.3 is an approximation of the volume of distribution of the bicarbonate, which is accounted for mostly by the extracellular fluid compartment. Higher factors have been used by some (up to 0.6, which approximates the volume of distribution of total body water), but these factors are not recommended because of the long time required for complete equilibration with the intracellular space and the possible overadministration of bicarbonate. This is discussed in the section on treatment of fluid imbalances.

If a blood-gas machine is not available, the measurement of total carbon dioxide determined by the Harleco CO_2 apparatus is a suitable alternative and gives a reliable measure of the bicarbonate excess or deficit.[12] The addition of acid to serum or plasma results in the liberation of free carbon dioxide, which is almost completely bicarbonate in origin:

$$\text{Total } CO_2 = \text{Dissolved } CO_2\ (Pco_2 \times 0.03) + HCO_3^- \text{ and}$$
$$\dfrac{HCO_3^-}{CO_2} = \dfrac{20}{1}$$

The bicarbonate, therefore, can be estimated by the following formula:

$$HCO_3^- = TCO_2 - \text{Dissolved } CO_2 = TCO_2 - 1.2\,mEq/L$$

This method is a convenient and economical way for the practitioner to plan and to monitor therapy for metabolic acidosis and to avoid overcorrection or undercorrection of the base deficit.

Although the situation of metabolic acidosis has been used to demonstrate the calculation of imbalances, clinical cases of metabolic alkalosis are identified in a similar manner. The bicarbonate excess is calculated from the base excess or bicarbonate levels using the same formula. If specific therapy is required, physiologic saline solution is administered, and the acid-base status is monitored until it returns to normal.

Blood gases alone will not enable one to detect the presence or severity of metabolic acidosis in horses with previous alkalinizing therapy or mixed acid-base disturbances. An estimate of the serum or plasma concentration of unmeasured ions allows detection of these cases. The anion gap or the simplified strong ion gap calculation may be used:

$$\text{Anion gap} = Na^+ - (Cl^- + HCO_3^-)$$
$$\text{Strong ion gap} = \dfrac{2.24 \times \text{Total Protein (g/dl)}}{1 + 10^{(6.65 - pH)}} - \text{Anion gap}$$

The anion gap is a measurement of the difference between the concentration of unmeasured anions and unmeasured cations in serum. The strong ion gap measures the difference between only the unmeasured strong anions and cations.[7] In horses with normal serum protein levels, the anion gap will provide an accurate estimate of unmeasured strong ion concentrations. A high anion gap (>24 mmol/L) will occur when the concentration of unmeasured anions in plasma (i.e., lactate) is elevated and is a reflection of lactic acidosis. However, in cases of metabolic alkalosis, elevated levels of serum protein can mask the detection of unmeasured anions. The simplified strong ion gap calculation should be used in these cases and will provide the most accurate calculation in horses of varying age and concentrations of albumin, globulin, and phosphate.[7]

An increased anion gap, even in the presence of a normal blood gas picture, can occur in, for example, a horse with L-lactic acidosis previously administered sodium bicarbonate or in mixed acid-base disturbance, such as in a horse with anterior enteritis and metabolic acidosis due to L-lactic acidosis and metabolic alkalosis due to gastric reflux.[13]

Diagnosis of Electrolyte Abnormalities

The electrolytes of principal concern in the fluid management of surgical patients are sodium, potassium, and chloride ions. The levels of these electrolytes are not evaluated routinely in every patient in which the need for fluid therapy is anticipated. In specific situations, however, evaluation of the status of these electrolytes is important. Sodium ion is an important electrolyte, and its concentration is intimately associated with fluid content in the body. Sodium and water are lost together (an isotonic loss) in surgical patients, and sodium ion is a routine component in replacement fluids; therefore, specific abnormalities in sodium are not of common concern unless there is a specific loss or gain of sodium. Hypernatremia may become a clinical problem in the patient that has received intensive fluid therapy and in which the addition of sodium bicarbonate to the balanced electrolyte solution has caused an excessive administration of sodium ion. This situation should be monitored in such patients.

A hyperkalemic state may occur during metabolic acidosis because of the redistribution of body potassium. Intracellular potassium moves out of the cells into the extracellular fluid as excess hydrogen ions move into the cells. Hyperkalemia usually is not a clinical problem in the nonanesthetized animal, except when the renal threshold is exceeded and potassium is lost from the body, resulting in a state of hypokalemia when the acidosis has been corrected. For this reason, potassium levels should be evaluated once acidosis has been corrected and equilibration of intracellular and extracellular potassium and hydrogen ions has recurred. Serum potassium levels under 3 mEq/L in the horse are indicative of significant hypokalemia.[4] Severe deficits of potassium also occur with diarrhea in horses. Thus, hypokalemia may be a clinical problem prior to surgery in a patient with such a history.

Calculation of the overall body deficit in potassium is difficult because the actual volume of distribution for the ion is uncertain. For convenience, an arbitrary volume of distribution of 40% of the body weight is used. In a 450-kg horse, for example, the potassium "space" may be considered $450 \times .4 = 180$ L. If a patient has a potassium level of 2.0 mEq/L, it is considered to have a deficiency of $180 \times (4 - 2) = 360$ mEq (normal potassium level is 4.0 mEq/L). The equivalent weight of potassium is 14. The patient is therefore deficient $360/14 = 26$ g potassium. If hyponatremia is encountered, a factor of 0.3 is used for the sodium space.

Decreases in chloride levels are observed in cattle with abomasal torsion. A significant correlation has been observed between postsurgical outcome and the presurgical serum chloride concentration.[19] Serum concentrations of sodium and potassium also decrease, but less dramatically.

Fluid Therapy in the Anesthetized Patient Undergoing Elective Surgery

In general, there are four essential principles of fluid therapy: the replacement of existing deficits, the fulfillment of maintenance requirements, the replacement of anticipated additional losses, and the monitoring of the patient's response to therapy. The routine surgical patient has no deficit at the time of anesthetic induction, but fluid should be administered during anesthesia in anticipation of maintenance requirements and metabolic changes during anesthesia.

A polyionic, isotonic solution with an alkalinizing effect should be administered during anesthesia. Lactated Ringer's solution, for example, is appropriate for this purpose (Table 2-14). In the uncompromised patient, metabolism of lactate by the liver yields a bicarbonate equivalent; the acetate and gluconate in Normosol-R are

metabolized by the muscle to yield a bicarbonate equivalent. An extracellular replacement fluid made at the Veterinary Teaching Hospital at Colorado State University contains sodium, potassium, chloride ions, and acetate as a bicarbonate precursor (composition in Table 2-14). Acetate, rather than lactate, is used mainly for convenience because it is available in a powder.

Fluids should always be administered intravenously, using an indwelling catheter or needles at least 5 cm in length and properly threaded in the vein. If intravenous catheters are used, an aseptic preparation should be made before insertion, and every precaution should be taken to avoid phlebitis. A rate of administration of 4.4 to 6.6 ml/kg/hr is sufficient to maintain the patient's hydration in elective cases;[17] however, the patient should be monitored continually to ensure that such maintenance therapy is adequate.

If a patient becomes compromised during surgery, the fluid therapy regimen should be changed immediately to satisfy any specific requirements.

Fluid Therapy in the Compromised Patient, According to Requirements

Fluid therapy in the compromised patient should be directed specifically at the volume deficits, acid-base imbalances, and electrolyte changes. At the same time, intensive monitoring is required to ensure that the therapy is satisfactory and to recognize developing needs.

Volume replacement is usually the most important and urgent requirement in the compromised large animal patient. Polyionic replacement fluids of the alkalinizing type are used, except in case of metabolic alkalosis. Because the rate of administration varies with the state of the animal, formulas for administration rate have little value in the compromised patient. Fluids are generally given rapidly, and the administration rate is dictated by changes in the clinical signs and the PCV and TPP. Rapid volume replacement is particularly urgent in shock patients, to maintain circulating blood volume. Untoward sequelae of overzealous volume replacement are rare unless the animal is recumbent or has a low TPP or kidney failure. The usual error in volume replacement in large

Table 2-14. Composition of intravenous fluids (mEq/L).

Polyionic Replacement Solutions	Na+	K+	Ca++	Mg++	Cl−	Bicarbonate Precursor
Ringer's solution	147.5	4	4.5		156	
Lactated Ringer's solution	130	4	3		109	28 (lactate)
Normosol-R	140	5		3	98	50 (acetate, gluconate)
Polysol	140	10	5	3	103	55 (acetate)
Extracellular replacement fluid	140	5			115	30 (acetate)
Physiologic saline solution	154				154	
5% Bicarbonate	600					600
Lactated Ringer's solution + 5 g/L NaHCO₃	190	4	3		109	87

animals is the administration of an inadequate volume of fluids or slow administration of the volume.

When monitoring massive fluid replacement, a continued decrease in TPP without evidence that the volume deficit is being replaced indicates a vital protein loss. A TPP of less than 4 g/dl is an indication for plasma administration. Plasma expanders such as dextran preparations are not used routinely; they are costly, and adverse reactions have been reported.

The specific treatment of metabolic acidosis is not so straightforward. In the past, any base deficit was treated immediately with sodium bicarbonate (often in bolus form with priority over volume replacement), and it was generally considered better to give too much than too little. Based on more recent information, this practice requires modification for several reasons. The first is that metabolic acidosis in the large animal surgical patient usually occurs secondary to hypovolemia and inadequate peripheral tissue perfusion. Rectification of the primary problems usually corrects any accompanying acidosis (at least mild acidosis) and makes the specific administration of sodium bicarbonate unnecessary. In addition, as volume and tissue perfusion are restored, the acetate, gluconate, or lactate in the polyionic replacement fluids acts as a source of bicarbonate (Table 2-14).

Opinions vary on the value of the lactate in lactated Ringer's solution as a bicarbonate source in the compromised patient. The conversion of lactate to bicarbonate requires a functioning liver and adequate perfusion to provide oxygen; consequently, immediate provision of bicarbonate by lactate cannot be anticipated in the patient in shock. As perfusion is restored, exogenously administered lactate does not accumulate, but acts as a bicarbonate source. In addition, the liver can still metabolize lactate when the blood flow to the organ is 20% of normal and oxygen saturation is 50%.[11] The other criticism of giving lactated solutions for the treatment of patients in shock has been that lactic acidosis already exists in these patients. Although lactate will not be converted to bicarbonate in these patients while they are in shock, there is no evidence that its presence causes any harm. Exogenous lactate, given in lactated Ringer's solution, does not increase blood lactate levels in normal or shock patients.[3] Additionally, studies in humans have shown that administering lactate Ringer's solution to patients in hemorrhagic shock does not exacerbate the lactate acidosis that occurs secondary to hypoperfusion.[8] However, lactated Ringer's solution may be contraindicated for animals with severe septicemia, endotoxemia, or liver disorders because the liver's ability to uptake and metabolize lactate may be compromised in these animals.[8]

For more severely compromised patients in which conversion of the bicarbonate precursors to bicarbonate is not anticipated, specific administration of bicarbonate is appropriate. Bicarbonate is indicated to treat cases of metabolic acidosis caused by either hyponatremia or hypochloremia.[8] Its use in the treatment of lactic acidosis is still controversial. Bicarbonate supplementation is certainly indicated when the base deficit is 10 mEq/L or greater. The amount administered is based on calculation of the deficit, as described previously. It is important to avoid overadministration. In the past, practitioners considered sodium bicarbonate a benign drug because excess bicarbonate could be excreted by the kidneys or converted to carbon dioxide and eliminated by the lungs.[5] Several potential hazards have been suggested, however: hypernatremia leading to hyperosmolality; iatrogenic alkalosis, which could interfere with neuromuscular function; and paradoxic acidosis of cerebrospinal fluid (CSF).[5] The last condition has been recognized in dogs and man.[1,2] The problem is best demonstrated by this equation:

$$HCO_3^- + H^+ \rightleftharpoons H_2CO_3 \rightleftharpoons H_2O + CO_2$$

Overadministration of sodium bicarbonate drives this reaction to the right, producing increased carbon dioxide. The carbon dioxide could potentially diffuse across the blood-brain barrier in preference to bicarbonate. The increased carbon dioxide in the CSF could cause the same reaction to be driven to the left, increasing hydrogen in the CSF and thereby leading to acidosis. The significance of this problem in large animals has yet to be substantiated, however.

Supplementary bicarbonate may be added to the polyionic replacement solution (if it does not contain calcium) or administered separately. If prolonged bicarbonate therapy is necessary, it may be desirable to give sodium bicarbonate in isotonic solution with sterile water or to substitute 5% dextrose solution for some of the sodium-containing replacement fluid, to minimize the development of hypernatremia.

If a patient has metabolic alkalosis (typically a cow with an abomasal disorder), physiologic saline solution is administered. This will replace lost volume and restore depleted chloride levels, which are the cause of the alkalosis. At the same time, surgical correction of the abomasal problem with cessation of chloride sequestration is an equally important part of the therapy. In man, the use of sodium chloride is not satisfactory for the treatment of severe cases of metabolic alkalosis.[22] If kidney function is decreased, hypernatremia becomes a problem; dilute hydrochloric acid, administered until the base excess is corrected, improves this condition.[22] This treatment may be appropriate in severe cases in animals.

In the patient with a recognized potassium deficit, potassium may be added to the intravenous fluids at a rate of up to 10 mEq/L,[20] with a total maximum of less than 100 mEq.[10] Higher rates (20 to 25 mEq/L) are used in the dog and man, but caution is advised when treating the horse. Correct levels of potassium may be achieved by the addition of 0.75 g of potassium chloride per liter of fluid. Administering this additional potassium intravenously is safe for horses with adequate renal function. In most cases, hypokalemia is recognized when the animal's condition is stabilized following a hypovolemic, acidotic crisis. In most of these cases, potassium replacement can be accomplished satisfactorily by administering 30 g of potassium chloride by stomach tube and repeating if necessary. Treatment of the other major electrolyte imbalances, hypochloremia and hypernatremia, has already been discussed.

The best indication of any fluid therapy protocol is the clinical response of the animal to the therapy. These observations should be accompanied by routine PCV and TPP estimations, acid-base status (blood gases or total carbon dioxide), and electrolyte assessment as appropriate. The animal's fluid status is dynamic, and the interval between measurement of these parameters depends on the individual clinical case. Because of the marked variability between cases and the need for continued monitoring, we have avoided quoting rates of administration.

Fluid Administration in the Compromised Patient without Preliminary Data

In certain field situations, the practitioner must initiate fluid therapy when the only preliminary data are those noted in the clinical examination. This practice is appropriate, but certain guidelines need to be followed. If volume replacement therapy is prolonged, PCV and TPP should be evaluated as soon as possible. If acid-base data are not available, 50 to 100 g of bicarbonate may be given empirically along with other fluids, in the case of the horse. Such empiric administration is not recommended in an anesthetized horse, however, because bicarbonate administration increases carbon dioxide production in a horse that is usually hypoventilating. Surgical conditions in cattle almost always result in metabolic alkalosis. Metabolic acidosis is usually seen only in adult cattle when they are terminally ill and can no longer maintain circulation. Therefore, in cattle, either saline solution or straight Ringer's solution should be used when acid-base information is unavailable. Electrolyte determination should be made before specific electrolyte disturbances are treated.

When performing volume replacement based on clinical examination alone, the clinician needs to have some concept of the volume of fluid necessary. Twelve to 20 L of fluid per hour have been given to horses in shock. When frequent or excessive urination occurs, the rate of the infusion should be decreased. After the initial rapid administration of fluids, the usual recommended flow rate is 3 to 5 L/hr.[4] A 450-kg horse needs 27 L of water per day for maintenance alone.[10]

References

1. Berenyi, K.J., Wolk, M., and Killip, T.: Cerebrospinal fluid acidosis complicating therapy of experimental cardiopulmonary arrest. Circulation, 52:319, 1975.
2. Bishop, R.L., and Weisfeldt, M.L.: Sodium bicarbonate administration during cardiac arrest. J. Am. Med. Assoc., 235:506, 1976.
3. Brasmer, T.H.: Fluid therapy in shock. J. Am. Vet. Med. Assoc., 174:475, 1979.
4. Carlson, G.P.: Fluid therapy in horses with acute diarrhea. Vet. Clin. North Am. (Large Anim. Pract.), 3:313, 1979.
5. Coffman, J.: Acid:base balance. VM/SAC, 75:489, 1980.
6. Constable, P.D.: Clinical assessment of acid-base status: comparison of the Henderson-Hasselbalch and strong ion approaches. Vet. Clin. Path., 29:115–126, 2000.
7. Constable, P.D., Hinchcliff, K.W., and Muir, W.W. III.: Comparison of anion gap and strong ion gap as predictors of unmeasured strong ion concentration in plasma and serum from horses. Am. J. Vet. Res., 59:881–887, 1998.
8. Corely, K.T.T.: Fluid therapy. In Equine Clinical Pharmacology. Edited by J.J. Bertone, L.J.I. Horspool. New York, W.B. Saunders, 2004, pp. 327–364.
9. Corley, K.T.T., and Marr, C.M.: Pathophysiology, assessment and treatment of acid-base disturbances in the horse. Eq. Vet. Educ., 10:255–265, 1998.
10. Donawick, W.J.: Metabolic management of the horse with acute abdominal crisis. J. S. Afr. Vet. Assoc., 46:107, 1975.
11. Garner, H.E., et al.: Postoperative care of equine abdominal crises. Vet. Anesth., 4:40, 1977.
12. Gentry, P.A., and Black, W.D.: Evaluation of Harleco CO2 apparatus: comparison with the Van Slyke method. J. Am. Vet. Med. Assoc., 167:156, 1975.
13. Gossett, K.A., French, D.D., and Cleghorn, B.: Laboratory evaluation of metabolic acidosis. In Proceedings of the Second Equine Colic Research Symposium. Athens, GA, University of Georgia, 1986, p. 161.
14. Green, R.A.: Perspectives in clinical osmometry. Vet. Clin. North Am. (Small Anim. Pract.), 8:287, 1978.
15. Haskins, S.C.: An overview of acid-base physiology. J. Am. Vet. Med. Assoc., 170:423, 1977.
16. Kohn, C.W.: Preoperative management of the equine patient with an abdominal crisis. Vet. Clin. North Am. (Large Anim. Pract.) 1:289, 1979.
17. Reibold, T.W., Goble, D.O., and Geiser, D.R.: Principles and Techniques of Large-Animal Anesthesia. East Lansing, Mich. State Univ. Press, 1978.
18. Siggaard-Anderson, O.: Blood acid-base alignment nomogram: scales for pH, pCO2, base excess of whole blood of different hemoglobin concentrations, plasma bicarbonate, and plasma total CO2. Scand. J. Clin. Lab. Invest., 15:211, 1963.
19. Smith, D.F.: Right-side torsion of the abomasum in dairy cows: classification of severity and evaluation of outcome. J. Am. Vet. Med. Assoc., 173:108, 1978.
20. Waterman, A.: A review of the diagnosis and treatment of fluid and electrolyte disorders in the horse. Equine Vet. J., 9:43, 1977.
21. Whitehair, K.J., Haskins, S.C., Whitehair, J.G., and Pascoe, P.J.: Clinical applications of quantitative acid-base chemistry. J. Vet. Intern. Med., 9:1–11, 1995.
22. Williams, D.B., and Lyons, J.H.: Treatment of severe metabolic alkalosis with intravenous infusion of hydrochloric acid. Surg. Gynecol. Obstet., 150:315, 1980.
23. Johnson, P.J.: Electrolyte and acid-base disturbances in the horse. Vet. Clin. Eq., 11:491–513, 1995.

Chapter 3

SURGICAL INSTRUMENTS

Objectives

1. Familiarize the inexperienced surgeon with some general instruments commonly used in veterinary surgical practice.
2. Serve as a reference for the instrumentation used in various techniques that are discussed in this chapter.

Use of Surgical Instruments

The most important aspect of instrumentation is knowing which instrument to use at which time; this is essential to good surgical technique. It ensures that the particular surgical procedure is undertaken with minimal trauma to the tissues, is performed in the minimal amount of time, and ultimately results in the least harm to the patient. In learning about this wealth of instruments, it helps to handle them and to use them in situations such as laboratory work and practical sessions whenever possible.

Scalpel

The scalpel is used for the sharp division of tissue with minimal damage to nearby structures. Today, scalpels come with a variety of blade configurations, each designed for a specific purpose. The blades are disposable, thereby avoiding the need to be sharpened. Scalpel handles come in different sizes; no. 3 and no. 4 are generally adequate for most large animal surgical procedures. For work in deep cavities, such as rectovaginal fistula repair and urine-pooling operations, longer-handled scalpels are essential.

The scalpel must be held so that it is under complete control. It is grasped between the thumb and the third and fourth fingers, with the index finger placed over the back. To cut, make a smooth sweep with the rounded portion of the blade, or *belly,* rather than with the point. The amount of pressure applied varies, but the aim is to produce a bold, single, full-thickness skin incision with a single sweep of the scalpel blade. The skin of the bovine flank, for example, is tough, and the neophyte surgeon usually does not apply enough pressure when making an incision in this area; the skin in the inguinal area of the horse, on the other hand, is thin, and a light stroke over the tissues with the middle of the blade is adequate.

Figure 3-1*A* shows the stroke made with nos. 10, 20, 21, and 22 scalpel blades. The handle should be at an angle of 30 to 40° to the surface incised. Figure 3-1*B* depicts the pencil grip with nos. 10, 20, 21, and 22 scalpel blades. The pencil grip is used for nos. 11 and 15 blades when more precise incisions are required (Figure 3-2*A*). Figure 3-2*B* shows the incorrect use of a no. 15 blade. The bistoury blade (no. 12) has a hook shape and is used for lancing abscesses. The bayonet tip blade (no. 11) can also be used for lancing abscesses and for severing ligaments.

When the scalpel blade becomes dull, the blade is removed carefully by grasping the blade with a needle holder or hemostat (Figure 3-3). The proximal end of the blade is then bent slightly to clear the blade from the hub of the handle. Then the blade is pushed up over the end of the scalpel handle. The reverse process is used to replace a scalpel blade. Although the blade may be too dull for a particular surgical procedure, the blade is still sharp enough to cause serious injury if care is not taken while removing it from the scalpel handle. The spent blade should be discarded appropriately.

To remove the new scalpel from its packet, the ends of the packet are grasped by the operating room nurse or nonscrubbed assistant and peeled open, exposing the end of the blade. The blade is carefully plucked out of the packet, contacting only the blade itself, to avoid a break in aseptic technique (Figure 3-4). Various types of scalpel blades and scalpel handles are illustrated later in this chapter.

Scissors

A variety of scissors are available and are used for such procedures as cutting tissues or dissecting between tissue

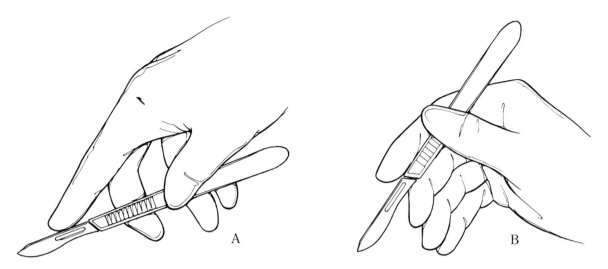

Fig. 3-1. Use of nos. 10, 20, 21, and 22 blades. A, Stroke. B, Pencil grip.

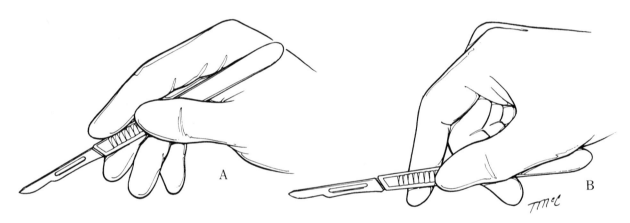

Fig. 3-2. A, Pencil grip for nos. 11 and 15 blades. B, Incorrect use of no. 15 blade.

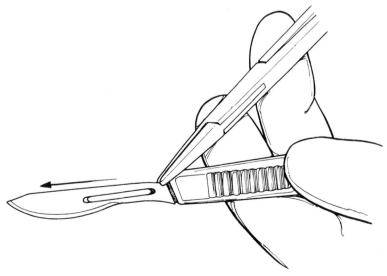

Fig. 3-3. Removing the used scalpel blade.

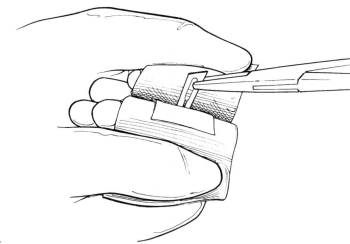

Fig. 3-4. Aseptic technique for handling new blade.

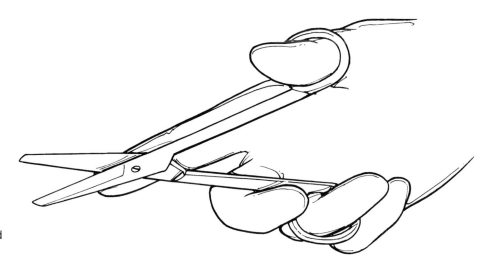

Fig. 3-5. Correct way to hold scissors.

planes. Generally speaking, scissors used for tissue are light and are made with precision in mind. They must be kept sharp or they will crush tissues rather than cut them. Mayo or Metzenbaum scissors are used for most tissues. They are available with curved or straight blades. Straight scissors are used for working close to the surface of the wound, whereas the curved scissors are used for working deeper in the wound. Scissors are also classified according to the shape of the tips, for example, sharp/sharp, sharp/blunt, and blunt/blunt. Some scissors are designed to cut wire. The heel of the wire-cutting scissors is used for this purpose. Various types of scissors are illustrated later in this chapter.

The scissors are grasped by placing the thumb and ring finger through the rings and setting the index finger against the blades. The index finger provides control of the tips of the scissors. The scissors must be kept near the last joint of the finger, and the fingers must not be allowed to slip through the rings of the handle (Figure 3-5). The end of the blade is used for cutting; however,

when tough structures are encountered, the heel of the blade is used. The scissors should not be closed unless the surgeon can see the tips of the blades; otherwise, vital structures may be endangered. For blunt dissection, insert the closed tips of the scissors into the tissue, and then open the points. Scissors used for tissue work should not be used for cutting suture material; one of the various types of suture scissors should be used instead.

Bandage scissors are an essential part of large animal surgery instrumentation, especially in equine limb surgery, in which the areas to be treated are commonly under bandage, and much of one's day may be spent changing bandages on horses' limbs. Some bandage scissors have slightly angled blades, and the lower blade has a small *button tip* on it to protect structures under the bandage. If bandage scissors are used against soiled or contaminated wounds, they must be sterilized after use to prevent transfer of infection to another wound or another patient.

Needle Holders (Needle Drivers)

During a large portion of an operation, the surgeon uses needle holders. The type of needle holder depends on individual tastes. Some needle holders, such as Olsen-Hegar or Gillies, have suture-cutting scissors incorporated into the jaws to enable the surgeon to cut sutures without reaching for suture-cutting scissors. These needle holders are useful in large animal practice where the surgeon is commonly on his own. Care must be taken to avoid cutting the suture accidentally during the procedure. There are many variations of width and serrations in the heads of the needle holders.

There are two different ways to hold needle holders. The first is to hold the needle holder as the surgeon would hold scissors, that is, with the thumb and the ring finger in the rings of the handles (Figure 3-6A). The other option is to *palm* the needle holder. Palming generally provides the surgeon with better control over the tip of the needle holder. The needles used with needle holders are curved; straight needles are held by hand only and are usually reserved for the skin and bowel. With the needle holder, the needle should be driven through the tissues in an arclike motion, following the curve of the needle. The needle holder is then removed and is reapplied to the protruding point of the needle, which is extracted from the tissue. The needle should be grasped by its thicker portion, rather than by the tip, because the tip may be easily bent or broken.

Some needle holders, such as the Mathieu, have a ratchet on the handle that releases when additional pressure is applied to the spring handles. These are time saving, but if the tissues resist passage of the needle, a firm grip cannot be applied to a needle without causing the needle holder to unsnap. Various types of needle holders are illustrated later in this chapter.

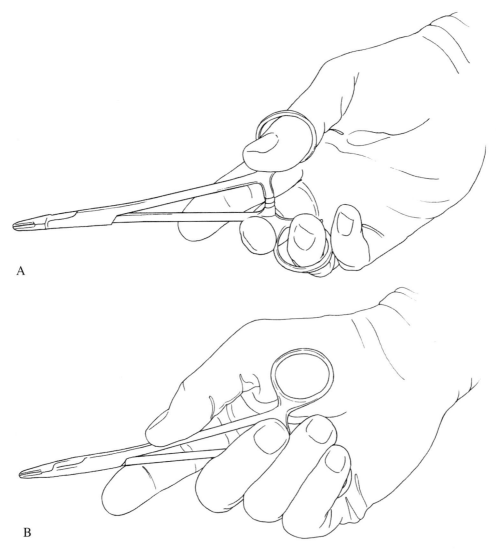

A

B

Fig. 3-6. A, Using rings to hold the needle holders. B, Palming the needle holder.

Thumb Forceps

Thumb forceps are used for grasping and holding tissues. They are held between the thumb and the middle and index fingers (Figure 3-7). It is common for the inexperienced surgeon to hold thumb forceps incorrectly, like a scalpel handle, especially toward the end of the operation when fatigue is setting in. Thumb forceps are usually held in the left hand while the right hand holds the scalpel or needle holder. Thumb forceps with teeth bite into tissue and prevent the instrument from slipping. Some surgeons consider these forceps too traumatic for use on hollow organs or blood vessels and reserve them for skin. Thumb forceps are illustrated later in this chapter.

Grasping Forceps

A variety of forceps used for larger portions of tissue maintain their hold with the use of a ratchet device on the handle. Allis tissue forceps have opposing edges with short teeth. They may be used for grasping tissues such as fascia and tendon, but they should not be used on skin edges or viscera. Vulsellum forceps are useful for grasping the uterine walls of the various large animal species, to stabilize the walls during closure. Sponge forceps are used in the inguinal approach for cryptorchidism, to grasp the vaginal process. Towel-holding forceps (clamps) are useful for grasping skin edges, as well as for holding drapes in position.

Hemostatic Forceps

Hemostatic forceps are used to clamp the ends of blood vessels and thereby to establish hemostasis. They vary not only in size; they also vary in the shape and direction of the serrations. Halsted mosquito forceps are used for clamping small vessels.

When larger vessels are encountered, Kelly forceps may be more suitable. The amount of tissue crushed should be kept to a minimum. Hemostatic forceps are frequently used in conjunction with electrocautery. When ligating bleeding points, the tips of the instruments should be elevated to facilitate passage of the ligature. Curved hemostats should be affixed with the curved jaws pointing upward. If a scrubbed assistant is present during an operation, he or she should pass the instruments by slapping them, handles first, into the hands of the surgeon (Figure 3-8).

It is not within the scope of this chapter to describe the applications of more than a few forceps. A variety of the forceps used in large animal practice are shown later in this chapter.

Retractors

Retractors are used to maintain exposure at various surgical sites. Handheld retractors are held by an assistant. If the surgeon does not have the luxury of an assistant, as is often the case in large animal practice, self-retaining retractors can be used. Self-retaining retractors anchor themselves against the wound edges by maintaining fixed pressure on the retractor arms. When abdominal or thoracic retractors are used, moist sponges or towels are placed between the retractor blades and the tissues to minimize trauma to the wound edges. Examples of handheld retractors are United States Army retractors, malleable retractors, Volkmann retractors, Jansen retractors, and Senn retractors. Among the self-retaining retractors,

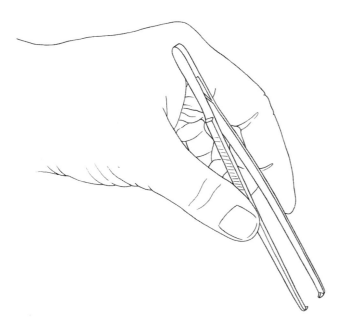

Fig. 3-7. Correct way to hold thumb forceps.

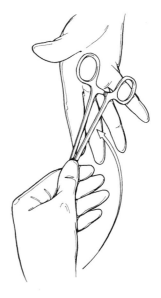

Fig. 3-8. Passing hemostatic forceps.

Weitlaner retractors and Gelpi retractors are useful for small incisions, such as laryngotomy and arthrotomy incisions in the horse. The large Balfour retractors are predominantly used in laparotomy incisions. Occasionally, if thoracotomy is indicated, Finochietto rib retractors are the instruments of choice. Retractors are illustrated later in this chapter.

General Surgery Pack

Listed below is a standard set of instruments routinely used by us. Such a set of instruments suffices for most basic procedures. In the remainder of the text, these standard instruments are included as a general surgery pack, and any additional instruments required will be noted individually. Instruments in this standard set are

16 Towel forceps
4 Curved mosquito hemostats
4 Straight mosquito hemostats
2 Curved Kelly/Crile hemostatic forceps
2 Straight Kelly/Crile hemostatic forceps
2 Allis tissue forceps
1 Curved Mayo scissors
1 Straight Mayo scissors
1 S/S operating scissors (sharp/sharp)
1 Curved Metzenbaum scissors
1 Straight Metzenbaum scissors
2 Needle holders (1 Mayo-Hegar or Olsen-Hegar)
2 Right-angle forceps
1 Curved 6″ Ochsner forceps
1 Straight 6″ Ochsner forceps
1 No. 3 scalpel handle
1 No. 4 scalpel handle
3 3″ × 4″ thumb tissue forceps
2 1″ × 2″ Adson tissue forceps
1 Sponge forceps (curved or straight)
1 Saline bowl
4 Towels
Sponges in inverted bowl

Preparation of Instruments

The classification of the surgical procedure as clean, clean-contaminated, contaminated-dirty may influence how the surgeon prepares the surgical instruments. To illustrate, we obviously do not advocate that the instruments used to castrate piglets all be individually wrapped and sterilized. Yet for some of the *clean* surgical procedures described in this book, the use of instruments that have been cold-sterilized may be construed as malpractice.

As part of overall planning, all the necessary instruments for the particular procedure should be obtained and prepared prior to the operation. In most cases, the surgeon must attend to his/her own needs for instruments and so must be able to anticipate the necessity for particular instruments.

Autoclaving, a sterilization technique using moist heat from steam, is the method of choice for preparing instruments for aseptic surgery. Once the packs are open, it is the surgeon's responsibility to be sure that the autoclaving process has reached all the instruments by observing the indicator system used to ensure sterility.

Gas sterilization, with ethylene oxide gas or hydrogen peroxide (Sterrad), is used for instruments that would be damaged by the heat of autoclaving. Materials that have been sterilized with ethylene oxide must be aerated for 1 to 7 days, depending on the material; otherwise, residual gas may diffuse from the goods and may irritate living tissues. Instruments sterilized with hydrogen peroxide can be used immediately.

Cold (chemical) sterilization is commonly used by large animal surgeons in practice for preparation of instruments. The instruments are soaked in one of the commercially available solutions for whatever time and at whatever concentration recommended by the manufacturer. Some of these solutions can be irritating to tissues, so care must be taken not to transfer excessive amounts of the solution into the surgical site. This method of instrument sterilization or disinfection is recommended for multiple surgical procedures, such as dehorning and castration.

Boiling the instruments is another method used by the large animal surgeon. Boiling can be used for contaminated and dirty surgery. In an emergency, it can be used for clean-contaminated surgery, but it is not recommended for clean surgery. The boiling process also dulls sharpened instruments, although with disposable scalpel blades this problem is not serious.

General Surgical Instruments

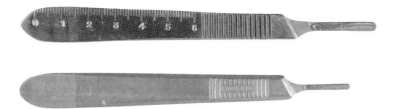

Scalpel handles.

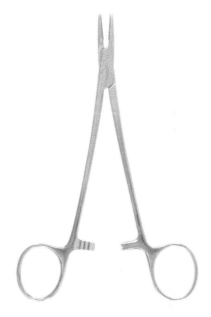

Mayo-Hegar needle holder.

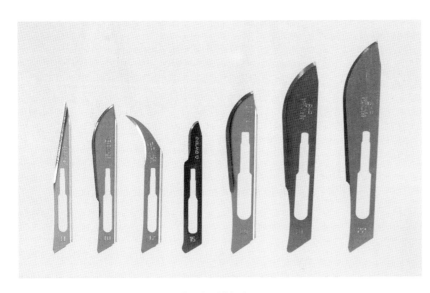

Scalpel blades.

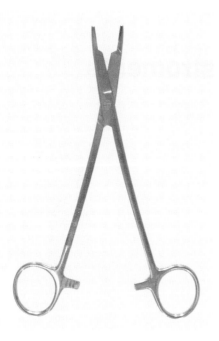

Olsen-Hegar combined needle holder and scissors.

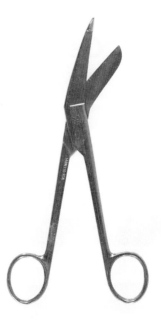

Lister bandage scissors.

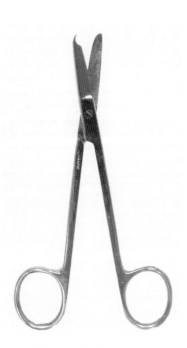

Littauer stitch scissors.

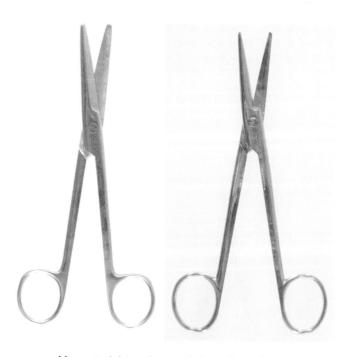

Mayo straight and curved dissecting scissors.

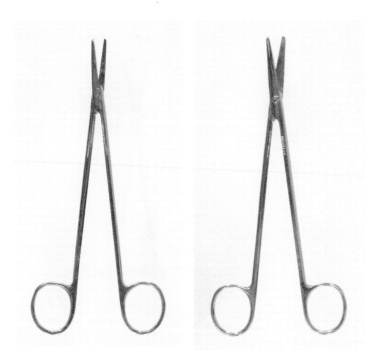

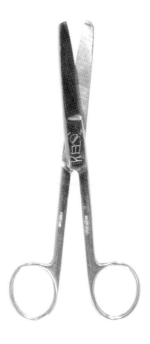

Operating scissors with blunt/blunt points.

Metzenbaum straight and curved scissors.

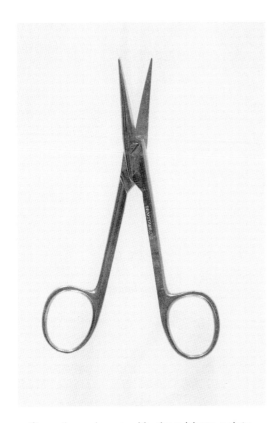

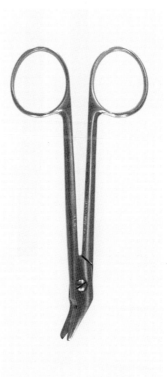

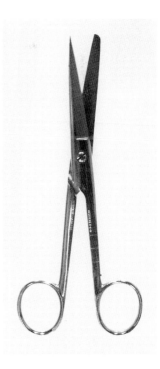

Operating scissors with sharp/sharp points.

Wire-cutting scissors.

Operating scissors with sharp/blunt points.

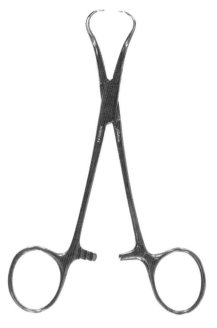

Backhaus towel clamp.

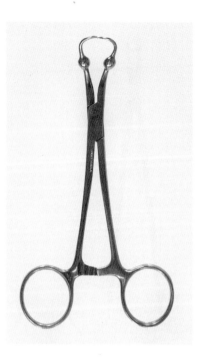

Roeder towel clamp.

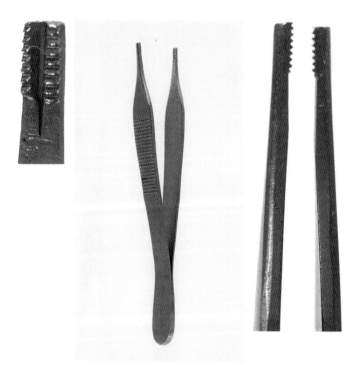

Brown-Adson forceps.

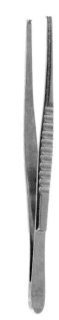

Tissue forceps.

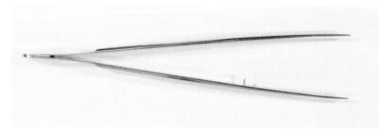

Adson forceps.

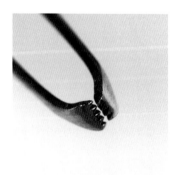

Allis tissue forceps.

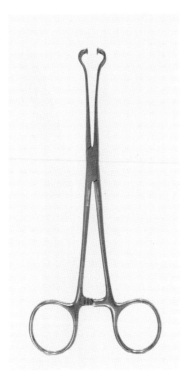

Babcock intestinal forceps.

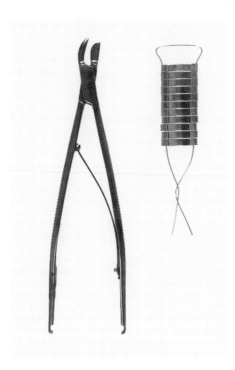

Michel clip applying-and-removing forceps.

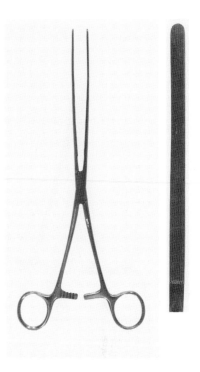

Doyen (Gillmann) compression forceps.

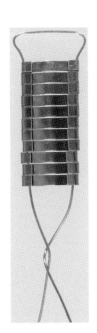

Michel clips.

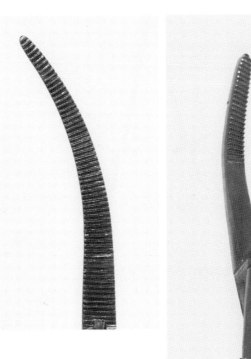

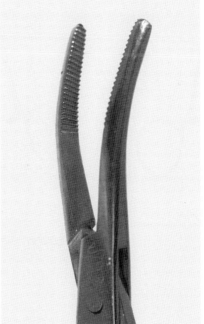

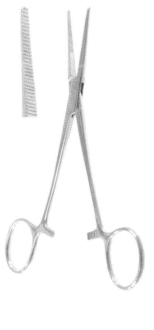

Crile straight and curved hemostatic forceps.

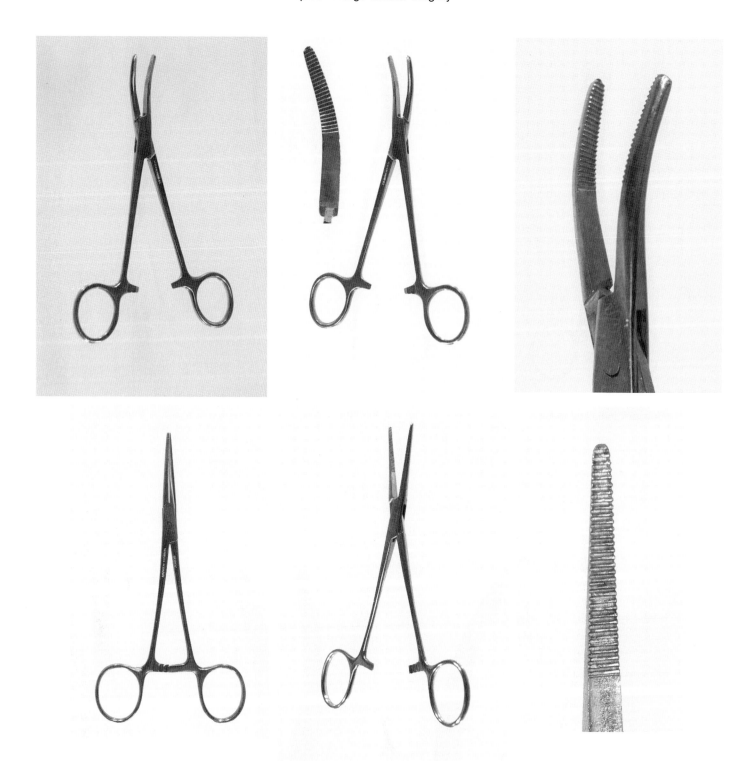

Kelly straight and curved forceps.

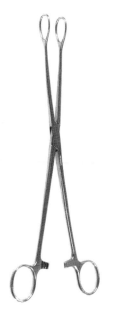

Foerster straight
sponge forceps.

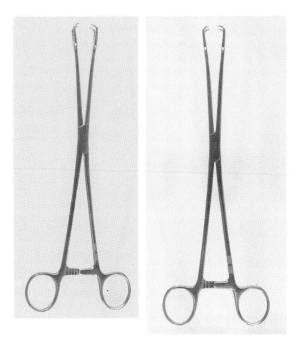

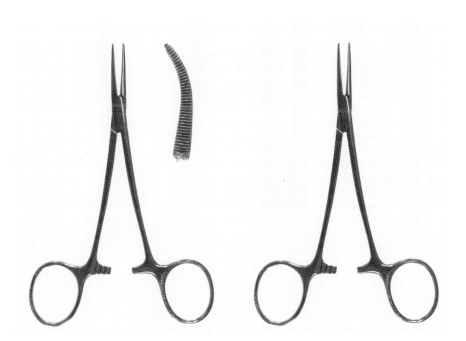

Vulsellum forceps.

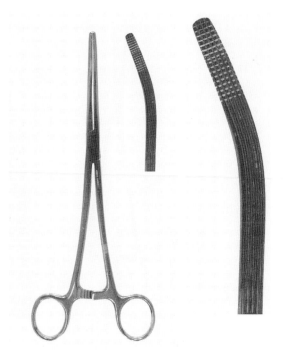

Rochester-Carmalt forceps.

Halsted mosquito straight and curved forceps.

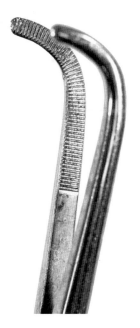

Mixter curved hemo-
static forceps.

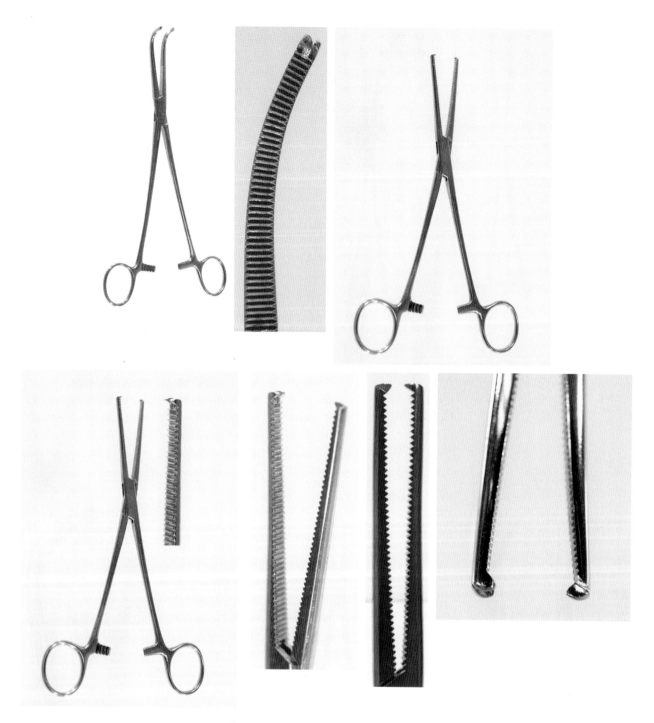

Ochsner straight and curved forceps.

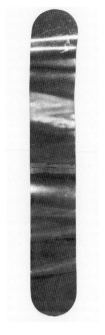

Malleable retractor.

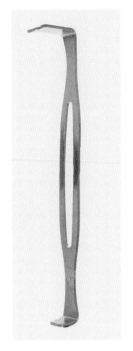

United States Army retractors.

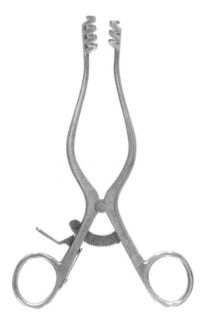

Weitlaner self-retaining retractor.

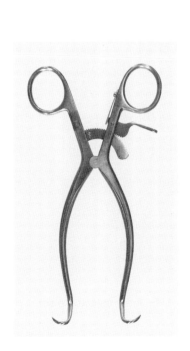

Gelpi self-retaining retractor.

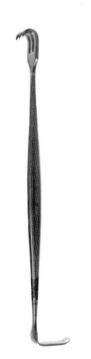

Senn retractor.

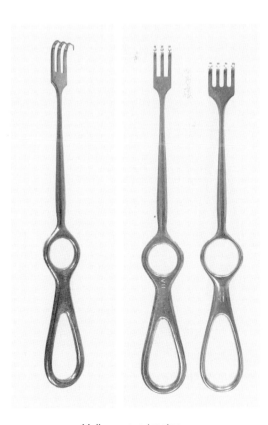

Volkmann retractor.

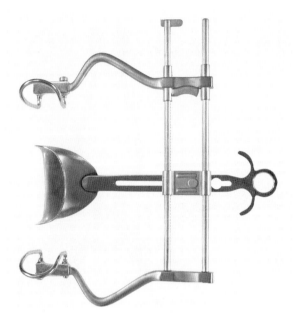

Balfour retractor.

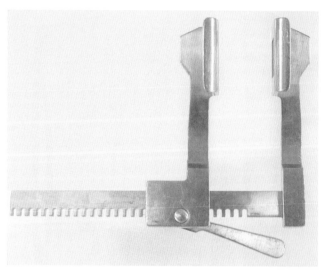

Finochietto rib spreader.

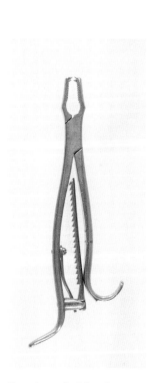

Kern bone-holding forceps.

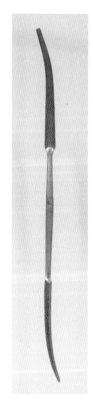

Putti double-ended bone rasp.

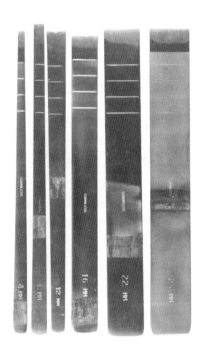

U.S. Army osteotome set.

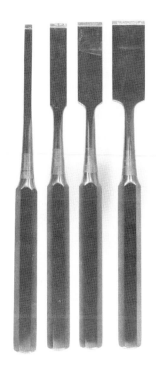

U.S. Army chisel set.

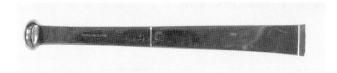

Alexander chisel.

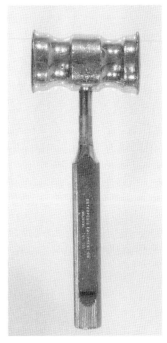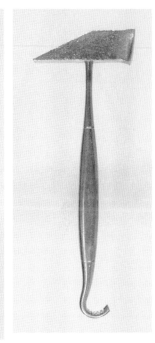

Mallet.

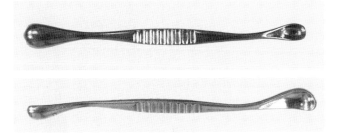

Volkmann double-ended curette.

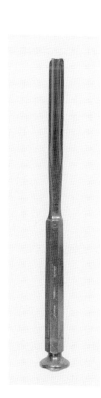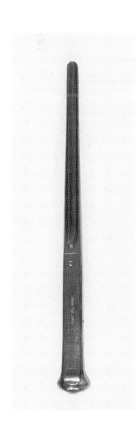

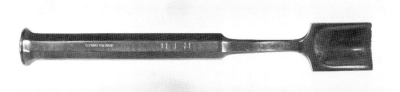

Hibbs gouge.　　　　　U.S. Army gouge.　　　Alexander gouge.

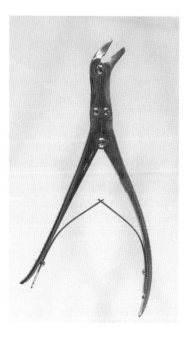

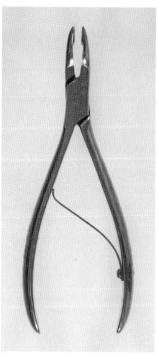

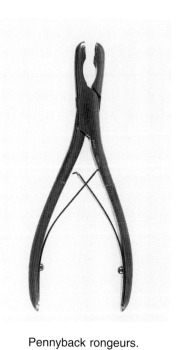

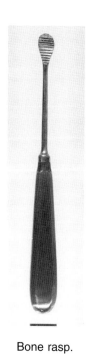

Pennyback rongeurs.

Bone rasp.

Still-Luer bone rongeurs.

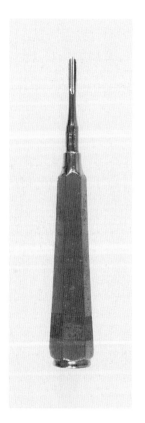

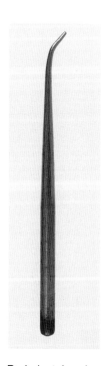

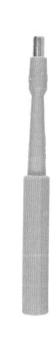

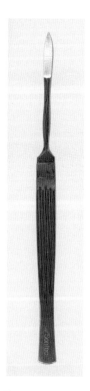

Dental elevator.

Periodontal probe.

Keyes skin punch.

Tenotomy knife.

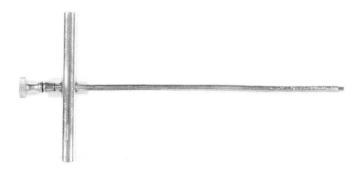

Michel trephine.

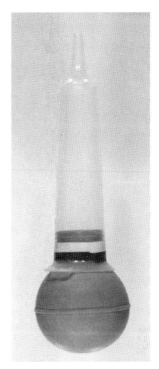

Bulb syringe.

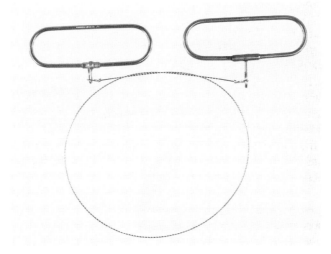

Gigli wire and handles.

Yankauer suction tip.

Instruments Used Specifically in Large Animal Surgery

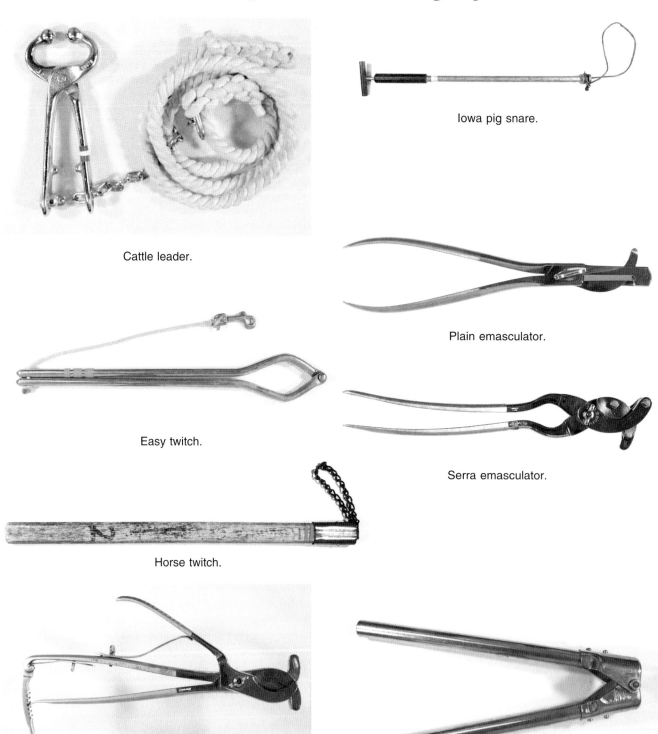

Iowa pig snare.

Cattle leader.

Plain emasculator.

Easy twitch.

Serra emasculator.

Horse twitch.

Reimer emasculator.

Barnes-type dehorner.

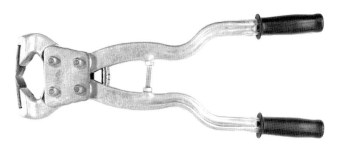

Keystone dehorner.

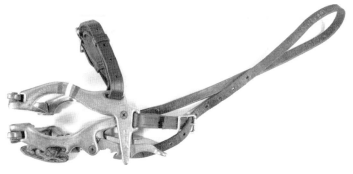

Gouge dehorner.

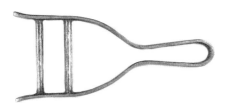

Heavy-swine mouth speculum.

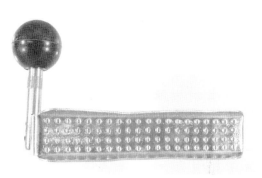

McPherson speculum.

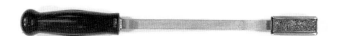

Dental float.

Bayer mouth wedge.

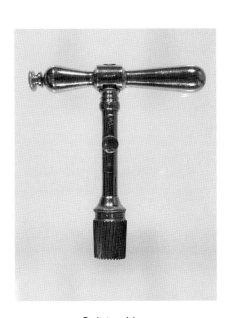

Galt trephine.

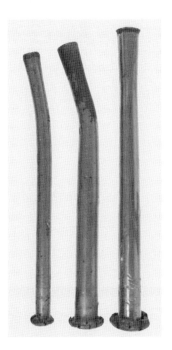

Dental punches.

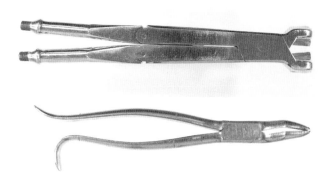

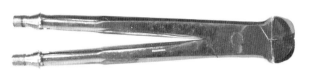

Closed, drop-jaw molar cutter.

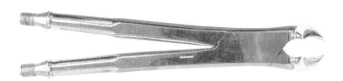

Equine molar forceps.

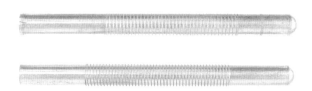

Interchangeable steel handles for foregoing dental instruments.

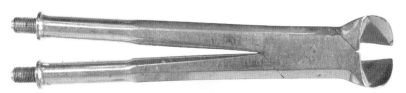

Drop-jaw multiple molar cutter.

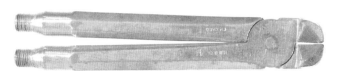

Half open, drop-jaw molar cutter.

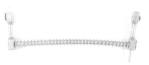

Open, drop-jaw molar cutter.

Canine mouth gag (for llama tooth extraction).

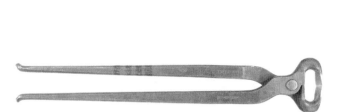

Hoof nippers.

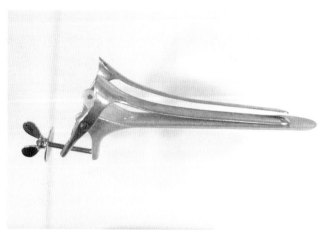

Thoroughbred vaginal speculum.

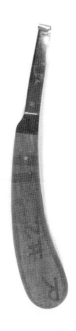

German hoof knife.

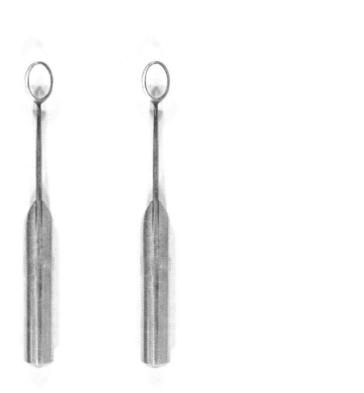

Hughes hoof groover.

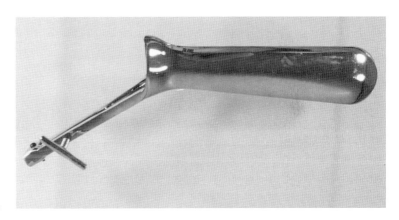

Bennett's speculum.

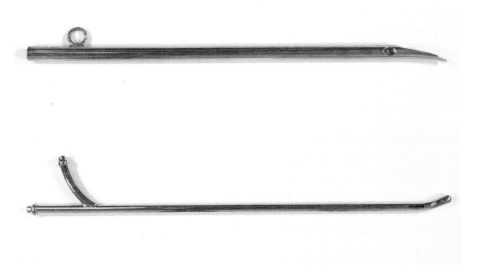

Cow catheters.

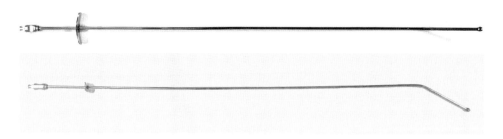

Mare catheter.

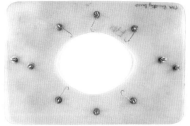

Rumentomy board.

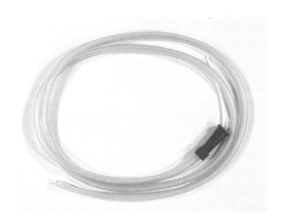

Stud catheter.

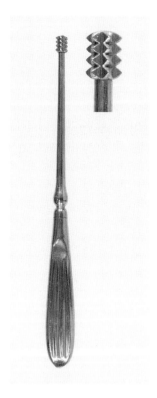

Hobday's roaring bur.

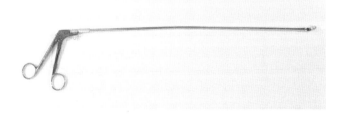

Jackson uterine biopsy forceps.

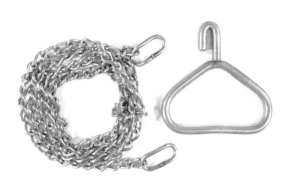

Obstetric chain handle.

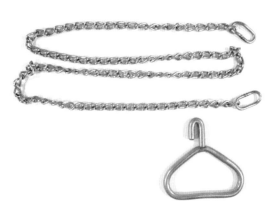

Obstetric chains.

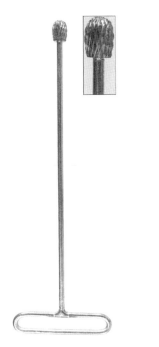

Strawberry roaring bur.

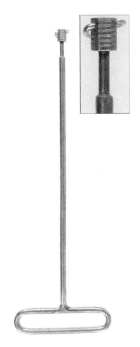

French-model roaring bur with hooks.

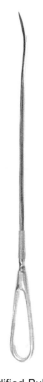

Modified Buhner
tape needle.

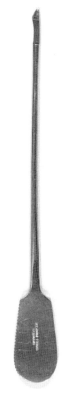

Udall teat bistoury.

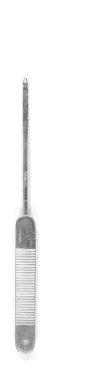

Cornell teat curette.

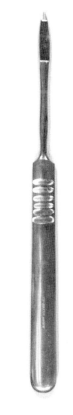

Lichty teat knife with
blunt point.

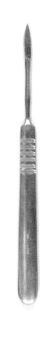

Lichty teat knife with
sharp point.

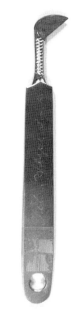

Hugs teat-tumor extractor.

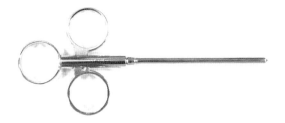

Teat slitter.

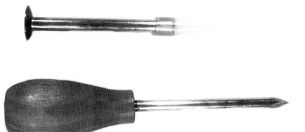

Wood-handle cattle trocar.

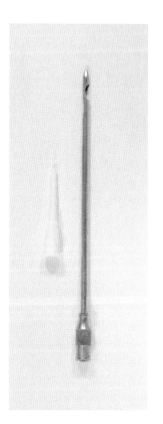

Udder infusion tube.

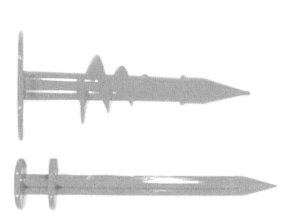

Corkscrew trocar.

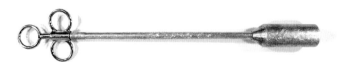

Standard balling gun.

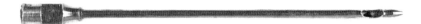

Teat cannula.

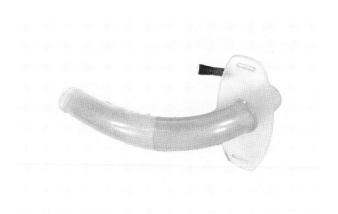

Endotracheal tube.

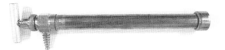

Stomach pump.

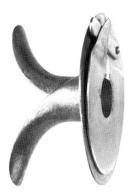

Tracheotomy tube.

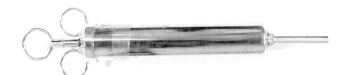

Dose syringe.

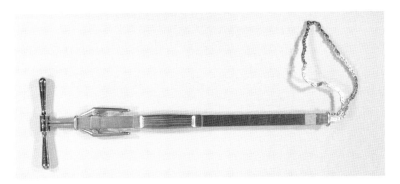

Écraseur.

Chapter 4

SUTURE MATERIALS AND NEEDLES

Objectives
1. Discuss the features, indications, and limitations of the commonly used sutures in large animal surgery.
2. Describe the advantages and disadvantages to different types of needles and the indications for each.

Suture Materials

Sutures and ligatures are fundamental to any surgical technique because they maintain approximation of tissues as the wound heals. All sutures should maintain their strength until the wound has healed and as a general rule should be as strong as the healthy tissue through which they are placed. The ideal suture material should

- Elicit minimal tissue reaction
- Not create a situation favorable for bacterial growth
- Be nonelectrolytic, noncapillary, nonallergenic, and noncarcinogenic
- Be comfortable for the surgeon to handle
- Hold knots securely without cutting or fraying
- Be economical to use

Needless to say, the ideal suture material has not been found and probably never will be; therefore, the surgeon must be familiar with the advantages and disadvantages of the various materials, and the selection of sutures should be based on suture-tissue interactions rather than habit or trade.

It is not the purpose of this chapter to present all the suture materials available, but rather to discuss the salient features of those commonly encountered in large animal practice. We have found that most surgeons, whether oriented to large or small animal practice, use a small variety of suture material. They learn the limitations, indications, and contraindications of these sutures, so they are able to adapt them to differing situations.

However, good surgeons are always watching to see whether there is a better material available that will provide more benefits to their patients.

Clinical Application of Sutures

The selection of suture type and size is determined by the purpose of the suture, as well as by its biologic properties in the various tissues. Suture materials have traditionally been divided into two categories: absorbable and nonabsorbable sutures. Absorbable sutures begin to be digested or hydrolyzed by the patient during healing of the wound and continue to disappear when the wound has healed. Nonabsorbable sutures retain their tensile strength for longer than 60 days and may remain in situ indefinitely, even though they may be altered slightly. Due to their persistence within tissues, nonabsorbable sutures are more likely to cause suture sinus formation.

Suture materials can also be subdivided into multifilament and monofilament sutures. In general, synthetic monofilament sutures induce less tissue reaction and exhibit less capillarity than multifilament or braided sutures. Multifilament sutures may also harbor bacteria and thus potentiate infection and suture sinus formation. Indeed, the prevalence of suture sinus formation has been shown to be higher following implantation of multifilament sutures than for monofilament sutures.

Veterinary surgeons deal with larger, more uncooperative patients than do their counterparts in human surgery; this often necessitates the use of a suture of greater durability and strength.[11] The surgeon must take into account the rate of healing of the particular tissue because wounds of different tissues achieve maximal strength at different times. For example, visceral wounds heal rapidly, as do superficial wounds around the head. The surgeon must also consider whether infection or drainage will be likely. Chromic gut, for example, disappears more rapidly in the face of infection because of an increase in the local phagocytic activity. On the other hand, a braided or multifilament synthetic material may actually harbor bacteria when an infection occurs. If strength is required for a long period of time—for example, during the healing of a fascial wound—the use of a nonabsorbable synthetic suture material may be necessary. The presence of crystalloids is also a factor in choosing a suture material; for example, a nonabsorbable suture used in the bladder wall represents a foreign body conducive to urinary calculus formation. An absorbable suture would be a better choice, but even some absorbable sutures initiate stone formation in certain species.[9] Other factors influencing the choice of suture are the surgeon's training, experience, judgment, and habits. However, habit is one of the poorest reasons to choose a suture material.

Once surgeons have chosen what they believe to be the best type of suture material, they must consider the size of the suture. The holding power of the tissue is the factor that usually determines the size of the suture material. Although all sutures enhance the development of infection, larger sutures retard wound healing and create a foreign-body reaction that is greater than the reaction caused by sutures with a smaller diameter. Consequently, the suture chosen should be just long enough to hold the tissue together.

The number of sutures placed in a wound is another consideration. As each new suture is placed in a wound, the stress on the other sutures decreases. In regard to wound healing, it is better to increase the number of sutures than to increase the size of the suture.[15] Sutures that are placed too far apart lead to poor apposition of the wound edges and contribute to dehiscence.[15, 20] Generally speaking, sutures should be as far from each other as the sutures are wide (tension sutures for secondary support are an exception); however, in thicker-skinned areas, the spacing between the sutures may be increased.[20] The sutures must include the correct amount of tissue and should not be placed too tightly. Too much tension with sutures delays wound healing by causing ischemia at the wound edges. If the bite in the tissue is too small, the suture will cut through the tissues, and dehiscence may occur.

Knotting the suture is the next important consideration. The knot is the weakest point of a suture loop and actually decreases the strength of the suture material. Variations in knot type are more important than variations in suture type and size.[21] Good-quality knots are essential to any surgical procedure; unfortunately, a surgeon's performance decreases with time because of boredom or fatigue.[14] The reader is referred to Chapter 5, "Knots and Ligatures." Table 4-1 summarizes commonly used suture materials.

Table 4-1. Commonly used suture materials.

Suture	Material	Qualities	Advantages	Disadvantages
Surgical catgut	Natural collagen from the submucosa of sheep intestine	Rapid absorption Digested enzymatically	Economical Good handling characteristics Some elasticity	Knot strength decreases when wet Loses strength within 3 to 7 days Tissue reaction
Collagen	From flexor tendons of steers	Similar to catgut Used primarily in opthalmic surgery	Smoother, more uniform than catgut Less tendency to fray	Same as catgut
Polyglycolic acid (Dexon)	Polymer of glycolic acid	Synthetic Braided Absorbable Hydrolyzed into natural metabolites	Nonantigenic Does not swell when wet Minimal tissue reaction Good knot security Handling characteristics	Some tissue drag Capillary action
Polyglactin 910 (Vicryl)	Polymer of glycolic acid and lactic acid in a ratio of 90:10	Synthetic Braided Absorbable Hydrolyzed into natural metabolites	Same as polyglycolic acid	Same as polyglycolic acid
Braided 9-1 lactomer (Polysorb)	Polyester of glycolide and lactide (derivatives of glycolic and lactic acids)	Synthetic Braided Absorbable Coated	Excellent knot security and tensile strength Softer than Vicryl, better knot security	Braided material
Polydioxanone (PDS)	Homopolymer of paradioxanone	Synthetic Monofilament Absorbable Hydrolyzed into natural metabolites	Less tissue drag Do not potentiate infection Persists longer in tissues High breaking strength	Brittle Tendency to break at knots

Table 4-1. *Continued.*

Suture	Material	Qualities	Advantages	Disadvantages
Polyglyconate (Maxon)	Copolymer of trimethylene carbonate and glycolide	Synthetic Monofilament Absorbable Degrade via hydrolysis	Same as polydioxanone	Less breaking strength, greater stiffness, inferior mechanical force compared to PDS
Glycomer 631 (Biosyn)	Polyester of 60% glycolide, 14% doxanone, and 26% trimethylene carbonate.	Synthetic Absorbable Monofilament	Less tissue reaction than braided suture More rapid absorption pattern Superior strength at implantation	More rapid absorption pattern
Poliglecaprone 25 (Monocryl)	Segmented block copolymer of caprolactone and glycolide	Synthetic Monofilament Absorbable Degraded by hydrolysis	Better handling characteristics than other monofilament absorbable sutures High initial tensile strength Increased pliability Good knot security Minimal tissue drag	Rapidly absorbed Maintains initial tensile strength for up to 2 weeks
Polyglytone 6211 (Caprosyn)	Polyester of glycolide, caprolactone, trimethylene carbonate, and lactide	Synthetic Absorbable Monofilament	Fast absorption Less tissue drag, better handling characteristics, and greater breaking strength than chromic gut	Very rapid absorption pattern, should be used only in the bladder, uterus, and subcutaneous tissue
Silk	Protein filament from silkworms	Slow absorption by proteolytic degradation within 2 years Natural material	Excellent handling qualities Good knot-holding properties	Potentially allergenic Capillary action
Cotton	Twisted yarn from cotton plant	Nonabsorbable	Good handling characteristics Economical for food animal use	Greater tissue reaction than silk Potentiates infection
Nylon (Dermalon, Ethilon, Supramid)	Long-chain polymer	Nonabsorbable Synthetic Available as monofilament (most cotton) or multifilament	Inert Maintains most of its initial strength	High memory Poor knot security Bulky knot
Polypropylene (Prolene: Ethicon, Surgipro: Kendall)	Similar to nylon	Nonabsorbable Synthetic Monofilament	Similar to nylon	Similar to nylon
Polymerized caprolactam (Supramid, Vetafil)	Related to nylon	Nonabsorbable Synthetic Braided and coated	Coating minimizes capillarity High tensile strength Minimal tissue reaction Economical skin suture	Some knot slippage Potentiation of infection
Polyesters (coated: Dacron, Polydek, Ethibond) (uncoated: Mersilene, Dacron)	Polymer of ethylene glycol and terapthalic acid	Synthetic Nonabsorbable Coated or uncoated	Inert Prolonged strength	Uncoated forms create capillarity and tissue drag Coating reduces knot security Potentiation of infection
Stainless steel	Iron alloy (iron-nickel-chromium)	Nonabsorbable Multifilament of monofilament forms	Strongest suture material Good knot security Inert Can be repeatedly sterilized Does not potentiate infection like other braided sutures	Difficult to handle Bulky knots Can cut tissues and surgical gloves

Absorbable Sutures

Surgical Gut (Catgut)

Catgut is a natural absorbable suture that consists mainly of collagen obtained from the submucosa of sheep intestine or from the serosa of beef intestine. It is packaged in at least 85% alcohol, is sterilized with gamma irradiation, and cannot be resterilized once the package is open. Many of the synthetic sutures have essentially replaced catgut because they cause significantly less tissue reaction and possess a greater tensile strength for the same diameter.

Catgut may be plain or chromic. *Plain catgut* loses its strength so rapidly that its use in certain regions may be contraindicated. *Chromic catgut* is produced by exposure to basic chromium salts. This process increases the intermolecular bonding and results in greater strength, decreased reaction in tissues, and slower absorption. Catgut is further classified according to the degree of chromicization: type A (plain) is untreated; type B has mild treatment; type C has medium treatment; and type D (extra chromic catgut) has prolonged treatment. Because the absorption pattern of gut is quite variable, newer synthetic sutures are better choices for most procedures. The subject's reaction to catgut is variable, but in general, plain catgut loses its strength in 3 to 7 days. Catgut is gradually digested by acid proteases from inflammatory cells and may be used when a suture is needed for only a week or two and absorption is desirable. The rate of absorption varies, depending on where the catgut is implanted and, to some extent, on the size of the suture. It is rapidly absorbed if it is implanted in regions with a greater blood supply. Similarly, it is absorbed rapidly if exposed to gastric juices or other organ enzymes. Catgut may be used in the presence of infection; however, the increased environment for enzyme digestion causes it to be absorbed rapidly.

Catgut handles well and possesses some elasticity. Three throws are required for knotting, and, when wet, the knot-holding ability decreases. The ends should be left slightly longer than other types of suture material to minimize the chances of untying. Despite the advent of synthetic absorbable sutures, catgut is still used in large animal surgery for purely economic reasons, which is not generally a good reason for selecting a suture material.

Collagen

Collagen is a suture material related to catgut. It is produced from the flexor tendons of steers, is smoother and more uniform than catgut, and has less tendency to fray. It is occasionally used in ophthalmic surgery.

Braided Absorbable Sutures

In our experience, the synthetic absorbable suture materials have, with few exceptions, replaced catgut. Synthetic suture materials are advantageous for their good knot security, handling characteristics, consistent absorption patterns, and minimal tissue reaction.[10]

These materials are polymers that are extruded as filaments and include polyglycolic acid (Dexon-Tyco), Polyglactin 910 (Vicryl-Ethicon), and lactomer 9-1 (Polysorb-Tyco). These compounds differ from catgut in their reaction in tissues. They are invaded by macrophages, yet their disappearance is independent of the local cellular reaction. These compounds are hydrolyzed into natural body metabolites, rather than absorbed by an enzymatic process. The breaking strength of these synthetic sutures diminishes more or less in a straight line, when compared to the almost exponential decline of the strength of catgut in tissues. This characteristic disappearance pattern was the main reason for the introduction of these synthetic materials, because they are more consistent and reliable in this regard than catgut. Because none of these suture materials contains protein, they are nonantigenic.[7] Unlike catgut, they do not swell when wet. These materials have a low coefficient of friction, and it is necessary to use a surgeon's knot with multiple throws to prevent slippage or untying of the knots. One disadvantage of these suture materials is that they tend to drag through tissues and cut soft organs; this property has prompted the manufacturers to coat them with an absorbable lubricant to make them smoother, to decrease pulling, and to improve overall handling.[2,6]

Polyglactin 910 is now coated with equal parts of a copolymer of glycolide and lactide (polyglactin 370) and calcium stereate (coated Vicryl). Polyglycolic acid is now constructed of filaments finer than the original suture to provide better handling and smoother passage through the tissues (Dexon-S). Polysorb is much softer and has better knot security than either Vicryl or Dexon. The newer designs of the suture materials have not altered their reactivity or other biologic properties. However, Vicryl is now available as a more rapid absorbing suture (Vicryl-Rapide) and an antimicrobial impregnated suture (Vicryl-Plus). Tissue drag can be considered an advantage in some situations, however, because the suture will not slide out of the tissue when the surgeon is placing continuous suture patterns. Polyglycolic acid has been used successfully for closure of skin wounds in man as well as in large and small animals.[11,13]

Absorbable Monofilament Sutures

Absorbable monofilament sutures minimize the tissue drag that occurs with the braided sutures and are not believed to potentiate infection. Because they are monofilament sutures, they are theoretically better in an infected wound because they are less likely to harbor bacteria.[5,12] Polydioxanone (PDS), a homopolymer of paradioxanone, and Polyglyconate (Maxon), a copolymer of trimethylene carbonate and glycolide, are two synthetic monofilament sutures with similar properties. Like polyglycolic acid and polyglactin 910, both are degraded by hydrolysis in a predictable manner, although more slowly. Studies show that polydioxanone has a superior breaking strength, longer-lasting mechanical performance over 28 days, and less stiffness compared to polyglactin.[8] Similarly, polyglyconate can withstand high immediate loads for up to 21 days before weakening due to absorption. Polyglyconate surpasses polydioxanone in strength up to 4 weeks after implantation and knot security.[10] Glycomer 631 (Biosyn) is a newer synthetic monofilament absorbable suture material that is similar to polyglyconate. It is stronger when implanted but loses its strength more rapidly.

Poliglecaprone 25 (Monocryl), a segmented block copolymer of caprolactone and glycolide, is a more recently developed absorbable monofilament suture designed to have the favorable properties of other monofilament sutures but with superior handling characteristics.[10] Poliglecaprone 25 has been shown to have the advantages of a greater initial tensile strength than polydioxanone, chromic gut, or polyglactin 910; increased pliability compared to polyglyconate, polydioxanone, or gut; less tissue drag than gut; and good knot security.[3,10] However, poliglecaprone 25 is absorbed faster than polyglactin 910 and polydioxanone, maintaining 20 to 30% of its initial tensile strength 2 weeks after implantation.[3] Polyglytone 6211 (Caprosyn) is another synthetic monofilament absorbable suture material with a rapid absorption pattern. These sutures should be limited to use in the bladder or uterus of large animals. They have been designed to replace gut suture materials.

Nonabsorbable Sutures

Silk

Silk, a continuous protein filament produced by silkworms, has traditionally been considered a nonabsorbable suture. However, the consensus in recent literature is that silk is indeed slowly absorbed in vivo at a rate dependent upon the type and condition of the tissue it is implanted in, the physiological status of the patient, and characteristics of the silk (virgin versus extracted black braided fibrion and the diameter of the silk fiber).[1] Research shows that silk fibers in vivo are susceptible to proteolytic degradation, lose tensile strength within a year of implantation, and are undetectable within 2 years.[1]

Silk fibrion fibers are usually braided, dyed, and coated with wax or silicone for use as sutures, which are referred to as *black braided silk*. Virgin silk is not commonly used due to its potential allergenic nature in some patients, although it is still commercially available. Silk suture has been widely used in human surgery although its use has declined with the availability of synthetic sutures. A similar trend has been seen in veterinary surgery. It is popular with some veterinary surgeons, however, and its superb handling quality is the standard for the producers of the synthetic suture materials. It has good knot-holding properties as well. Silk possesses capillary action, which means it should not be used in the presence of infection because it will provide a refuge for bacteria and will result in a nidus of infection. Silk is still used for vascular surgery, although the newer synthetic sutures are better for this purpose.

Cotton

The most common application of cotton in large animal practice is as umbilical tape. *Cotton* is the twisted yarn from the filament of the cotton plant. It handles well, but it produces more tissue reaction than silk. Cotton potentiates infection because it can harbor bacteria, and the fistulation that may result resolves only when the offending suture material has been removed. Nevertheless, cotton is a useful, economical suture material in a variety of situations, especially those involving food animals. It has been used as a suture in the perineal region for prolapses of the uterus, vagina, and rectum, where the suture will be removed.

Nylon

Nylon (Dermalon, Ethilon, Supramid) is a long-chain polymer available in monofilament and multifilament forms. It is most commonly used in the monofilament form. Nylon is a stiff suture that should be stretched out following its removal from the manufacturer's packet. It has significant *memory,* which is defined as the suture's ability to resist bending forces and to return to its original configuration. As a result, nylon and, to a lesser extent, polypropylene are difficult to knot securely. The additional throws required for security produce a bulky knot. Nylon is relatively inert when implanted in tissues; a thin connective tissue capsule is produced around the suture, and this characteristic is one of its major advantages when it is used as a buried suture. Nylon loses a slight amount of strength initially, after which no appreciable diminution in strength is noted. Because there are no interstices to harbor bacteria, the monofilament form of nylon fares better than multifilament sutures in the presence of infection.

Nylon is available in multifilament forms (Nurolon). Braiding this suture gives it some roughness to provide better knot retention and better handling characteristics than the monofilament form.

Polypropylene and Polyethylene

Polypropylene (Prolene and Surgilene) and *polyethylene* are polyolefins that are usually available in monofilament form. These sutures are relatively biologically inert and lose little strength in situ over a 2-year period. However, knot security has been shown to be inversely proportional to the memory and size of the suture, and because these sutures have very high memory, their knot retention is poor compared to the smaller monofilament alternatives. Multiple knots are required to ensure knot security, which could enhance tissue irritation. The first throw of a knot with polypropylene tends to slip unless tension is maintained. Both these suture materials are more suitable for use in infected wounds than the braided synthetic materials. Polypropylene has been recommended for closure of abdominal incisions in patients that are predisposed to developing postoperative infection because of its high tensile strength. However, due to its mechanical properties and persistence in the tissues, polypropylene is associated with suture sinus formation following equine abdominal wall closure.[22] The amount of tissue incorporated in the suture loops, suture tension, and knot volume should be minimized to reduce the risk of sinus formation.[22] The slower-degrading, synthetic, monofilament sutures, such as polyglyconate and polydioxanone, may be better options for equine abdominal wall closure.

Polymerized Caprolactam

Polymerized caprolactam (Supramid, Vetafil) is a synthetic suture material used extensively in large and small animal practice. It is available for veterinary use only. The twisted fibers are made from a material related to nylon and coated to minimize capillarity.[18] Compared to catgut or silk, the material has a high tensile strength and causes little cellular reaction in tissues. Polymerized caprolactam is packaged in plastic dispenser bottles in which it is chemically sterilized; in this form, it is suitable for use in skin closure. Because of its smoothness, some knot slippage occurs with this material, and at least three knots are required for a safe tie.[20] In general, the material behaves like the other braided synthetics. The suture should not be used in the presence of infection, nor should the suture material be buried without its having been autoclaved. Either of these events can lead to the formation of a chronic draining tract that will not resolve until the suture is removed. For this reason, this material has been used primarily for skin suture. From the standpoint of economics, polymerized caprolactam has a useful place in large animal practice. Surprisingly, little has been written about its behavior in the tissues of domestic animals.

Polyesters

Polyesters consist of Dacron, a polymer of ethlylene glycol and terapthalic acid, that has been coated or impregnated with various finishes. Tevdek and Ethiflex are Teflon-impregnated Dacron, whereas Polydek is Teflon-coated Dacron. Ethibond is Dacron coated with polybutylate, and Ticron is silicone-impregnated Dacron. The suture is also available in uncoated forms (Mersilene and Dacron), but these sutures naturally have more tissue drag than the coated forms.[18] Coating or impregnating the suture decreases capillary action and tissue drag, but also reduces knot-holding ability. These materials need four throws, all squared, or five throws (two slip and three squared).[14] The knot-holding ability varies within the group. These suture materials are unreactive when implanted in tissues, but the shedding of the Teflon coat increases the inflammatory response.[16] It is not known whether the shedding of the Teflon coat in the tissues of large animal species

has any clinical significance; if it does, it is probably minor.

The polyesters are strong sutures and are used when prolonged strength is required. Because of the multifilament nature of this material, bacteria and tissue fluids can penetrate the interstices of the polyester sutures. This can produce a nidus of infection, converting contamination to infection. Immobile bacteria have been transported inside the suture material; this is more significant than the spread of infection on the surface of the suture material.[4] Consequently, these suture materials must be used under aseptic circumstances, circumstances that unfortunately may not always exist in large animal practice.

Stainless Steel

Stainless steel is an alloy of iron (iron-nickel-chromium) and is available in multi- or monofilament forms. It is difficult to handle because it is easily kinked; yet it is the strongest of all suture materials. Stainless steel holds knots well, but the knots tend to be bulky. It is one of the most unreactive suture materials and can be repeatedly sterilized, but it has a tendency to cut tissues as well as surgeons' gloves. Unlike the braided synthetics, stainless steel does not harbor bacteria and can be used in the presence of infection. Its use in large animal practice is infrequent.

Michel Clips

Michel clips are short, malleable clips with points on the ends that are used to appose wound edges. A special pair of forceps is used to bend them; however, they do tend to pucker the skin once they are applied. These clips are used infrequently in large animal practice, but have been used for Caslick's operation in mares.

Skin Stapling Devices

Disposable *skin stapling devices* (Proximate) have become available for use in man and horses. They are commonly used for closing the skin of horses following laparotomy for the surgical correction of colic. One advantage of the device is its speed: the instrument closes skin incisions that are up to 2 feet long in a minute or so. This factor is important when the survival of animals could be adversely affected by a longer anesthetic time. One study showed that the use of staples saved an average of 15.5 minutes of closing time per incision.[17] Although the staples are well tolerated by horses and can remain in the skin almost indefinitely, it is best to remove them in 2–3 weeks before the hair grows back.

Skin staples have been shown experimentally to be more resistant to abscess formation than percutaneous sutures. Because they are metallic, they do not provide an environment conducive to bacterial growth and they do not penetrate as deeply into the relatively avascular subcutaneous tissue plane. We have noticed excellent wound healing in uninfected wounds. In abdominal surgery in which the intestinal tract has been opened, the skin incision may have received an inoculum of bacteria prior to closure, and therefore skin staples would be of benefit.[19] A small pair of forceps is available for removal of the staples once the wound has healed. We have used staples in a variety of other skin incisions in horses and found them equally acceptable. The only limitation of the device is cost, although we have used it in situations such as colic surgery, in which the cost of the staples is a small part of the total bill. We have also used skin staples in calves, other small ruminants, and llamas, although economy is a limiting factor in these species. They are particularly useful in wound closure where there is no tension. They can be applied with the use of a twitch in show horses where sedation of local anesthesia cannot be used.

References

1. Altman, G.H., Diaz, F., Jakuba, C., Calabro, T., et al.: Silk-based biomaterials. Biomat., 24:401–416, 2003.
2. Artandi, C.: A revolution in sutures. Surg. Gynecol. Obstet., 150:235, 1980.
3. Bezwada, R.S., Jamiolkowski, D.D., In-Young, L., Vishvaroop, A., et al.: Monocryl suture, a new ultra-pliable absorbable monofilament suture. Biomat., 16:1141–1148, 1995.
4. Blomstedt, B., Osterberg, B., and Gergstrand, A.: Suture material and bacterial transport. Acta Chir. Scand., 143:71, 1977.
5. Chusak, R.B., and Dibbell, D.G.: Clinical experience with polydioxanone monofilament absorbable sutures in plastic surgery. Plast. Reconstr. Surg., 72:217, 1983.
6. Conn, J., and Beal, J.M.: Coated Vicryl synthetic absorbable sutures. Surg. Gynecol. Obstet., 150:843, 1980.
7. Craig, P.H., et al.: A biological comparison of polyglactin 910 and polyglycolic acid synthetic absorbable sutures. Surg. Gynecol. Obstet., 141:1, 1975.
8. Fierheller, E.E., and Wilson, D.G.: An in vitro biomechanical comparison of the breaking strength and stiffness of polydioxanone (sizes 2,7) and polyglactin 910 (sizes 3,6) in the equine linea alba. Vet. Surg., 34:18–23, 2005.
9. Kaminski, J.M., Katz, A.R., and Woodward, S.C.: Urinary bladder calculus formation on sutures in rabbits, cats and dogs. Surg. Gynecol. Obstet., 146:353, 1978.
10. Kawcak, C.E., and Baxter, G.M.: Surgical materials and wound closure techniques. Vet. Clin. Equine, 12:195–205, 1996.
11. Larsen, R.F.: Polyglycolic acid sutures in general practice. N. Z. Vet. J., 26:258, 1978.
12. Lerwick, E.: Studies on the efficacy and safety of polydioxanone monofilament absorbable suture. Surg. Gynecol. Obstet., 156:51, 1983.
13. Mackinnon, A.E., and Brown, S.: Skin closure with polyglycolic acid (Dexon). Postgrad. Med. J., 54:384, 1978.
14. Magilligan, D.J., and DeWeese, J.A.: Knot security and synthetic suture materials. Am. J. Surg., 127:355, 1974.
15. Price, P.B.: Stress, strain and sutures. Ann. Surg., 128:408, 1948.
16. Postlethwait, R.W.: Five-year study of tissue reaction to synthetic sutures. Ann. Surg., 190:53, 1979.
17. Ramey, D.W., and Rooks, R.L.: Consider the use of skin stapling equipment to expedite equine surgery. Vet. Med., 80:66, 1985.
18. Stashak, T.S., and Yturraspe, D.J.: Considerations for selection of suture materials. Vet. Surg., 7:48, 1978.
19. Stillman, R.M., Marino, C.A., and Seligman, S.J.: Skin staples in potentially contaminated wounds. Arch. Surg., 119:138, 1984.
20. Swaim, S.: Surgery of Traumatized Skin: Management and Reconstruction in the Dog and Cat. Philadelphia, W.B. Saunders, 1980.
21. Tera, H., and Aberg, C.: Strength of knots in surgery in relation to type of knot, type of suture material, and dimensions of suture thread. Acta Chir. Scand., 143:75, 1977.
22. Trostle, S.S., and Hendrickson, D.A.: Suture sinus formation following closure of ventral midline incisions with polypropylene in three horses. J. Am. Vet. Med. Assoc., 207:742–746, 1995.
23. Trostle, S.S., Wilson, D.G., Stone, M.C., and Markel, M.D.: A study of the biomechanical properties of the adult equine linea alba: a relationship of tissue bite size and suture material to breaking strength. Vet. Surg. 23:435–441, 1994.

Needles

Surgical needles are essential for the placement of sutures in tissues. They must be designed to place the suture in the tissue with a minimum of trauma; they should be rigid enough to prevent bending, yet flexible enough to prevent breaking; and they must be sharp enough to penetrate tissues with the minimum of resistance. Naturally, they must be clean and resistant to corrosion. Of the many different types of needles available, the selection of the needle is determined by the type of tissue to be sutured, its location and accessibility, and the size of the suture material.

Surgical needles have three basic components: the eye, the body (or shaft), and the point. The eye is usually of two types, *closed eye* or *swaged (eyeless)*. The closed eye is similar to a household sewing needle, and the eye itself is available in a variety of shapes. Swaged-on needles are permanently attached to the suture (Figure 4-1). The suture and needle are of approximately the same diameter. The outstanding advantage of a swaged-on needle is that tissues are subjected to less trauma, because only a single strand, rather than a double strand, of suture is pulled through the tissue. In addition, handling of the suture and needle is minimal, and it is ready for immediate use. At the end of surgery, the needle and the remaining piece of suture are discarded, and dull needles are continually culled. Tying the suture to the eye of the needle lessens the possibility of separation, but further increases the trauma as the suture material is drawn through the tissue. With a suture needle named Control Release, the suture material can be rapidly separated from the needle.

Needles are usually curved, although some surgeons prefer to use straight needles, especially when suturing skin or bowel. Needles have a variable curvature, and they may be 1/4-, 3/8-, 1/2-, and 5/8-circle and half-curved (Figure 4-2). Selection of a needle depends on the depth of the region to be sutured. When suturing deep in a wound, for example, the needle will have to "turn a sharp

corner." In this case, a 1/2-circle or 5/8-circle needle would be most suitable. Curved needles must be used with needle holders.

The body of the needle is available in a number of different shapes: round, oval, flat, or triangular. Flat and triangular bodies have cutting edges; round or oval-bodied needles usually taper from the small diameter at the point to a larger diameter at the eye.

Needles are also available with varying types of points (Figure 4-3). Cutting needles are designed to cut through dense, thick, connective tissue, such as bovine skin. Cutting needles can be reverse cutting, where the cutting edge is provided along the convex side of the needle, rather than on the concave surface. The purpose of a reverse-cutting needle is to minimize the excessive cutting of transfixed tissue. Another modification of the cutting needle combines the cutting point with a round needle shaft so that the needle will readily penetrate the dense tissue but not cut through it; this has been called a *taper cut needle*. One company manufactures a needle of similar concept that is useful in tough, dense tissues such as cartilage (K-point needle). This needle readily penetrates the cartilage of the equine larynx.

Noncutting needles, or round needles, have no edges and are less likely to cut through tissues (Figure 4-3). They are used for abdominal viscera, connective tissue, vessels, and other fragile tissues. Round (atraumatic)

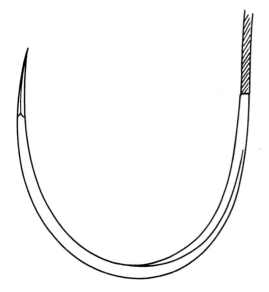

Fig. 4-1. A swaged-on needle. The suture and needle have approximately the same diameters.

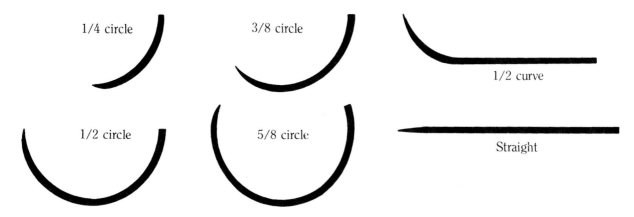

1/4 circle   3/8 circle   1/2 curve

1/2 circle   5/8 circle   Straight

Fig. 4-2. Various needle shapes.

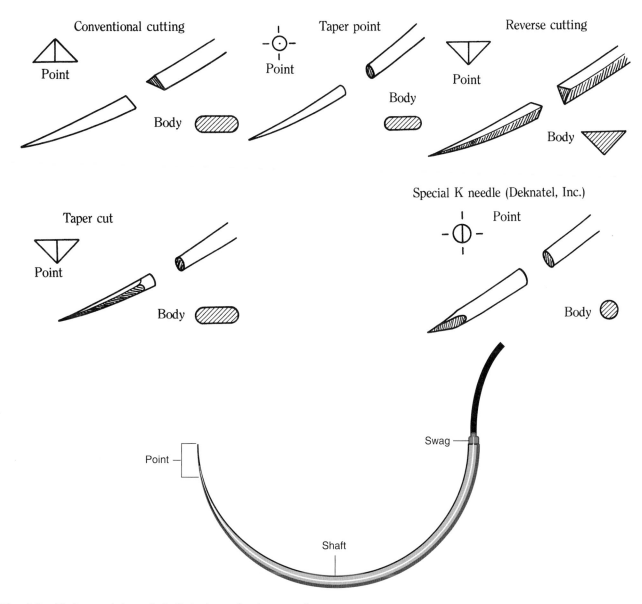

Fig. 4-3. Various points and shaft designs of suture needles.

needles are actually round behind the tip, but the remaining portion of the shaft is oval. This design prevents angular or rotational displacement of the needle within the jaws of the needle holder.

Long-stemmed needles are also used in food animal practice. They are useful for placing heavy suture materials into the tissues, such as in vaginal prolapse in cattle.

Chapter 5

KNOTS AND LIGATURES

Objectives

1. Learn basic knotting techniques for the square knot, granny knot, and surgeon's knot.
2. Describe the applications of ligatures and two ligature techniques: the transfixation ligature and the three-forceps method of tissue ligation.

Principles of Knot Tying

The following are several important principles of knots and ligatures that the surgeon should consider:

- The amount of friction between the strands of suture determines knot security.
- Suture size and type impact the amount of friction between strands and thus knot security; the smallest size suture and knot that will not jeopardize wound strength should be used.
- Monofilaments create less friction against one another and the tissue. They have been designed to deform when tied to provide increased knot security.
- The length to which the suture ends should be cut depends on the security of the knot. For example, catgut suture tends to swell and untie when exposed to moisture, so the surgeon should leave the suture ends slightly longer than other sutures.
- Studies show that regardless of suture type, maximum knot security is reached at a maximum of two additional throws to the starting square knot (four throws total). Additional throws will exacerbate tissue irritation and impede healing. They should be used when a surgeon's knot or slip knot is used.[1]
- If instruments such as clamps are to be applied to the suture, as in herniorrhaphy in foals and calves, they should not be applied to those parts of the suture material that will remain in situ.

Knotting Techniques

The *square knot* is the knot used most in surgery (Figure 5-1). The knot is usually tied with needle holders, which should remain parallel to the wound, whereas all movements are made perpendicular to the wound. Uniform tension to the ends of the suture ensures that the knot ends up as a square and not as two half-hitches (slip knot). Two half-hitches result from unequal tension on the two ends during tying (Figure 5-1).

The *granny knot* is a slip knot that will not hold, especially if the strain on the ends is unequal, and its use is not recommended (Figure 5-1).[6] Knots that tighten when the second throw is pressed home, as well as knots that end a continuous suture in which two strands are tied to one, are also prone to slippage.[4]

Knots stay tied because of the friction of one component against another. At least three separate throws are required to achieve the minimum amount of friction with the square knot. Monofilament suture materials, such as nylon, polypropylene, and braided synthetics, especially those that are Teflon coated, have poor knot security. With these materials, the first throw may loosen before the next throw is applied. Knotting technique warrants careful attention when using such suture materials. However, newer monofilament suture materials are designed to deform when the knot is tightened to improve knot security beyond that of braided suture. The surgeon can ensure knot security with braided synthetics with four throws, all squared (a double square knot) or with a knot with five throws, two slip and three squared.[3] Care must also be taken with steel because it also is prone to slippage if the knots are poorly placed. The reader is referred to Chapter 4, "Suture Materials and Needles."

A *surgeon's knot* is used when the first throw of a square knot cannot be held in position because of excessive tension on the wound edge (Figure 5-1). The surgeon's knot is basically the same as a square knot, except the first suture consists of two throws. The surgeon's knot should be further reinforced by four additional throws (Figure 5-1). The *Miller's knot* is very useful for ligating pedicles. There are two encircling wraps of suture to increase

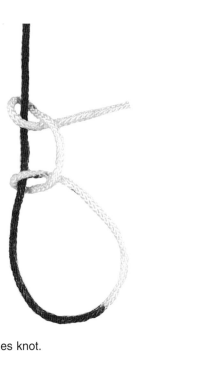

Two half-hitches knot.

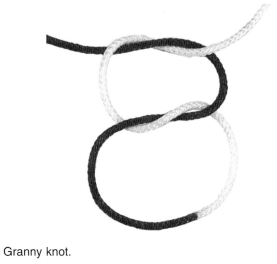

Granny knot.

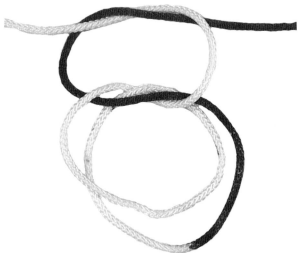

Miller's knot.

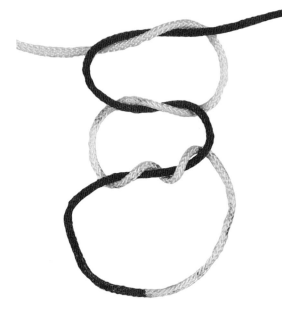

Reinforced knot.

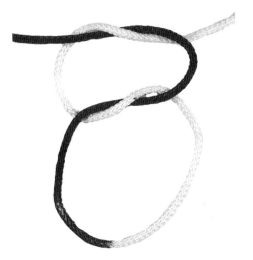

Square knot.

Fig. 5-1. Surgical knots.

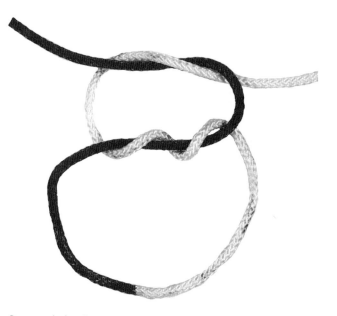

Surgeon's knot.

72

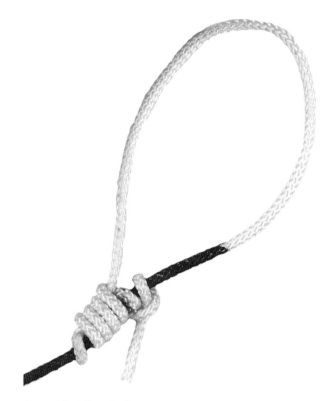

4-S modified Roeder knot.

Fig. 5-1. *Continued.*

friction between the suture and pedicle (Figure 5-1). The knot should be finished with four throws, all squared. In locations where tying knots is difficult, such as deep in the abdomen, or in laparoscopy, a 4-S modified Roeder knot can be very helpful (Figure 5-1). It is essentially a slip knot that uses friction to keep from loosening. The knot is tied, the loop placed over the structure to ligate, and the knot is pushed down with a knot pusher to tighten.

Tying with the Needle Holder

In most instances, knots are tied with the aid of a needle holder (Figure 5-2A to F). The instrument tie is recommended for most surgery because of its adaptability and because it is economical, when compared with the one-hand or two-hand tie. It is possible to use short pieces of suture material and still grasp the suture firmly.

The technique for an instrument tie is as follows: a loop of the long end of the suture is made around the end of the instrument with the instrument in front of the suture (Figure 5-2A). The short end of the suture is grasped by the needle holder, which is then pulled through the loop, setting the knot down securely (Figure 5-2B and C). Traction must be applied in the same plane as the knot (Figure 5-2D) while keeping the instrument and hand with suture close to the tissue. The second throw is begun by wrapping the long end of the suture around the instrument,

but in the opposite direction (Figure 5-2E). It is important to not lift the suture ends or the first throw will loosen. The short end of the suture is grasped and pulled through the loop (Figure 5-2F). The surgeon's knot is made using essentially the same procedure, except the first loop is doubled by placing a double loop around the needle holder.

Knots should be tied with the correct tension. Excessive tension results in strangulation of the tissues, which leads to necrosis and delayed wound healing. Similarly, the wound should not be allowed to gape, because of either too few sutures or lack of tension. To relieve the tension on individual sutures, the number of sutures used to close the incision should be increased; the underlying principle is that when sutures are uniformly spaced, the tension is distributed equally among the sutures.

Ligatures

A *ligature* is a loop of suture used for occluding a blood vessel either before or after it is severed. Ligature loops are frequently used in laparoscopy for structures within the abdominal cavity. Laparoscopic ligatures, such as the 4-S modified Roeder knot, are usually formed using a knot pushing device and a slip knot. These techniques are covered in depth elsewhere.[2,5]

To prevent slipping, a ligature can be converted to a *transfixation ligature* by passing it through the middle of the vessel. It is tied around half the vessel and then around the entire vessel. Transfixation ligatures can be used to ligate several blood vessels within tissues (Figure 5-3). As little tissue as possible should be left distal to the ligature because the stump so created will become necrotic and will have to be absorbed by the animal. Care must be taken not to cut the stump too short or the ligature may slip over the end and result in the loss of fixation. Double loops are stronger than single loops because of the distribution of friction and tensile forces. In addition, the bursting strength of a loop is inversely proportional to the volume that it encloses. In other words, the tension on the suture is proportional to the volume. Practically speaking, mass ligation of tissue is more apt to break than are ligatures around small bleeding points or isolated vessels.[3] Furthermore, vessels can recanalize within a large mass of ligated tissue.

When large amounts of tissues must be ligated, the *three-forceps method* can be used. The forceps are placed on the pedicle, as shown in Figure 5-4. Forceps A are distal and forceps C are proximal. The pedicle is divided between forceps A and B, and the ligature is placed proximal to forceps C. The first throw on the ligature is made, and, as forceps C are removed, the ligature is tied into the crease left by forceps C. Further throws are then placed on the ligature, and forceps B are loosened to check for hemorrhage. This is a good time to use a Miller's knot.

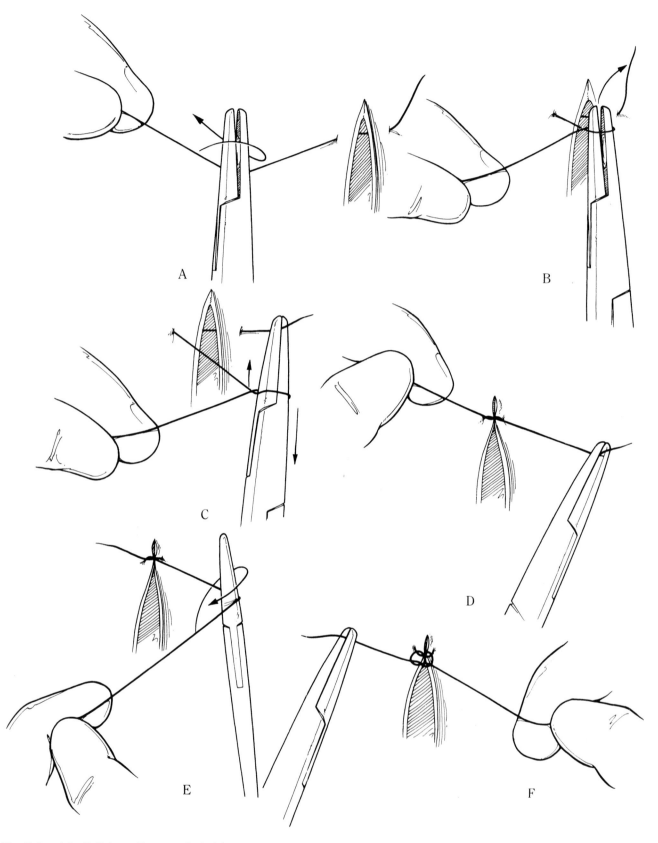

Fig. 5-2. A to F, Tying with a needle holder.

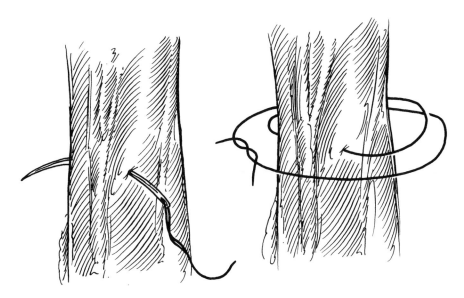

Fig. 5-3. Transfixation ligature.

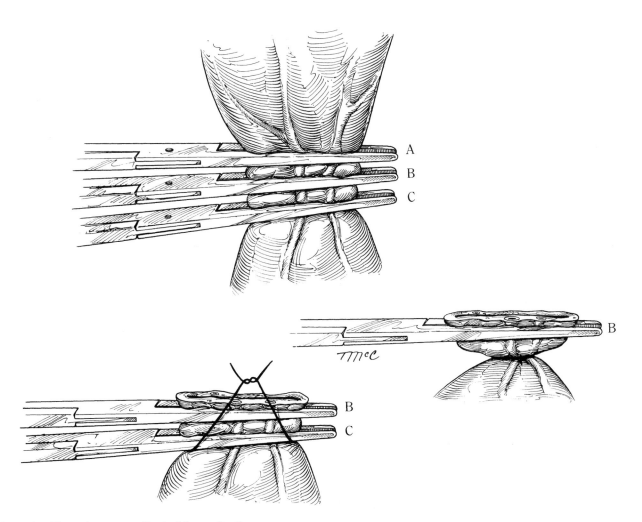

Fig. 5-4. Three-forceps method of tissue ligation.

References

1. Brown, R.P.: Knotting techniques and suture materials. Br. J. Surg. *79*:399–400, 1992.
2. Carpenter, E.M., Hendrickson, D.A., James, S., Frank, C., et al.: A mechanical study of ligature security of commercially available pre-tied ligatures versus hand tied ligatures for use in equine laparoscopy. Vet. Surg., *35*:55–59, 2006.
3. Magilligan, D.J., and DeWeese, J.A.: Knot security and synthetic suture materials. Am. J. Surg., *127*:355, 1974.
4. Price, P.B.: Stress, strain and sutures. Ann. Surg., *128*:408, 1948.
5. Shettko, D.L., Frisbie, D.D., and Hendrickson, D.A.: A comparison of knot security of commonly used hand-tied laparoscopic slipknots. Vet. Surg., *33*:521–524, 2004.
6. Swaim, S.: Surgery of Traumatized Skin: Management and Reconstruction in the Dog and Cat. Philadelphia, W.B. Saunders, 1980, p. 269.

Chapter 6

SUTURE PATTERNS

Objectives

1. Provide an overview of the indications for and uses of different suture patterns.
2. Detail the technique for the following basic suture patterns:
   - Simple interrupted
   - Simple continuous
   - Interrupted horizontal mattress
   - Continuous horizontal mattress
   - Vertical mattress suture
   - Near-far-far-near suture
   - Subcuticular suture
   - Cruciate (cross mattress) suture
   - Continuous lock stitch (Ford interlocking suture)
3. Describe suture techniques that are most advantageous for the closure of hollow organs, tendon repair, and the closure of wounds under high tension.

Basic Suture Patterns

A wide variety of suture patterns for use under different circumstances is available to the surgeon. Each pattern will have some good points and some detrimental points. It is important to choose the appropriate combination of suture pattern, suture type, suture size, and knot type to provide the best outcome for the patient. If one pattern does not produce optimum results, a new technique must be mastered. Suture patterns are divided into interrupted or continuous patterns, and the following patterns are important to the large animal surgeon.

Simple Interrupted Suture

The simple interrupted suture is the oldest and most widely used suture pattern. It is easy and relatively rapid to perform. However, because each suture must be tied individually it often takes longer to close an incision when using a simple interrupted pattern. The technique of insertion depends on the thickness of the tissue apposed. The needle and suture are inserted a variable distance from one side of the incision, across the incision at right angles, and are inserted through the tissue on the other side. For a right-handed surgeon, this would be accomplished from right to left, and the reverse would apply for a left-handed surgeon (Figure 6-1). The knot should be offset, so as not to rest against the incision. If this suture is used for skin closure, the point of insertion will vary, depending on the thickness of the skin. This may be 1 cm in bovine skin or 2 to 3 mm for the thin skin on the inguinal area of a foal. The simple interrupted suture should appose the wound margins, but it may invert them if it is pulled too tightly or if the insertion and exit points are too far from the cut edge. The spacing between the sutures depends on the tension on the wound edges. Gaping of the wound edges should be avoided.

Simple Continuous Suture

This continuous suture is made up of a variable number of simple bites and is tied only at the ends (Figs. 6-2 and 6-3). It is used in tissues that are elastic and will not be subjected to a lot of tension. The bites in the edges of the wound are made at right angles to the edges of the wound, but the exposed part of the suture passes diagonally across the incision. This suture pattern can be applied rapidly. Ending the suture depends on whether a swaged-on needle or a needle with an eye is used. To end the suture with an eyed needle, the needle is advanced through the tissues, and the short end of the suture is held on the proximal end of the needle passage. A loop of suture is pulled through with the needle, and the loop is tied to the single end on the opposite side (Figure 6-2). When a swaged-on needle is used, the needle end of the suture is

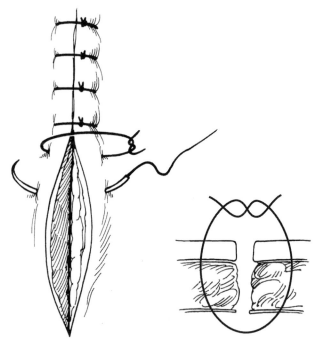

Fig. 6-1. Simple interrupted suture with cross section of suture bite.

tied to the last available loop of suture material that is exterior to the tissues (Figure 6-3). If any one of the sutures in a continuous suture pattern fails, the strength of the suture line will be lost. If one suture fails in an interrupted suture pattern, the remaining sutures have a better chance of maintaining the strength of the suture line.

Interrupted Horizontal Mattress Suture

The interrupted horizontal mattress suture is illustrated in Figure 6-4A. The external parts of the suture lie parallel to the wound edges. To prevent eversion, the needle should be angled through the skin, and the wound edges should oppose each other gently. This suture can be used in conjunction with pieces of rubber tubing or with buttons to act as a tension suture (Figure 6-4B). In this situation, the suture is placed some distance from the skin edges. Another pattern of sutures, such as the simple interrupted suture, is used to coapt the incision line more precisely. Because of the geometry of the horizontal mattress suture, the sutures have a tendency to reduce the blood supply to the wound edges. The horizontal mattress suture is probably best reserved for muscle belly reapposition (Figure 6-4C).

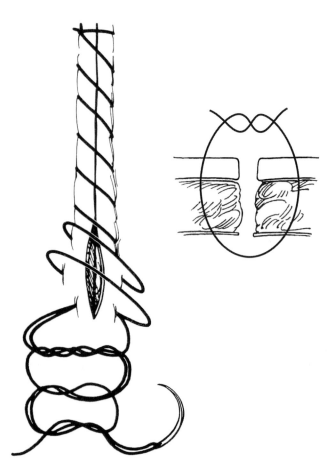

Fig. 6-2. Simple continuous suture with cross section of suture bite (eyed needle).

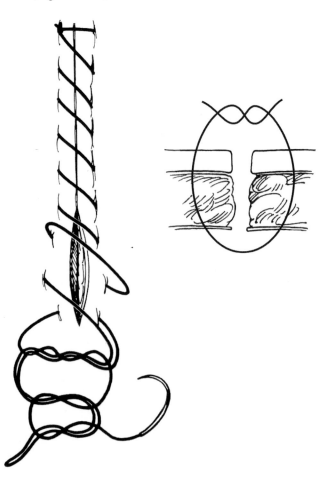

Fig. 6-3. Simple continuous suture with cross section of suture bite (swaged-on needle).

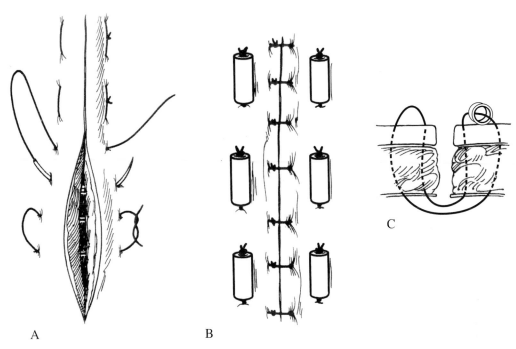

Fig. 6-4. A, Interrupted horizontal mattress suture. B, Interrupted horizontal mattress sutures as tension-relieving sutures, using pieces of rubber. C, Cross section of horizontal mattress.

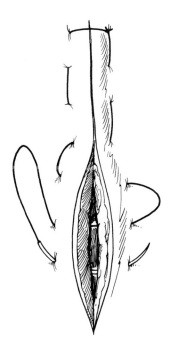

Fig. 6-5. Continuous horizontal mattress suture.

Continuous Horizontal Mattress Suture

The continuous horizontal mattress suture, illustrated in Figure 6-5, is similar to the horizontal mattress pattern, except it is continuous. Its main advantage is speed, and it is not often used in large animal surgery.

Vertical Mattress Suture

Initially, the suture and needle make a superficial bite close to the wound edge and then pass across the incision to take a small bite on the opposite side (Figure 6-6A). The needle is then reversed in the jaws of the needle holder and is returned to the opposite side, where it takes a larger bite. If this suture is used as the sole method of skin closure, a partial skin-thickness superficial bite of the suture pattern will ensure adequate approximation of the wound edges; if used as tension-relieving sutures some distance from the wound, simple interrupted sutures can accurately coapt the wound edges (Figure 6-6B).

Compared with the horizontal mattress pattern, the geometry of this suture allows better circulation to the wound edges and thereby decreases the chances of necrosis of the margins of the wound. The only disadvantages of this suture are that it uses slightly more suture material and may take longer to insert.

The vertical mattress suture is popular in repairing traumatic lacerations of the skin of equine limbs, where the blood supply may already be compromised. Like the horizontal mattress suture, it can also be used as a tension suture in conjunction with pieces of rubber tubing or with buttons. Pieces of rubber or buttons minimize tissue cutting by the suture material (Figure 6-6C and D).

Near-Far-Far-Near Suture

This suture, illustrated in Figure 6-7, is a tension suture often used in large animal surgery. The first bite is made close to the wound and then passes under the wound

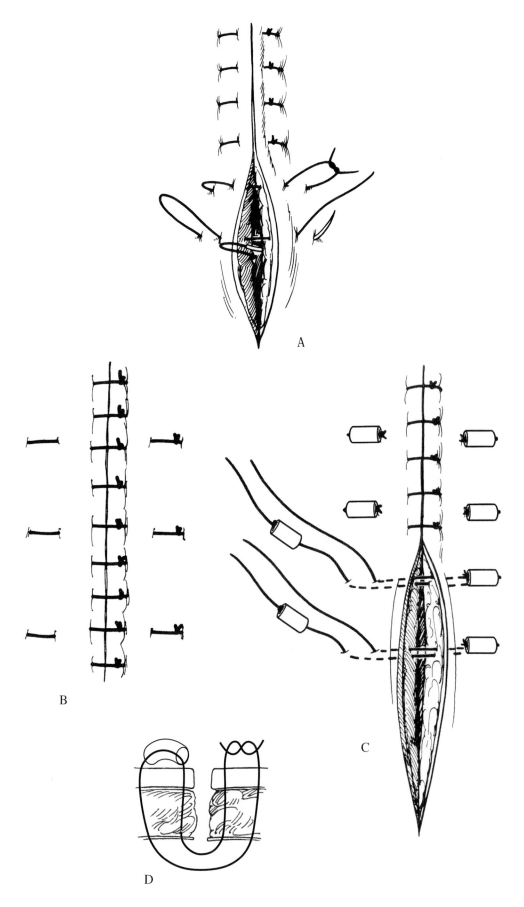

Fig. 6-6. A, Vertical mattress suture. B, Vertical mattress suture as tension-relieving sutures. C, Vertical mattress suture using pieces of rubber. D, Cross section of vertical mattress.

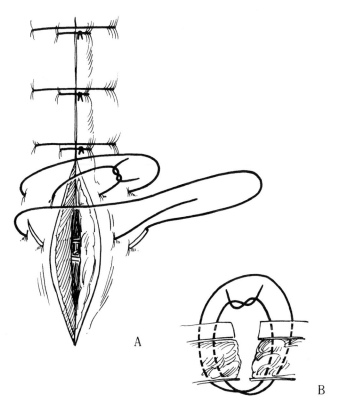

Fig. 6-7. A and B, Near-far-far-near suture.

across its edges at right angles to emerge at a greater distance from the wound edge. The next part of the suture consists of crossing over the wound to the original side and inserting the needle and suture at a distance farther from the edge than the original entry point. The suture is then directed into the wound perpendicular to the edges of the wound, crosses the wound, and emerges close to the wound edge. Then the suture ends are tied. The suture is less time consuming to insert than the vertical mattress and is an excellent tension suture. This suture has been used to close the linea alba of horses whenever tension on the wound edges is excessive. One of the main benefits of this tension-relieving suture is that the needle is always placed "forehand" and never needs to be reversed.

Subcuticular Suture

This suture is used to eliminate the small scars produced around the suture holes of the more common patterns. The first part of the suture is placed by directing the needle up into the apex of the incision in the opposite direction of the incision (Figure 6-8). The needle is then reversed and is directed down the incision. The knot is tied and, in this way, will be subcutaneous. The remainder of the suture pattern is placed like a horizontal mattress suture, with the needle crossing the incision at right angles, but advancing underneath the dermis parallel to the incision. A knot similar to the one used in the simple

continuous pattern finishes the suture. The needle is then reversed and is directed back along the incision; the knot at this end should also be subcutaneous. The suture material used for this pattern should be a synthetic absorbable and should be relatively unreactive and sterile. The suture bites are taken parallel to the incision where there is little dead space (Figure 6-8C), and perpendicular to the incision when there is more dead space (Figure 6-8D).

Cruciate (Cross Mattress) Suture

The cruciate suture, illustrated in Figure 6-9, is commenced by inserting the needle from one side to the next, as one would place a simple interrupted suture. The needle is then advanced without penetrating the tissue, and a second passage is made parallel to the first. The suture ends are then on opposite sides of the wound and form an "x" on the surface of the wound. This suture pattern is used by some surgeons if the skin edges are under tension.

The cruciate suture is used to close the small hole made by a hypodermic needle that is used for deflating a gas-distended bowel. The suture is often used as a skin-closure technique after arthroscopy or laparoscopy. It has some tension-relieving properties and takes almost half the time to place when compared to a simple interrupted pattern in an incision.

Continuous Lock Stitch (Ford Interlocking Suture)

The continuous lock stitch is a modification of the simple continuous suture (Figure 6-10). In this continuous pattern, the needle is passed perpendicularly through the tissues in the same direction. Once the needle is passed through the tissues, it is drawn through the preformed loop and is tightened. Each subsequent stitch is locked until the end of the incision is reached. To end the lock stitch, the needle should be introduced from a direction opposite the insertion of the previous sutures, and the end should be held on that side. The loop of suture is formed, and the single ends are tied. The interlocking suture is commonly used in the skin of cattle following a laparotomy. Good approximation of the skin edges can be obtained, especially with the thick skin on the flanks of cattle.

Suture Patterns Used for Closure of Hollow Organs

A suture pattern used for a hollow organ must be placed meticulously because of the disastrous consequences possible if infectious material should leak. In the intestinal tract, for example, gas, solid, and liquid feces propelled

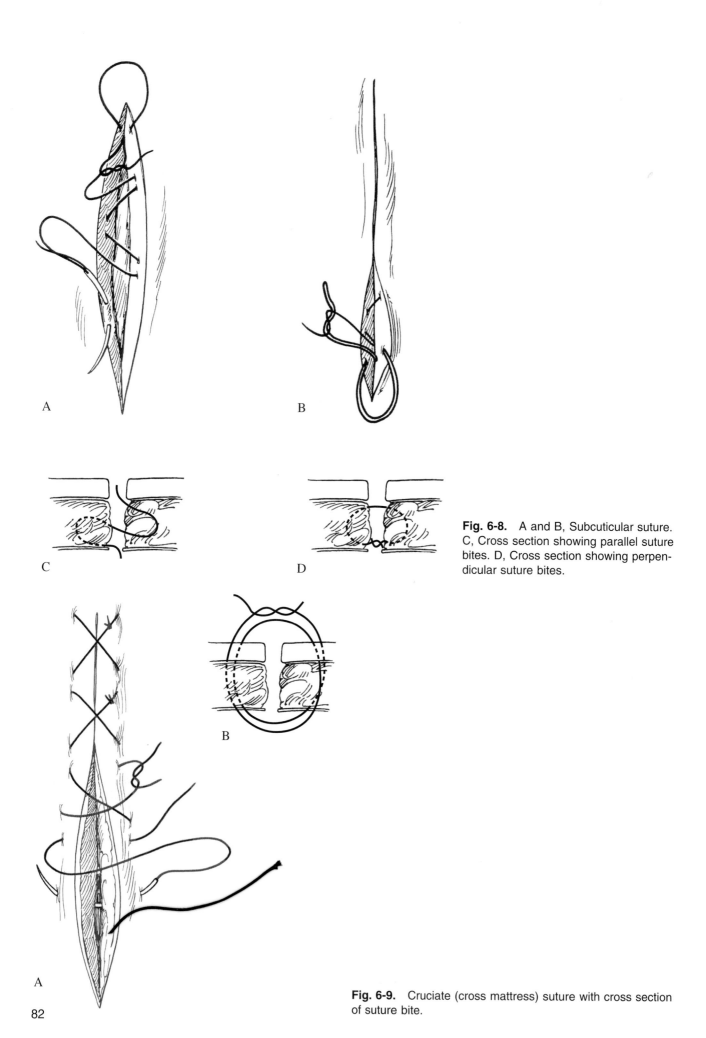

A

B

C

D

Fig. 6-8. A and B, Subcuticular suture. C, Cross section showing parallel suture bites. D, Cross section showing perpendicular suture bites.

B

A

Fig. 6-9. Cruciate (cross mattress) suture with cross section of suture bite.

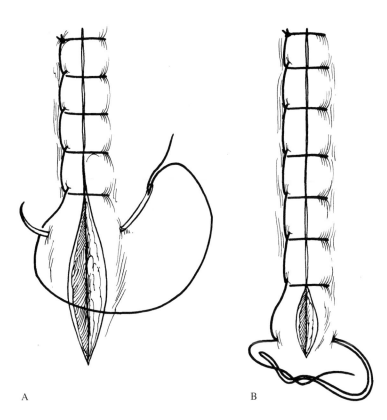

Fig. 6-10. A and B, Continuous lock stitch (Ford interlocking suture).

A   B

by peristalsis place strain on the suture line. Fortunately, the walls of the healthy gastrointestinal tract are tough, pliable, and easy to manipulate. On the other hand, the friable uterus of a cesarean patient with a decomposing fetus may be difficult to suture. Another advantage of surgery of hollow organs is that the organs generally heal quickly and are remarkably secure in as short a time as a week to 10 days after surgery.

A watertight closure was once thought to be mandatory when suturing a hollow organ; however, any technique that opposes the wound edges well is satisfactory because a fibrin clot provides an almost immediate seal. Eversion of the mucosa, however, is detrimental and can lead to the leakage of septic contents, resulting in peritonitis.

Classically, suture patterns used on hollow organs have been inverting sutures or opposing sutures. This section presents the inverting patterns, followed by some of the opposing patterns. When suturing the intestinal tract, the strength of a suture depends on its grasp of the tunica submucosa or fibromuscular layer. Absorbable or nonabsorbable sutures may be used to close the gastrointestinal tract. Needles used for hollow-organ surgery should be round-bodied (noncutting), with the suture material swaged on to reduce the size of the hole made on the organ wall. Noncutting needles are less likely to lacerate suture material that may have been placed in a deeper layer.

Interrupted or continuous sutures can be used in hollow-organ surgery. Interrupted sutures have been thought to be safer because, if one knot becomes untied,

the integrity of the entire suture line will not be jeopardized. By using interrupted sutures, the tension on each suture can be adjusted, thereby ensuring an optimum blood supply to the wound edges. However, the use of interrupted sutures requires more knots and consequently more suture material, leaving more foreign material. In most instances, two to three runs of a continuous pattern are used for bowel closure.

Interrupted Lembert Suture

The Lembert suture is a commonly used suture in gastrointestinal surgery (Figure 6-11). The suture is directed through the tissue from the outside, toward the cut edge of the incision. It penetrates the tunica serosa, muscularis, and submucosa, but not the mucosa. The suture exits on the same side and emerges close to the edge of the incision. It is reinserted close to the incision edge, passes laterad through the tunica serosa, muscularis, and submucosa and is brought up again through the tunica muscularis and serosa. The wall of the viscus automatically inverts as the knot is tied. The knot should not be so tight as to strangulate the tissues. At no stage does the suture penetrate the lumen of the viscus; it is considered a safe and useful stitch in gastrointestinal surgery and can be used as a one-layer closure. It is also suitable for use in the uterus and the rumen of large animals. The main drawback of the Lembert suture pattern is the amount of inversion. It should not be used where lumen diameter is already compromised.

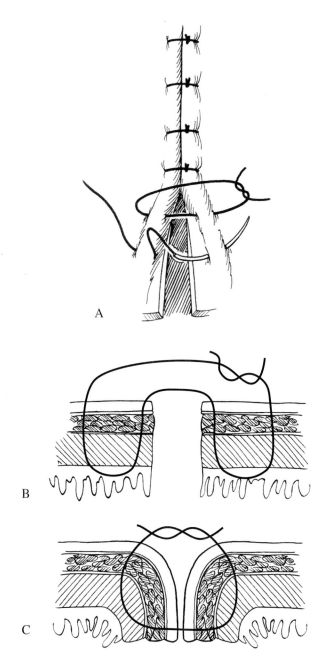

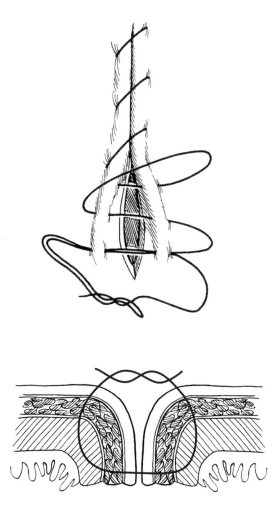

Fig. 6-12.   Continuous Lembert suture.

Fig. 6-11.   A, Interrupted Lembert suture. B, Lembert suture before tightening. C, Lembert suture after tightening.

Continuous Lembert Suture

The Lembert suture can be performed in a continuous pattern (Figure 6-12). The same spacing is used as in the interrupted suture, and the continuous suture is tied to itself at its proximal end and again at its distal end. The suture is commonly used in both intestinal and uterine closures and requires less time than the interrupted suture.

Cushing Suture

This is a method of continuous suturing in which the bites are made parallel to the edges of the wound (Figure

6-13). As the suture is placed, it penetrates the tunica serosa, muscularis, and submucosa, but does not pass through the mucous membrane; hence, it does not enter the lumen of the viscus. The suture crosses the incision at right angles and is tied to itself at the proximal end and at the distal end. The Cushing suture inverts the tunica mucosa and approximates the serosa. It is generally used as the outer tier on a double-layer closure and can be executed rapidly. The main benefit is that it is a minimally inverting pattern. The main disadvantage is that the suture run is perpendicular to the blood supply.

Connell Suture

The Connell suture resembles the Cushing suture, but the suture material penetrates all layers of the gut wall (Figure 6-14). The suture is tied when the first stitch has been taken and is tied again at the far end of the incision. Once outside the serosal surface, the needle and suture cross the incision and are reinserted in the tunica serosa of the opposite side at a point that corresponds to the preceding exit site. The directions of the Connell and Cushing suture are the same, and both sutures invert tissue. The Connell pattern is rarely used.

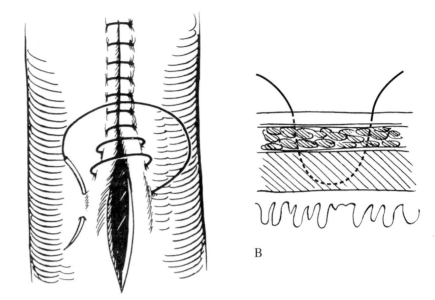

Fig. 6-13. A, Cushing suture. B, Cross section of Cushing suture.

A

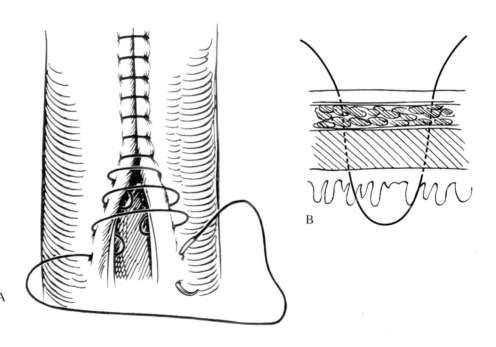

Fig. 6-14. A, Connell suture. A B, Cross section of Connell suture.

Parker-Kerr Oversew

This suture is a modification of the Lembert and Cushing patterns, and it is used to close the stump of a hollow viscus (Figure 6-15). It is essentially a Cushing pattern oversewn by a Lembert pattern. The first layer of the suture pattern, which is a Cushing pattern, is performed over a pair of forceps placed on the end of the stump (Figure 6-15A and B). The forceps are withdrawn slowly

as the suture is pulled in both directions; this inverts the wound edges without opening the lumen, which would result in contamination (Figure 6-15C). A continuous Lembert suture is then used as an oversew using the same suture (Figure 6-15D). The needle end of the suture is brought back as the second layer to be tied at the origin of the first layer (Figure 6-15E). The suture patterns can be reversed in this technique, using a Lembert for the pattern directly over the forceps and oversewing this with

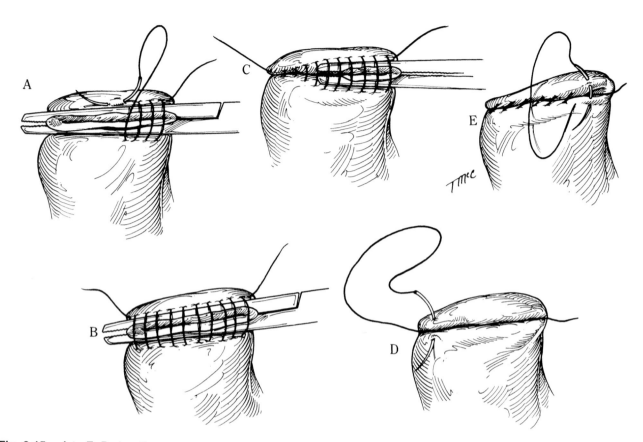

Fig. 6-15. A to E, Parker-Kerr oversew.

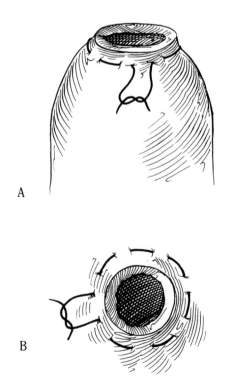

Fig. 6-16. A and B, Purse-string suture.

the Cushing, when the forceps have been withdrawn. The most common application of this suture pattern in large animal surgery is in the jejunocecal anastomosis in the horse.[2,6] This pattern is used in the stump of the terminal ileum.

Purse-String Suture

This pattern comprises a continuous suture placed in a circle around an opening; however, the suture is tied when the entire circumference of the circle has been followed (Figure 6-16). To aid inversion of the suture, an assistant should grasp that part of the purse string that is exactly opposite the knot and should exert upward traction. The purse string is then tightened following the release of the tissue forceps. Like the Cushing suture, the suture does not penetrate the lumen. Another layer of sutures may be used over the purse string, either in the form of another purse string or in a series of Lembert sutures. The purse-string suture is used to oversew an opening that evacuates gas in the gastrointestinal tract that is made by a needle or trocar puncture. It can also be used to stabilize permanent indwelling fistulae or cannulae.

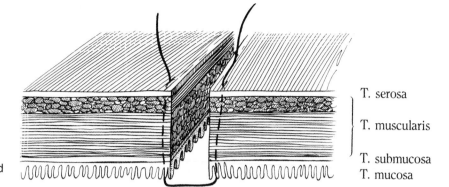

Fig. 6-17. Simple interrupted suture used in bowel.

T. serosa

T. muscularis

T. submucosa
T. mucosa

Simple Interrupted Suture

The simple interrupted suture can be used successfully to close the intestinal tract. It should be used to gently oppose the wound edges, thereby causing minimal interference to the blood supply. In Figure 6-17, the suture is placed through all the layers approximately 3 to 4 mm from the wound edges. The suture is then tightened. Conversely, the suture can be placed through all layers except the mucosa. This pattern is best reserved for end-to-end anastomosis of bowel with significant differences in lumen diameter.

Gambee Suture

The Gambee suture pattern is used for intestinal anastomosis as a single-layer closure (Figure 6-18). The suture and needle are introduced like a simple interrupted suture and pass from the tunica serosa, through all layers, except the mucosa. The needle is then directed back through the tunica submucosa. The suture crosses the incision, passes through the submucosa and out through the submucosa, muscular, and serosal layers. The suture is tied firmly, so that the tissue compresses on itself. Although it takes longer than a simple interrupted pattern, the Gambee pattern is useful in equine gastrointestinal surgery because it inverts the mucosa into the lumen. When this technique was evaluated experimentally in horses, it caused minimal adhesion formation and stenosis.[8,9]

Double-Layer Inverting Patterns

A two-layer inverting pattern (using Cushing, Connell, or Lembert) produces an anastomosis with higher initial tensile and bursting strength.[4] The incidence of adhesions is lower, but internal cuff formation may potentially produce intraluminal obstruction.

For end-to-end anastomosis of the small intestine a double-layer inverting anastomosis composed of a simple continuous mucosal layer and a continuous Lembert seromuscular layer has been advocated.[1] This technique inverts only one layer and results in a minimum reduc-

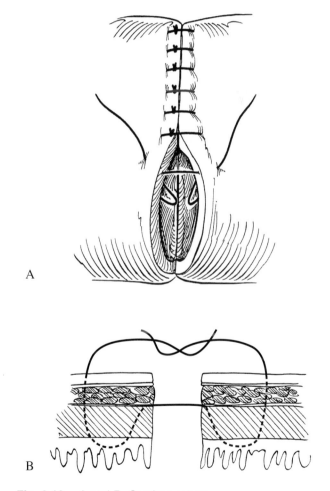

A

B

Fig. 6-18. A and B, Gambee suture.

tion of lumen diameter. The incidence of fibrosis and suture tract inflammation is higher with this technique than with Gambee and crushing patterns; however, adhesions were not present in six horses when this technique was used, as compared to a 50% adhesion incidence with the other two techniques.[1] The author prefers a simple continuous appositional pattern followed by a minimally inverting Cushing pattern. Further details of intestinal resection, anastomosis, and gastrointestinal stapling are available in *McIlwraith's and Turner's Equine Surgery: Advanced Techniques.*[4]

Stent Bandages (Tie-Over Dressings)

These dressings are used over areas that are difficult to apply pressure bandages to, such as the proximal regions of the limbs and the torso. As well as applying some localized pressure and minimizing postoperative swelling, this bandage helps keep dirt and bedding away from the skin incision. These dressings also can assist in the elimination of dead space, such as the throatlatch region following modified Forssell's operation for cribbing. They have been used to cover skin incisions following the closure of the linea alba for celiotomy.

For smaller incisions, a sterile gauze bandage is used. For larger incisions, a rolled hand towel is used. The bandage material should be long enough that the ends slightly overlap the ends of the incision. Following closure of the skin incision, an assistant holds the towel firmly in position. Using synthetic monofilament suture material, we insert a continuous horizontal mattress suture or

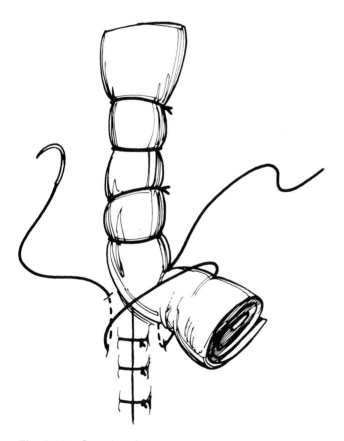

Fig. 6-19.   Stent bandage.

interrupted horizontal mattress sutures (Figure 6-19). As the sutures are tied, slight tenting of the skin may occur. This will disappear when these sutures are removed. The stent is usually removed 4 to 7 days after surgery, depending on the procedure. The bandage helps keep the incision dry because of its wicking effect, but it should not become moist enough to allow excessive fluid to adhere to the incision. The stent should be removed if excessive moisture persists.

Suture Patterns for Severed Tendons

Frequently, the large animal surgeon is presented with a traumatic wound involving severed tendons. If the tendon ends are not in approximate alignment, suturing may be indicated.

One has to weigh the advantages and disadvantages of suturing tendons. To appose the tendon ends properly with suture material, the tendon must be subjected to additional trauma. Nonabsorbable materials are generally used because of their ability to maintain strength during the protracted course of tendon healing. In the face of infection or contamination, these materials may potentiate infection, or a chronic draining tract may form. Nevertheless, tendon repair can be indicated to approximate the ends and to facilitate healing. This is especially true in horses, where traumatic laceration of the flexor tendons occurs frequently. Research suggests that when possible, performing tenorrhaphy greatly increases the prognosis of the horse returning to riding status. If a tendon is sutured, some form of external support will be necessary to minimize extreme forces placed on the repair.

Locking-Loop Tendon Suture

Based on tendon surgery in man, the traditional suture pattern for repair of severed tendons in the horse was the Bunnell pattern or variations on this pattern. Because of the extreme loads placed on equine tendons, this pattern was prone to failure. The suture would tear out of the fiber bundles by cutting or pulling through the weak interfibrous connections. It also was believed to compromise fragile vascularity within the tendon. Improved suture patterns have since been developed. One of the commonly used patterns is the locking-loop tendon suture (modified Kessler pattern) shown in Figure 6-20. This suture is strong, causes minimal interference with tendon blood supply, and exposes little of the suture material.[7]

The needle is inserted into the severed end of the tendon and emerges from the surface of the tendon (Figure 6-20*A*). The needle is then passed transversely through the tendon just superficial to the longitudinal part of the suture (Figure 6-20*B*). This results in a loop

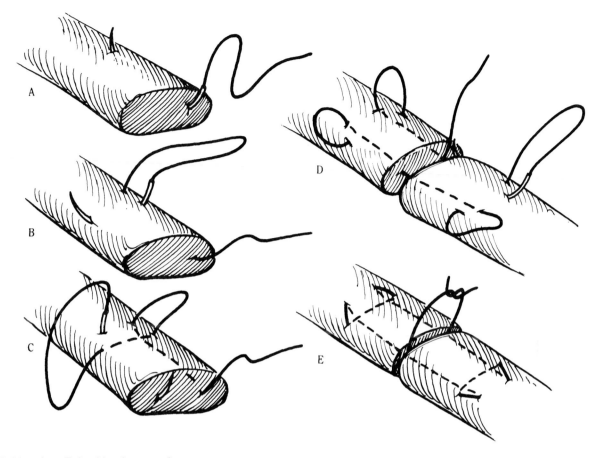

Fig. 6-20. A to E, Locking-loop tendon suture.

of suture locking around a small bundle of tendon fibers. When more tension is applied to the repair site, the grip of the suture loop on these fiber bundles becomes tighter. The needle is then reinserted in a longitudinal direction and passes under the transverse portion of suture material (Figure 6-20C); this process is repeated on the other piece of tendon (Figure 6-20D). After placement of the suture, all the loops should be tightened in turn and the suture tied snugly, so slight "bunching" occurs at the junction (Figure 6-20E).

Monofilament nylon or polypropylene is the recommended suture material for this pattern. Rough-surfaced sutures (braided or twisted) do not have sufficient glide or elasticity to permit longitudinal strain to be transmitted into locking tension. Wire is not flexible enough for this suture pattern and is not recommended.[7] The largest-diameter monofilament nonabsorbable suture should be used. At this time, the largest commercially available suture material of this type is no. 2 nylon. A single locking-loop suture pattern with this material in equine tendon is insufficient to prevent gap formation during weight bearing,

even when the area is immobilized with a cast. In vitro biomechanical studies have shown that a double locking-loop pattern should be used because it is twice as resistant to gap formation and failure as a single locking-loop pattern. Three locking-loop patterns can be used, but they may be technically difficult and time consuming to apply.[3]

Carbon fiber is not recommended for use in this pattern. Despite some earlier enthusiasm for carbon fiber for tendon repair in horses, research has shown that nylon suture is superior to carbon in the reestablishment of tension-resisting capacity.[5]

Another good tendon repair suture pattern is the three-loop pulley pattern (Figure 6-21). The suture is inserted across the diameter of the severed tendon (Figure 6-21A) and then moved to the other portion of the tendon and inserted in the same plane (Figure 6-21B). This is repeated two more times, dividing the tendon into three planes (Figure 6-21C). The sutures are then tightened and the knot tied (Figure 6-21D). Similar suture materials and external coaptation as for the locking loop pattern should be used.

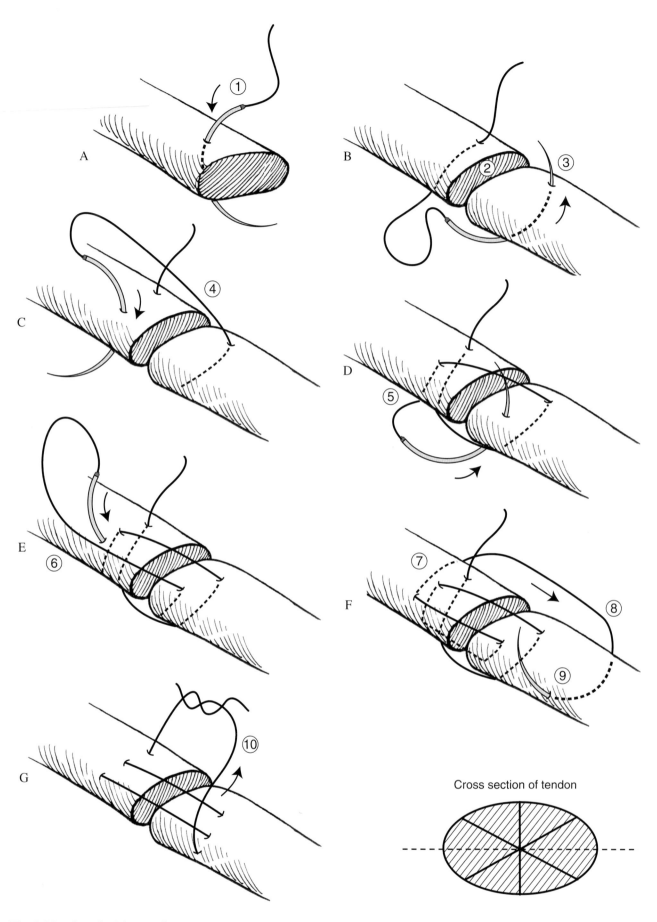

Fig. 6-21. A to G, 3-loop pulley suture.

References

1. Dean, P.W., and Robertson, J.T.: Comparison of three suture techniques for anastomosis of the small intestine in the horse. Am. J. Vet. Res., *46:*1282, 1985.

2. Donawick, W.J., Christie, B.A., and Stewart, J.V.: Resection of diseased ileum in the horse. J. Am. Vet. Med. Assoc., *159:*1146, 1971.

3. Easley, K.J., Stashak, T.S., Smith, F.W., and Van Slyke, G.: Mechanical properties of four suture patterns for transected equine tendon repair. Vet. Surg., *Mar–Apr;19(2):*102–106, 1990.

4. McIlwraith, C.W., and Robertson, J.T.: McIlwraith's and Turner's Equine Surgery: Advanced Techniques, 2nd Ed. Baltimore, Williams & Wilkins, 1998.

5. Nixon, A.J., et al.: Comparison of carbon fiber and nylon suture for repair of transected flexor tendons in the horse. Equine Vet. J., *16:*93, 1984.

6. Owen, R.R., et al.: Jejuno or ileocecal anastomosis performed in seven horses exhibiting colic. Can. Vet. J., *16:*164, 1975.

7. Pennington, D.G.: The locking-loop tendon suture. Plast. Reconstr. Surg., *63:*648, 1979.

8. Reinertson, E.L.: Comparison of three techniques for intestinal anastomosis in equidae. J. Am. Vet. Med. Assoc., *169:*208, 1976.

9. Vaughan, J.T.: Surgical management of abdominal crisis in the horse. J. Am. Vet. Med. Assoc., *161:*1199, 1972.

Chapter 7

PRINCIPLES OF WOUND MANAGEMENT AND THE USE OF DRAINS

Objectives

1. Describe the fundamental principles of wound management and healing in large animals.
2. Discuss factors that impact wound healing and how they may be used to predict the wound environment.
3. Describe techniques for wound exploration and debridement.
4. Describe the indications for antimicrobial therapy in wound management.
5. Describe basic principles and appropriate wounds for primary closure, second-intention healing, and delayed primary closure.
6. Provide indications and applications for the use of drains in wound management.

Wound Management

There are three main methods of wound management and healing; primary closure, second-intention healing, and delayed primary closure (tertiary intention). Primary closure describes the initial closure of wounds. Second-intention healing describes wounds that are left to heal without surgical correction via wound contraction and epithelialization. Wound contraction is an active process characterized by the centripetal movement of the whole thickness of the surrounding skin, which results in diminished wound size. It is the major process for reestablishment of skin continuity in wound healing by secondary intention, with the exception of the distal limbs. In the distal limbs, epithelialization plays the major role in skin closure, and the resulting fragile epithelium is devoid of hair follicles and sweat glands. Finally, delayed primary closure entails a period of open wound management to establish a healthy wound bed until the wound edges can be approximated. An understanding of the basic physiological processes involved in wound healing will aid the practitioner in developing the best treatment regimen for traumatic wounds.

Most of the discussion in this chapter is directed at horses because the incidence of traumatic wounds is highest in this species, but the basic principles are the same for ruminants and swine. Emphasis is placed on wounds of the distal limbs, where wound healing can be a difficult and frustrating process.

Assessment of Traumatic Wounds

The initial assessment of a traumatic wound enables the practitioner to evaluate the blood supply to the wound, viability of surrounding tissues, and any other factors that may inhibit or retard wound healing or increase the wound's susceptibility to infection. The characteristics of the wound—including the type, degree of contamination, location, size, and surrounding vascular supply—can be readily evaluated upon presentation. The type of wound—laceration, abrasion, puncture, etc.—is a good indication of the wound's blood supply and contamination, as well as the viability of the surrounding tissue. Wounds can also be categorized by their degree of contamination; clean, clean-contaminated, contaminated, or infected. Clean and clean-contaminated wounds are suitable for primary or delayed primary closure. Traumatic wounds are generally contaminated or infected wounds, which are not suitable for primary closure. Contaminated and infected wounds can be converted to a clean wound and closed primarily through debridement and lavage, or they can be healed via secondary or tertiary intention.

The location of the wound is important to take into account because certain areas have physiological advantages or disadvantages that affect wound healing as well as anatomical structures. In horses, wounds on the body heal well via second intention, whereas wounds on the distal limb are prone to developing exuberant granulation tissue, hypertrophic scarring, and cell transformations.[5] Research has shown that the distal limb wound environment is very different from that of wounds on the body; profibrotic growth factor expression and fibroblast proliferation is prolonged, collagen synthesis is increased, myofibroblasts fail to organize as they do in bodily wounds, and collagen degradation is decreased.[6,7,9,12,13] These studies coincide with the in vivo observations that wounds of the distal limb exhibit persistent inflammation, increased retraction, retarded epithelialization, and decreased contraction, making healing difficult and frustrating in many cases.[4,11] The distal limb lacks the underlying musculature and vascular supply that the trunk has, which undoubtedly accounts for many of these physiological limitations of wound healing. Other anatomical considerations associated with the location of the wound include structure involvement, cosmetic importance, movement (wounds over joints versus the trunk), and underlying bony prominences. All of these have implications for the wound's vascular supply; physiological factors associated with wound healing; and, subsequently, the best method of management for the wound.

Information from the client, such as the mechanism and time of injury and any prior treatment that may have been administered, is beneficial in determining the wound environment and identifying any underlying factors that might compromise healing. For example, many topical ointments and systemic treatments inhibit or retard wound healing. Shearing injuries, as opposed to crushing injuries, generally have a better surrounding vascular supply and are more amenable to closure. The initial care of traumatic wounds has a large impact on the outcome; therefore, it is beneficial to familiarize clients with first aid and the use of nonirritating cleansing solutions, sterile dressings, and pressure bandaging.

Wound Preparation

Because of the environment in which large animals reside, contamination may be so extensive that some trauma patients will require a complete hosing down, especially in the winter and spring when barnyards are muddy. In these cases, tap water is the only practical answer, although its application directly onto the wound should be minimized.

To prepare the wound itself, the edges of the wound should be clipped and, in most instances, shaved. An ample area around the wound should be clipped in case additional exposure to deeper parts of the wound is required. To prevent the introduction of hair into the wound, a sterile water-soluble lubricating gel such as K-Y can be used to protect the wound. Once the wound is clipped, the gel can be rinsed off with sterile saline or water.

Wound cleaning should be minimally traumatic and the agents used should be relatively noncytotoxic. The cleansing agent can be delivered by gravity or by low pressure with the aid of a bulb syringe. Wounds can be cleaned by scrubbing with woven or nonwoven gauze, or by lavage. Scrubbing causes significant mechanical trauma to the wound, so it is important to weigh the benefits of this method against the trauma it causes to the wound bed. High-pressure lavage units are more effective in removing bacteria than conventional techniques; they do not, as it was once believed, force bacteria deeper into the wound or cause significant tissue injury.[1] They can be equally traumatic though if caution is not used to maintain the pressure below 15 pounds per square inch (psi). To attain pressure below 15 psi, it has been shown that a 35-ml syringe can be used with a 25-, 21-, and 19-gauge needle. When the size of the syringe is decreased to 6 or 12 ml, the pressure exceeds 15 psi. Low-pressure lavages can be achieved by punching holes in the top of a saline bottle with a 16 gauge needle. Normal or isotonic saline is an effective agent for mildly contaminated wounds and can be used in a lavage or as a cleaner. Tap water will suffice for grossly contaminated wounds, although it is hypotonic and causes edema of the tissues. The wound microenvironment is usually acidic, so a final rinse with physiological sodium bicarbonate following wound cleaning has been recommended in an effort to restore the tissue to normal pH.[2] This may help ensure the maximal efficacy of topical antibiotics and the host's local immune responses.

Antiseptic agents are used for skin preparation, wound cleaning, and lavage, but they are not effective against bacteria deep in the wound tissue and most are cytotoxic. Their use is best reserved for skin surrounding the wound and in some cases, antiseptic agents are indicated to remove necrotic debris or tissue in the wound. Povidone-iodine scrub and chlorhexidine can be used on periwound tissue, whereas strong antiseptics such as hydrogen peroxide, acetic acid, and Dakin's solution are reserved only for grossly contaminated wounds. A 0.05% solution of chlorhexidine gluconate and a 1% povidone-iodine solution are recommended because they have been shown to be less cytotoxic than other alternatives and still effective at reducing bacterial loads.[2,8] Hydrogen peroxide (3% solution) can be useful for its effervescent action, which can lift debris from the wound, but is not very bactericidal and is relatively cytotoxic.[2] Soap solutions should also be avoided because they are irritating to the tissues. If contamination of the wound is massive, however, the advantages gained by the action of the soap may outweigh the disadvantage of irritated tissues. Newer surfactant-based wound cleansers have been shown to be very effective in mildly contaminated wounds.

Wound Exploration

Traumatic wounds should always be thoroughly explored to rule out the possibility of a foreign body. A foreign body left undetected in a wound reduces the number of organisms needed for infection to start, inhibits or prolongs wound healing, and can result in a poor cosmetic outcome. Depending on the temperament of the horse, chemical restraint may be necessary. For most traumatic wounds where there may be significant blood loss, tranquilizers should be avoided because of their vasodilation effects, which may enhance hypovolemia or produce shock.[14] Xylazine and detomidine are recommended to allow basic evaluation of the wound. Morphine or butorphanol may be added to the injection if increased analgesia is required.[14] Direct infiltration of the wound with a local anesthetic along its edges should be avoided if possible. This method of desensitizing the wound drives contamination deeper into the wound and may even open up new tissue planes; therefore, the use of regional analgesia is preferable. General anesthesia is indicated if the injury is so extensive that a local anesthetic is impractical or if the animal is too fractious. It is also indicated if extensive debridement and cast application are to be performed. The reader is referred to Chapter 2, "Anesthesia and Fluid Therapy," for details on anesthesia and restraint.

Wound exploration can be accomplished via manual palpation of the area, surgical exploration, ultrasound, and radiography. Contrast agents can be useful for identifying and following draining tracts to their source. When exploring wounds that might involve synovial structures, thorax, or abdomen, it is crucial that the practitioner use strict aseptic technique. If it is suspected that the wound may communicate with a synovial structure, a needle may be inserted into the synovial cavity at a distant site and fluid withdrawn for cytology and culture and sensitivity testing. Sterile saline should be injected into the cavity to see whether it communicates with the wound and determine whether the joint capsule or tendon sheath has indeed been penetrated.

Excision and Debridement of the Wound

In some instances, contaminated and infected traumatic wounds can be converted to clean wounds through debridement of the wound. Debridement promotes contraction and epithelialization in a wound and is used to remove necrotic tissue and foreign material, reduce bacterial numbers that potentiate infection, and excise excess granulation tissue to facilitate closure. Horses are particularly susceptible to developing exuberant granulation tissue in wounds of the distal limb. Debridement can be accomplished by a number of ways, including mechanical, chemical, and natural methods. Mechanical methods such as sharp excision, application of wet-to-dry and dry-to-dry dressings, hydrotherapy, and scrubbing of the wound are common in equine practice. Sharp excision using either a scalpel or tissue scissors, such as Metzenbaums, is the least traumatic and most frequently used of these methods and therefore will be the only method discussed in detail here. Dead tissue (fascia, adipose tissue, muscle) should be selectively excised from the wound, as well as small, detached fragments of bone, contaminated

skin edges, and edematous tissue. If possible, nerves, blood vessels, and tendons that appear viable should be left. If the wound is heavily contaminated, an initial preparation and debridement may be followed by a second preparation and debridement, with a change of gloves and instruments.

Antimicrobial Therapy

Antimicrobial therapy is indicated to reduce the bacterial load in traumatic wounds, especially those on the distal limb where the degree of contamination is usually high and anatomical factors impede local immune defenses. Disadvantages to their use, however, include superinfection, adverse reactions in the patient, and bacterial resistance. The practitioner should consider the location and type of wound, tissue involved, and level of structure involvement when determining whether antimicrobial therapy is necessary for a wound and the most appropriate regime.[2,3] Tetanus prophylaxis is always indicated in the horse.

The use of topical antibiotics or antibacterial agents has been controversial. Exudate on the wound can prevent effective contact of the agent with the microorganisms, and many topical antibacterial agents can inhibit wound healing. However, there is evidence that topical antibiotics, when used correctly, can be effective at reducing bacterial numbers in wounds. Topical antibiotics should not be applied longer than 2 weeks.

A wound culture and sensitivity test will establish which organism(s) are infecting the wound and, in conjunction with the appearance of the wound and response from the horse, will allow the practitioner to ascertain whether antimicrobial therapy is necessary. Gram-negative aerobic enteric species, anaerobic bacteria, S. aureus, and S. pyogenes are the most common organisms found in traumatic wounds.[2] Quantitative bacteriology can also be used to determine the necessity of antimicrobial therapy. Wound healing may not be adversely affected by bacteria if there are fewer than 10^5 organisms per gram of tissue. If a foreign body exists in the wound, the level of bacteria is decreased to 10^4 organisms per gram of tissue.

Systemic antibiotics are used often during the treatment of grossly contaminated traumatic wounds in large animals. To be effective, antibiotic administration needs to be initiated as soon as possible, and adequate dosage levels need to be maintained. Systemic antibiotics should not be applied topically to reduce the risk of bacterial resistance.

Other Therapies

Other than antibiotics and tetanus prophylaxis, the judicious use of nonsteroidal, antiinflammatory drugs should be considered. Drugs such as phenylbutazone are often indicated, especially for horses. Unlike high dosages of corticosteroids, these drugs have little to no effect on the course of wound healing. They diminish pain from inflammation, improve the overall well being of the horse, encourage ambulation, and thereby stimulate circulation, especially in the limbs. Corticosteroids are not usually used in the treatment of traumatic wounds unless the surgeon is treating a separate problem.

References

1. Brown, L.L., et al.: Evaluation of wound irrigation by pulsatile jet and conventional methods. Am. J. Surg., *187*:170, 1978.
2. Brumbaugh, G.W.: Use of antimicrobials in wound management. Vet. Clin. Eq., *21*:63–75, 2005.
3. Brumbaugh, G.W.: Antimicrobial therapy of adult horses with emergency conditions. Vet. Clin. Eq., *10*:527–534, 1994.
4. Cochrane, C.A., Pain, R., and Knottenbelt, D.C.: In-vitro wound contraction in the horse: differences between body and limb wounds. Wounds, *15*:175–181, 2003.
5. Knottenbelt, D.C.: Equine wound management: are there significant differences in healing at different sites on the body? Vet. Dermatol., *8*:273–290, 1997.
6. Schwartz, A.J., Wilson, D.A., Keegan, K.G., Ganjam, V.K., et al.: Factors regulating collagen synthesis and degradation during second-intention healing of wounds in the thoracic region and the distal aspect of the forelimb of horses. Am. J. Vet. Res., *63*:1564–1570, 2002.
7. Theoret, C.L., Barber, S.M., Moyana, T.N., and Gordon, J.R.: Expression of transforming growth factor beta (1), beta (2), beta (3), and basic fibroblast growth factor in full-thickness skin wounds of equine limbs and thorax. Vet. Surg., *30*:269–277, 2001.
8. Van den Boom, R., Wilmink, J.M., O'Kane, S., et al.: Transforming growth factor-β levels during second intention healing are related to the different course of wound contraction in horses and ponies. Wound Rep. Regen., *10*:188–194, 2002.
9. Viljanto, J.: Disinfection of surgical wounds without inhibition of normal wound healing. Arch. Surg., *115*:253, 1980.
10. Wilmink, J.M., Nederbragt, H., Van Weeren, P.R., Stolk, P.W.T., and Barneveld, A.: Differences in wound contraction between horses and ponies: the in vitro contraction capacity of fibroblasts. Eq. Vet. J., *33*:499–505, 2001.
11. Wilmink, J.M., Stolk, P.W.Th., Van Weeren, P.R., and Barneveld, A.: Differences in second intention wound healing between horses and ponies: macroscopic aspects. Eq. Vet. J., *31*:53–60, 1999.
12. Wilmink, J.M., Van Weeren, P.R., Stolk, P.W.Th., Van Mil, F.N., and Barneveld, A.: differences in second intention wound healing between horses and ponies: histological aspects, Eq. Vet. J., *31*:61–67, 1999.
13. Wilmink, J.M., and Van Weeren, P.R.: Second-intention repair in the horse and pony and management of exuberant granulation tissue. Vet. Clin. Eq., *21*:15–32, 2005.
14. Wilson, D.A.: Principles of early wound management. Vet. Clin. Eq., *21*:45–62, 2005.

Methods of Closure and Healing

Primary Closure

Appropriate Wounds

Primary wound closure is suitable only for wounds with sufficient surrounding tissue so that the skin edges can be approximated with minimal tension. Wounds that are grossly contaminated or infected or that contain foreign material should not be closed primarily. Time since injury should be taken into account but the "golden period" for primary closure, usually 6 to 8 hours after injury, is not a reliable indicator for when primary closure should be ruled out necessarily. More important factors to consider are those discussed previously: the vascular supply to the wound, anatomical considerations, wound characteristics, and degree of contamination. For example, a wound on the head may heal with first intention even after a 24-hour delay, whereas a wound on the distal limb may not respond to primary closure after several hours.

Suturing Traumatic Wounds

An important factor relating to whether a wound can be closed primarily is the tension that is created by approximating the skin edges. The wound needs to be closed without undue tension. It is preferable to leave some of the wound edges apart rather than to apply sutures under tension, because those sutures will produce ischemia of the wound edges and a larger defect than before. Tension-relieving suture patterns, such as the vertical and horizontal mattress patterns, may be used in combination with stents to minimize local ischemia in the wound edges. In the skin edges themselves, the author prefers to use the near-far-far-near pattern (see Chapter 6, "Suture Patterns").

Dead space should be closed whenever possible; this can be accomplished by deep closure with absorbable suture material or by using a pattern that will pull the skin down onto the defect. Braided synthetic materials should be avoided in the deeper layers. If used in the face of contamination, they can become infected and harbor this infection until they are removed by the surgeon or extruded by the animal. Synthetic absorbables, such as polyglyconate (Maxon), glycomer 631 (Caprosyn), and lactomer 9-1 (Polysorb) (see Chapter 4, "Suture Materials and Needles"), are useful for this purpose; if infection does result, they will maintain tensile strength longer than a material such as catgut. Noncapillary, nonreactive synthetic material, such as nylon or polypropylene, should be used for tension-relieving sutures that can be applied to the wound edges. Use sutures that are just large enough to hold the tissue together to reduce the amount of foreign material in the wound.

Drains are indicated in the treatment of traumatic wounds in which unobliterated dead space or the likelihood of fluid accumulation exists. The use of drains is detailed later in this chapter.

Secondary-Intention Healing

Appropriate Wounds

Wounds that are grossly contaminated, have extensive tissue loss, or contain a significant amount of debris or necrotic tissue should be healed via second intention. Wounds that are on the body heal well, and are cosmetically satisfactory, by secondary intention. However, distal limb wounds in horses are not always suitable for second-intention healing because they are particularly prone to developing excessive granulation tissue, hypertrophic scarring, and cell transformations.

Moist Wound Healing

A moist wound environment is now known to produce the most optimal environment for wound healing and minimizes pain. Moist wound healing allows the exudate to remain in contact with the wound to enhance the host's immune response and speed healing. Wound fluid contains enzymes, growth factors, and various chemokines and cytokines that promote the influx of phagocytic cells and leukocytes to the wound for natural debridement of necrotic tissue and debris. Growth factors and cytokines also stimulate fibroblasts, epithelial cells, and angiogenesis, promoting the growth of new tissue.

During second-intention healing, the goal is to maintain a moist wound environment without letting the wound exudate become so abundant that the periwound tissue is macerated. Recent advances in veterinary wound care products have made it possible to adapt the dressing and bandage regime to best suit the needs of the wound at various stages in the healing process.

Wound healing by this process needs constant attention if one wants to obtain the best functional and cosmetic results. Although the wound is "granulating in," it should receive regular cleansing with a minimally toxic surfactant-based wound cleanser. The intact skin that is ventral to the wound should be protected from serum scald with a bland ointment, such as petrolatum jelly. Once the granulation bed has become established, topical antibiotics are unwarranted because of the innate resistance to infection of this tissue. Parenteral antibiotics are used only in the initial stages of healing, unless signs of diffuse infection develop.

Other Considerations

For wounds on the distal limb that are healed by secondary intention, excessive granulation tissue ("proud flesh") can become a major problem. Prevention consists of avoiding irritating and oil-based ointments, minimizing movement, and maintaining the wound under a pressure bandage or cast. If excess granulation tissue exists, it must be removed until it approximates the level of the surrounding skin; otherwise, the migration of epithelium will be severely retarded. Excision of granulation tissue with a sharp scalpel, while being careful not to disrupt the advancing epithelium at the wound edge, is the treatment of choice. Caustics and astringents are still popular, but their action is not selective, and they remove the delicate epithelium along with the granulation tissue.

If bone or tendon is exposed, as it often is in traumatic wounds of large animals, it must be covered by granulation tissue before epithelium covers the defect. Sequestration of bone usually results if the periosteum has become dried or if the initial injury has chipped off a piece of bone. As soon as it is identified, the sequestrum should be removed; this may mean incising through the already-formed bed of granulation tissue. Skin grafting is indicated in wounds in which a large defect exists or slow skin healing is anticipated. This is discussed in detail in Chapter 8, "Reconstructive Surgery of Wounds."

Tertiary-Intention Healing

Appropriate Wounds

Delayed primary closure (tertiary-intention healing) is used for wounds that cannot be closed immediately due to excessive swelling or contamination. It is often appropriate for distal limb wounds in the horse to reduce the healing time and achieve a greater cosmetic outcome. The wound is allowed to heal to a certain point by secondary intention. Excess granulation tissue may be allowed to form so that the skin expands over the defect. Following sharp excision of the granulation tissue, there is adequate skin to close the wound without excessive tension.

Wound Care and Closure Techniques

Prior to closure, the wound is managed as described in the previous section on second-intention healing. The wound should be cleansed, debrided if necessary, and managed with appropriate dressings. After a healthy wound bed has been established and if the edges may be approximated without undue tension, the wound is prepared to be sutured closed. The wound edges should be sharply excised to freshen the wound and undermined to facilitate closure. Debridement of the most superficial layers of granulation tissue covering the wound is always indicated because it dramatically reduces the bacterial load and the risk of infection. However, overzealous debridement and undermining will compromise the blood supply to the wound, cause local ischemic necrosis, and can lead to incisional dehiscence. The wound is sutured the same as by primary intention. Dead space and tension should be minimized as much as possible, and drains may be indicated.

Use of Drains

Indications

The basic purpose of drainage is to facilitate healing by obliterating dead space or by removing unwanted material from a particular location. The simplest method of wound drainage is the open technique, in which the skin is left unsutured. This technique is commonly used in large animal surgery when a primary closure cannot be performed.

When a primary closure is performed and drainage away from the incision is desired, some form of artificial drainage is necessary. Artificial drains may be classified as either *passive* or *active*. Passive drains, such as the Penrose drain, rely on gravity and capillary action to remove fluid, whereas active drains are closed-suction systems that remove fluid by negative pressure.

The indications for drainage cannot be sharply defined and indeed are controversial. Drains are beneficial in postoperative situations in which seroma formation is a potential problem or when the complete obliteration of dead space is not possible, which can occur after the internal fixation of fractures, for example. Contaminated wounds, especially those involving the thoracic and peritoneal cavity, or instances where infection or contamination of these cavities is a potential problem are common indications for drainage as well. However, the general philosophy of "when in doubt put a drain in" has yielded to a more cautious approach, with a careful analysis of the benefits and disadvantages.

The widespread use of drains has given rise to complications in both human and veterinary patients. Potentiation of parietal abdominal wound infections has been demonstrated in both clinical cases and experimental situations.[5,7] Both latex (Penrose) and Silastic drains potentiate infection. The problems caused by using Penrose drains for peritoneal drainage following abdominal surgery have also been emphasized.[10] Many valid indications for the use of drains still exist, but one should be more critical of the type of drain used, the number of times it is used, the duration of use, and how it is used. With regard to any drain, one should pay careful attention to aseptic technique at the time of placement and the postoperative management of the drains. Drainage should not be used as a substitute for meticulous debridement or careful closure of a wound.

Passive Drains

Passive drains, such as Penrose and bandage drains, are indicated for wounds that cannot be closed without creating subcutaneous dead space. At present, the latex Penrose drains and the perforated tube drains of plastic or Silastic (Redi-Vacette Perforated Tubing) are the most commonly used drains in large animal surgery. The Penrose drain is a thin, latex tube usually 7 to 12 mm in diameter (2.5-cm

diameter drains are also available); it functions by capillary action and gravity flow, with drainage occurring around the drain rather than through the lumen. Fenestration of these drains for passive drainage is contraindicated, because it decreases the surface area of the drain.

The advantages to using Penrose drains are their ease of insertion and need for less maintenance than suction drains. In many cases, the use of a Penrose drain in a wound is sufficient to minimize the postoperative accumulation of blood or fluid. Penrose drains become walled off from the wound rapidly, however, with a decrease in their efficacy, and they also predispose the depths of the wound to retrograde infection from airborne and skin contamination. Additionally, Penrose drains are not indicated for drainage of the peritoneal cavity because they may potentiate infection and should be restricted to wounds and the obliteration of subcutaneous dead space.

In a typical wound closure, the drain is inserted with the ends exiting in the most dependent location remote from the incision, and the incision is sutured. The dependent end of the drain is sutured to the skin. The stab incision through which the drain exits should be of sufficient size to allow drainage to occur around it. The drain should be inserted so that only one end emerges from the wound, and the deep end of the drain is retained within the wound by a suture that can be removed later (Figure 7-1). A dependent region for the emergence of at least one

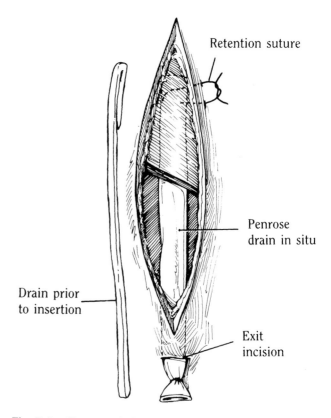

Fig. 7-1. Penrose drain with one end emerging from wound. The retention suture can be removed later and the drain extracted from the exit incision.

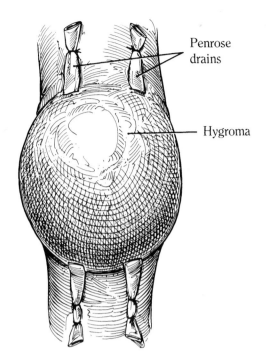

Penrose
drains

Hygroma

Fig. 7-2. Penrose drain used for treatment of hygroma.

end of the drain should be selected. The drain should not be brought out through the primary incision, because it encourages drainage through the incision. Daily cleansing of the drain, and bandage covering if possible, should be performed to minimize the occurrence of retrograde infection. In addition, retrograde infection is time related, and the drain should be removed as soon as it is considered nonfunctional. The drain itself acts as a foreign body, and a daily drainage of fewer than 50 ml/day may be purely drain induced.[3]

Use of Penrose Drains to Treat Hygromas

Penrose drains can be used effectively in the treatment of hygromas in which fluid removal by drains can facilitate obliteration of the cavity by granulation tissue. It is also believed that the foreign-body effect of the drains may be advantageous in stimulating a granulation response in these cases. Stab incisions are made dorsally and ventrally into the hygroma, using aseptic technique. Fibrin and debris within the cavity are removed, and the drains are inserted (Figure 7-2). The drains may be left in place 10 days to 2 weeks.

Active Drains

Active drains are usually indicated only for deep traumatic wounds when more than overflow drainage is necessary. When these drains can be managed appropriately and it is possible to maintain the negative pressure appa-

ratus on the animal, the use of sealed, continuous suction drainage is definitely superior to the use of Penrose drains.[2] These drains should not be used as a substitute for hemostatic control and atraumatic technique during surgery, however.

Fenestrated Tube Drain

A fenestrated tube drain is laid in the wound and exited through the skin by using a trocar (Figure 7-3A) to form a tight seal around the drain (Figure 7-3B). Constant suction can then be applied externally, and fluid can be evacuated from a deep tissue space. It is important that wound closure be airtight. Various evacuators are available commercially, but a simple and economical technique is the use of a syringe, as illustrated in Figure 7-3. The three-way stopcock is used to reduce further the possibility of retrograde infection when the syringe is emptied and suction is reapplied. The drains are heparinized prior to insertion; however, the suction pulls tissue into the holes in the drain, and clogging eventually results. The drains are generally effective long enough to eliminate the acute accumulation of serum following orthopedic surgery and for other procedures in which the dead space cannot be completely obliterated. Patency of tube suction drains can be prolonged by inserting a soft rubber section into the drainage system and regularly stripping the catheter.[7]

Peritoneal Drainage

Peritoneal drainage following laparotomy in large animals can be indicated in instances such as peritonitis, intra-abdominal abscesses, hemorrhage, and to remove leakage from anastomosis or lavage fluid following equine abdominal surgery.[4,9] Active abdominal drainage and lavage has been successfully used in horses to treat peritonitis and to prevent septic peritonitis and abdominal adhesions following intestinal surgery or abdominal contamination.[4,9] When used in conjunction with lavage, abdominal drainage may reduce the incidence of abdominal adhesions by removing excess fibrin and inflammatory cells and facilitate the mechanical separation of bowels.[4,9]

The authors perform peritoneal drainage for a few hours after equine abdominal surgery if any amount of lavage fluid has been left in the abdomen at closure. In this case, a centrally fenestrated tube drain is placed with the nonfenestrated ends and exits cranially and caudally. The drain is removed within 12 hours. With peritoneal drainage of longer duration, the fenestrations of a tube drain will become clogged by fibrin, adhering omentum, or viscera. The ideal method for peritoneal drainage is the use of a sump-Penrose combination. A sump drain is a double-lumen, fenestrated tube drain that incorporates a smaller air vent. The air vent allows air to enter the drained region with the object of displacing fluid into the drain (an example of this is the Shirley wound drain).[10]

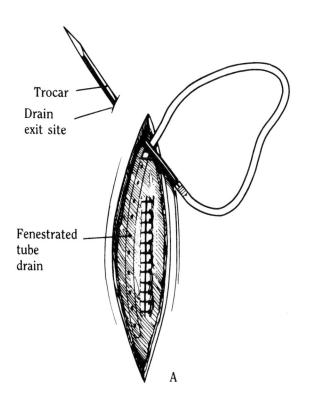

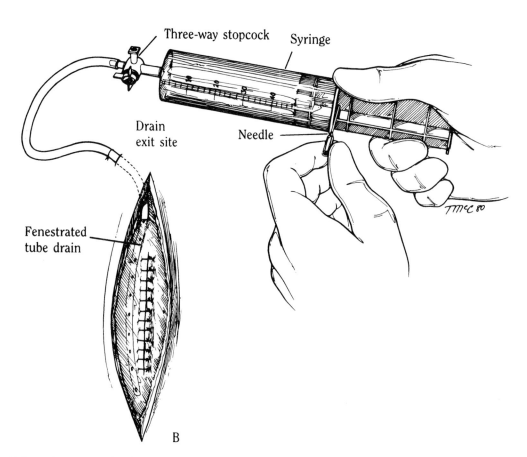

Fig. 7-3. A, Using a trocar to exit a fenestrated drain. B, Syringe technique for suction drainage.

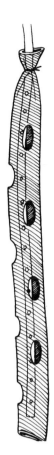

Fig. 7-4. Sump-Penrose drain combination.

By placing such a drain within a Penrose drain (Figure 7-4), occlusion of the fenestrations of the central tube drain is delayed, and drainage efficiency is increased. The placement of gauze around the sump drain prior to insertion within the Penrose drain is another modification claimed to increase efficiency.[11]

Sophisticated, intraabdominal sump drains, which also allow sterile irrigation, have been developed for man.[1,5] Whenever air or fluid ingress systems are used, careful technique is mandatory to prevent the introduction of infection. Bacterial filters should be used with the air channel of sump drains. If any ingress flushing system is to be combined with drainage, it is recommended that the flushing or irrigation be performed through a separate tube positioned through a separate entry site.

References

1. Formeister, J.F., and Elias, E.G.: Safe intra-abdominal and efficient wound drainage. Surg. Gynecol. Obstet., *142:*415, 1976.
2. Fox, J.W., and Golden, G.T.: The use of drains in subcutaneous surgical procedures. Am. J. Surg., *132:*673, 1976.
3. Golovsky, D., and Connolly, W.B.: Observations on wound drainage with a review of the literature. Med. J. Aust., *1:*289, 1976.
4. Hague, B.A., Honnas, C.M., Berridge, B.R., et al.: Evaluation of postoperative peritoneal lavage in standing horses for prevention of experimentally induced abdominal adhesions. Vet. Surg., *27:*122–126, 1998.
5. Hanna, E.A.: Efficiency of peritoneal drainage. Surg. Gynecol. Obstet., *131:*983, 1970.
6. Higson, R.H., and Kettlewell, M.G.W.: Parietal wound drainage in abdominal surgery. Br. J. Surg., *65:*326, 1978.
7. Jochimsen, P.R.: Method to prevent suction catheter drainage obstruction. Surg. Gynecol. Obstet., *142:*748, 1976.
8. Magee, C., et al.: Wound infection by surgical drains. Am. J. Surg., *131:*547, 1976.
9. Nieto, J.E., Snyder, J.R., Vatistas, N.J., Spier, S.J., and Hoogmoed, L.V.: Use of an active intra-abdominal drain in 67 horses. Vet. Surg., *32:*1–7, 2003.
10. Parks, J.: Peritoneal drainage. J. Am. Anim. Hosp., *10:*289, 1974.
11. Ranson, J.H.C.: Safer intraperitoneal sump drainage. Surg. Gynecol. Obstet., *137:*841, 1973.
12. Stone, H.H., Hooper, C.A., and Millikan, W.J.: Abdominal drainage following appendectomy and cholecystectomy. Ann. Surg., *187:*606, 1978.
13. Zacarski, L.R., et al.: Mechanism of obstruction of closed-wound suction tubing. Arch. Surg., *114:*614, 1979.

Chapter 8

RECONSTRUCTIVE SURGERY OF WOUNDS

Objectives

1. Provide an overview of some reconstructive procedures that are used to alleviate tension in large wounds, facilitate primary closure, or increase the cosmetic outcome of the wound.
2. Describe how to use undermining and tension relief incisions to close large wounds that cannot be closed primarily without creating excessive tension
3. Describe the indications for z-plasty and its application as a relaxation procedure for elliptical defects and as a scar revision procedure.
4. Describe techniques of skin grafting and full-thickness sliding skin flap procedures.

Elliptical Excision Undermining for Repair of an Elongated Defect

In some cases an elongated defect will be too wide for its edges to be sutured without excess tension. Using scissors, the surgeon undermines the adjacent skin in an elliptical fashion using a combination of sharp and blunt dissection (Figure 8-1A). The mobilized skin flaps can then be moved toward each other to allow a primary closure (Figure 8-1B). The use of tension sutures in addition to the row of simple interrupted sutures may be indicated.

Wound Closure Using Tension-Relieving Incisions

Also known as the *mesh expansion technique*, this procedure utilizes small, tension-relieving skin incisions made adjacent to the wound to facilitate wound closure or, at least, to decrease the healing time for the primary defect.[1,2]

The skin adjacent to the defect is undermined to a depth according to the vascular supply of the location of the wound.[1] Wounds on the trunk should be undermined to the panniculus muscle to retain the cutaneous vasculature, whereas wounds on the distal limb should be undermined along the plane between the subcutaneous tissue and deep fascia.[1] Following undermining, a series of stab incisions is made parallel to and approximately 1 cm from the skin edge (Figure 8-2A). Three rows of stab incisions are made on each side of the wound in a staggered fashion, with the adjacent rows approximately 1 cm apart (Figure 8-2A). The size of the stab incisions varies. In the initial description of the technique, the use of 10-mm stab incisions allowed sufficient expansion in fresh wounds and resulted in more rapid healing than when 7-mm tension-relieving incisions were used. In older wounds, however, with fibrosis and thickening of the surrounding skin, longer incisions (approximately 15 mm) are recommended. When the stab incisions have been made, the original wound edges are drawn into apposition and are sutured (Figure 8-2B). Tension relieving sutures such as the near-far-far-near pattern using large-diameter sutures have been recommended for closure.[1] It can be helpful to approximate the wound edges to ensure that the relief incisions are made in the correct location.

Wounds are managed postoperatively with bandaging or casting, depending on the individual case. The need for adequate postoperative support of the suture line should be recognized. Based on previous work, undermining can be performed for at least 4 cm on either side of the wound, without detrimental effects.[2] The release of blood and exudate through the stab incisions may facilitate the success of the technique by aiding revascularization and preventing hematoma and seroma formation.

Sliding H-Flap

This technique is used for the repair of rectangular or square defects. As illustrated in Figure 8-3A, two flaps are generally created; however, if skin is not available on both sides, half of the H-plasty may be used.[12] The actual defect serves as the crossbridge of the letter *H*, and two arms are

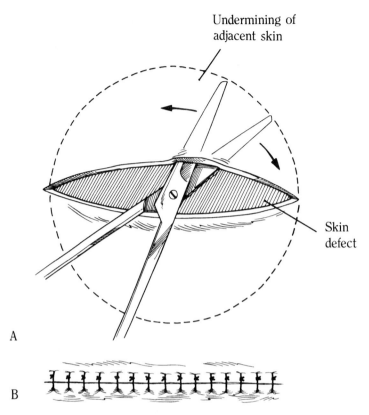

Undermining of
adjacent skin

Skin
defect

A

B

Fig. 8-1. A and B, Elliptical excision undermining for repair of an elongated defect.

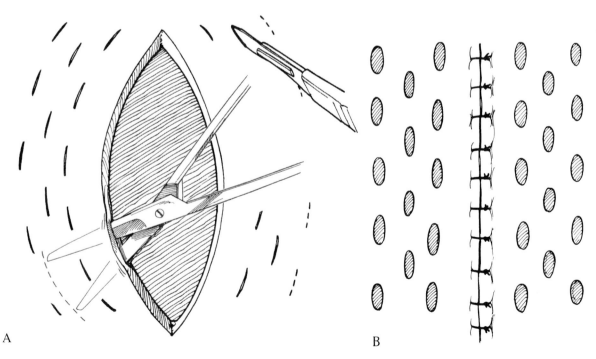

A

B

Fig. 8-2. A and B, Use of tension-relieving incisions to facilitate wound closure.

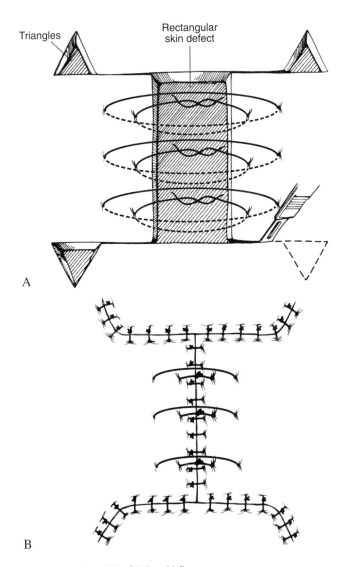

Fig. 8-3. A and B, Sliding H-flap.

The use of Z-plasty as a relaxation procedure for elliptical incisions is illustrated in Figure 8-4. A Z-incision is made adjacent to the elliptical defect (Figure 8-4A). The central incision of the Z (AB) should be perpendicular to the elliptical defect and centered over the area of greatest tension. The two triangles created by the incision should be equilateral; that is, having angles of 60°. The triangles are undermined to create two skin flaps. These skin flaps are then interchanged (Figure 8-4B), and they are sutured in place (Figure 8-4C). The principle behind this technique is that the interchange of the two flaps lengthens the original line (AB) by 50%.

In the second situation, illustrated in Figure 8-5, a linear scar (AB) has excessive tension along its longitudinal axis that results in an acquired ectropion of the upper eyelid (Figure 8-5A). If a Z-plasty is performed in the previous manner, with AB as the central arm of the Z, tension will be relieved, and the upper eyelid will be relaxed (Figure 8-5B).

Removal of Excessive Scar Tissue

A cross section of a typical situation in which exuberant granulation tissue of scar tissue coexists with incomplete skin closure is illustrated in Figure 8-6A. A dotted line indicates the incision for removal of the excess tissue, which is removed with sharp dissection (Figure 8-6B); this allows the primary closure of the skin over the dead space (Figure 8-6C). Placement of a subcutaneous drain is appropriate in this situation.

Skin Grafting

Skin grafting is indicated for wounds that are not amenable to closure or will not yield satisfactory healing via secondary intention. In equine practice, skin grafting is most beneficial in healing wounds with extensive tissue loss or in areas of cosmetic importance, locations where wound healing is impaired such as the distal limb, or where wound contracture could interfere with function, such as near the eye.

Several methods of free-skin grafting are available, including full- and split-thickness mesh grafts and sheet grafts.[3,9,11] Full-thickness grafts are comprised of the epidermis and dermis, whereas split-thickness grafts include only a portion of the dermis. Split-thickness grafts tend to have better success than full-thickness grafts, but the procedure is complicated and requires additional equipment, such as a dermatone, and will not be discussed here. Meshed grafts are considered superior to sheet grafts because of their higher tolerance for motion and less incidence of seroma formation. Nonmeshed grafts are rarely used in equine procedures, although sheet grafts can be effective on fresh wounds with no granulation tissue. Pedicle grafting is not commonly used in the horse.

created (Figure 8-3A). Triangles are cut at either end of each arm to prevent puckering of the skin when the flaps within the H are undermined and are slid together (Figure 8-3A). Near-far-far-near, or *vertical mattress sutures*, are preplaced in the undermined flaps to act as tension sutures. The two flaps are then brought together and are sutured in a simple interrupted pattern (Figure 8-3B). When performed correctly, sliding the flaps together closes the triangular defects. These incision lines are also sutured in a simple interrupted pattern (Figure 8-3B).

Z-Plasty

Z-plasty has two major indications. It may be used as a relaxation procedure for elliptical defects, and it can be used for scar revision of the palpebra when scar formation has produced acquired ectropion.

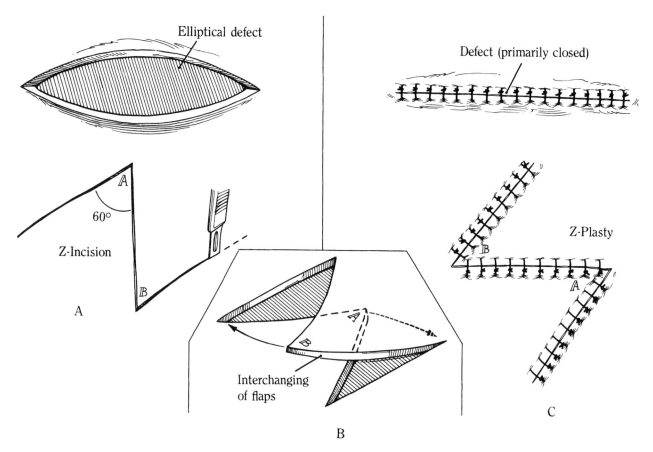

Fig. 8-4. A to C, Z-plasty as relaxation procedure.

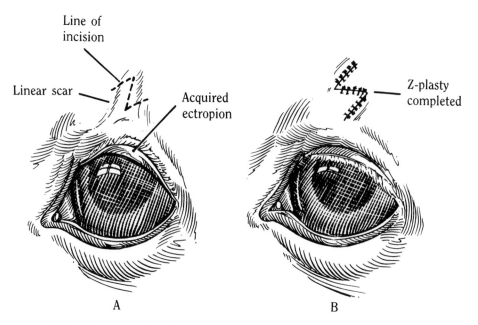

Fig. 8-5. A and B, Z-plasty to relieve ectropion of eyelid.

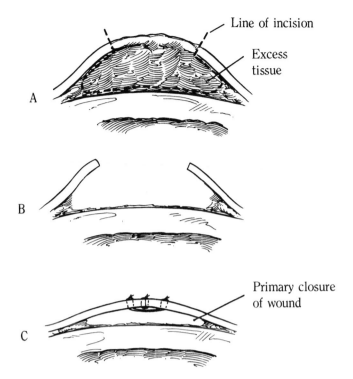

Line of incision

Excess
tissue

A

B

Primary closure
of wound

C

Fig. 8-6. Removal of excessive scar tissue (debulking) to allow primary closure of a wound.

Split-thickness and full-thickness mesh expansion grafts have been shown to yield the most cosmetic healing and quickest epithelialization rates in equine limb wounds. However, these procedures are often not practical for use in the field and require specialized tools and general anesthesia, and are limited to certain wounds. Pinch grafts, followed by punch grafts, have the slowest epithelialization rates and result in significantly less cosmetic healing than the mesh expansion grafts.[7] These wounds tend to heal with a cobblestone-like appearance and may have random hair growth patterns. However, the pinch- and punch-grafting techniques described here are the most economical option for the equine patient because they do not require anesthesia, can be performed in the field, and do not require special equipment. They may be successful in the presence of a hostile grafting bed and when prevention of limb motion is not as critical.[10] Even if the graft does not take, its presence seems to stimulate epithelialization from the periphery. However, prior to performing a pinch- or punch-grafting procedure, it is important to inform the client of the cosmetic outcome of these procedures, which may not be satisfactory for a show horse.

The last grafting procedure discussed in this section is the tunnel graft. It can be used in areas of high mobility, such as the limb, where other grafts may not take due to excessive movement. This procedure can be performed using strips of either full-thickness or split-thickness grafts. For the purpose of this book, the use of full-thickness grafts is described because they can be harvested in the field and do not require additional equipment.

Recipient Bed Preparation

To ensure acceptance of the graft, it is imperative that the recipient bed has a good blood supply and healthy tissue, and the area can be effectively immobilized. A splint may be indicated for wounds located near or on joints and can be incorporated into the bandage following the grafting procedure. Debridement of recipient site prior to graft placement may also be necessary. Ideally, the granulation bed should be healthy, free of infection, and level with edges of the skin prior to the skin graft.

Pinch-Skin Grafting

Skin grafts may be harvested from multiple locations on the horse; however, for cosmetic reasons they are usually taken from the ventral abdomen or beneath the mane on the neck. In the standing sedated horse, the graft donor site is usually the neck. The area is anesthetized by the subcutaneous administration of local analgesic solution in the shape of an inverted *L*. Because granulation tissue is devoid of nerves, analgesic infiltration of the recipient site is unnecessary. This site is prepared with dilute povidone-iodine solution (Betadine Solution) in sterile saline solution using sterile sponges.

When both the wound and the donor site have been prepared, the author prefers to harvest the grafts from the donor site first by elevating small pinches of skin (7 mm × 7 mm) with a needle or forceps and excising the pinches of skin with a scalpel blade (Figure 8-7C). The excised pinches of skin are transferred to a damp gauze moistened with saline solution or blood. The recipient bed is prepared by making a series of small, shallow "pockets" in the granulation tissue bed with a number 15 or 11 scalpel blade. The openings of the pockets should point proximally while the deepest end of the pocket is most distal. The pockets should be made in parallel rows 1 to 2 mm below the surface of the wound (Figure 8-7A), with approximately 1 cm between each pocket over the whole granulation bed (Figure 8-7B). When all the pockets have been made, it is beneficial to apply pressure to the wound for 3 to 4 minutes to reduce the hemorrhage from the newly created pockets in the granulation bed.

The pinches of skin are flattened as necessary and are inserted in each pocket of the granulation bed, just as one would insert a coin into a watch pocket (Figure 8-7D).[10]

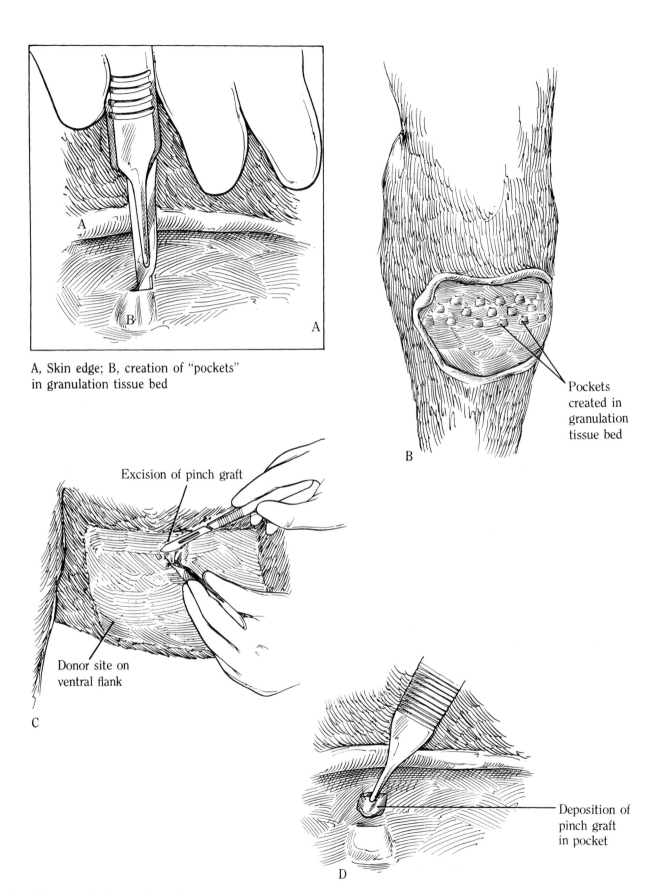

A, Skin edge; B, creation of "pockets" in granulation tissue bed

Pockets created in granulation tissue bed

B

Excision of pinch graft

Donor site on ventral flank

C

Deposition of pinch graft in pocket

D

Fig. 8-7. A to D, Pinch-skin grafting.

Naturally, the graft is inserted with the epithelial side facing out. This procedure is repeated until all the pockets have been filled. The wound is carefully dried, ensuring that the grafts are not extruded from their pockets, and bandaged.

Punch-Skin Grafting

Punch-skin grafting is similar to pinch-skin grafting, except cylindrical plugs of skin are inserted into cylindrical holes in the granulation tissue.[13] The advantages to punch grafting parallel those of pinch grafting. Punch-skin grafting is preferred by some clinicians. The technique can be applied to a thinner granulation tissue bed than pinch grafts, which require a certain depth to create tissue pockets.[13] It is also believed that a more cosmetic result may be obtained.

The general principles of recipient and donor site preparation are the same as in pinch grafting. When the recipient site has been aseptically prepared, small circular holes are made in the granulating bed using a 6-mm biopsy punch (Figure 8-8A). These recipient holes are spaced about 7 mm apart in every direction over the entire surface of the wound. Blood clots forming in the recipient areas are removed prior to placement of the grafts or are prevented by filling the recipient holes with cotton swabs.[13]

Donor grafts are taken from the ventrolateral abdominal area using an 8-mm biopsy punch (Figure 8-8B). The donor grafts are then placed one at a time into the recipient site (Figure 8-8C). The 8-mm donor grafts have a tendency to contract and therefore fit snugly into the 6-mm diameter recipient holes. The subcutaneous tissue should be removed from the plugs prior to insertion. A sterile nonadherent dressing is placed on the wound after surgery, and a bandage is applied.

Tunnel Grafting

In this procedure, strips of full-thickness grafts are placed inside tunnels that are created in the granulation tissue of the recipient bed (Figure 8-9). The strips can be excised by making parallel incisions into the subcutaneous tissue of the donor site or they can be cut from a full-thickness sheet that is already harvested from the donor site, which is closed primarily following graft removal. The strips are generally 2 to 3 mm wide and should be slightly longer than the wound to facilitate suturing of the grafts at the end of each tunnel. A simple interrupted suture is used for securing the grafts in place. The granulation tissue of the recipient bed can be allowed to extend slightly over the level of the surrounding skin so that when the grafts are placed through the tunnels, which are excised approximately 5 mm below the surface of the granulation tissue surface, they are flush with surrounding skin. A cutting

needle, flattened Kirschner wire with trocar point, a straight teat blade, or malleable alligator forcep can be used to form the tunnel in the granulation bed.[6] The tunnels should be formed 1 to 2 cm apart from each other to avoid potential disruption from adjacent tunnels where the graft may fail. Small forceps are used to pull the graft through the tunnel. An alternative method has been described that uses adhesive tape attached to the haired side of the graft to facilitate placement of the strip in the tunnel. The strip of graft and tape are threaded through the eye of a half-curved or straight cutting needle (10 to 12 cm), which is used to guide the strip through the tunnel with the haired side of the graft facing outward.[6] With this technique, multiple passes of the needle through the tunnel or smaller graft strips can be used when the wound exceeds the length of the needle. After 6 to 10 days, the granulation tissue should be excised from over the top of and between the grafts. Compared to pinch and punch grafting, tunnel grafting places a greater volume of skin into the wound without requiring additional specialized equipment.

Bandaging and Postgrafting Care

The author prefers to cover the grafted area with a semi-occlusive foam dressing secured by antimicrobial gauze. An elastic adhesive dressing can be used to maintain pressure over the graft site, although care must be taken to not impede blood supply to the area. A cast or pressure bandage is also applied to minimize movement. It is also recommended that the horse be confined to a box stall to ensure minimal movement at the surgical site. The first bandage should be left on for 1 week and subsequent bandage changes should be performed as needed. Minimizing the amount of bandage changes will reduce displacement of the grafts and the amount of new bacteria introduced into the graft site. During bandage changes, any exudates on the graft site should be carefully wiped off with sterile, saline-soaked sponges. The grafts can usually be identified in 2 to 3 weeks; failure to identify grafts at this time does not necessarily imply an unsuccessful result. As noted before, the procedure typically enhances the rate of epithelialization at the periphery of the wound and reduces healing time.

Random Pattern Flaps

In equine practice, random pattern flaps are used more commonly than axial patterns due to their superior skin perfusion and response to tension.[4,5] The suggested method of flap elevation is sharp dissection because research indicates that although it is more time consuming than other modalities, it yields the most satisfactory closure of the defect. Sharply dissected flaps are reported

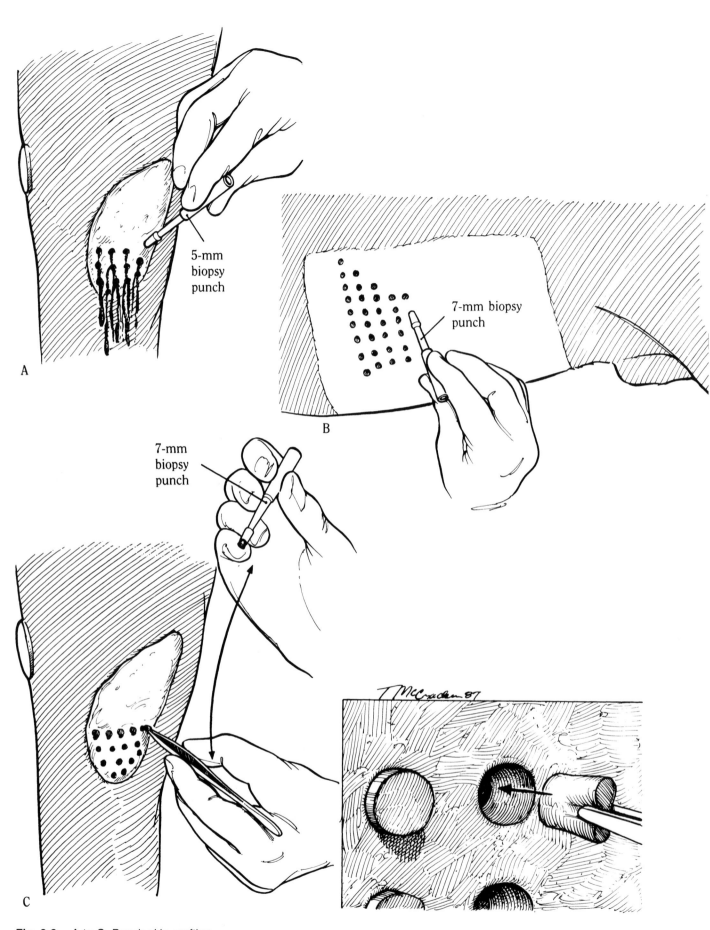

Fig. 8-8. A to C, Punch-skin grafting.

to have greater bursting strengths, less drainage postoperatively, higher collagen content and fibroblast infiltration, and a decreased infiltration of polymorphonuclear leukocytes.[4,8]

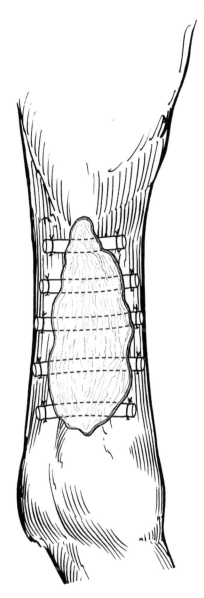

Fig. 8-9. Tunnel grafting.

References

1. Bailey, J.V.: Repair of large skin defects on the limbs of horses. Wien. Tierarztl. Mschr. *78*:277–278, 280–282, 1991.
2. Bailey, J.V., and Jacobs, K.A.: The mesh expansion method of suturing wounds on the legs of horses. Vet. Surg., *12*:78, 1983.
3. Boyd, C.L.: Equine skin autotransplants for wound healing. J. Am. Vet. Med. Assoc., *151*:1618, 1967.
4. Bristol, D.G.: Skin grafts and skin flaps in the horse. Vet. Clin. Eq., *21*:125–144, 2005.
5. Bristol, D.G.: The effect of tension on perfusion of axial and random pattern flaps in foals. Vet. Surg., *21*:223–227, 1992.
6. Carson-Dunkerley, S.A., and Hanson, R.R.: Equine skin grafting: principles and field applications. The Compendium, *19*:872–882, 1997.
7. French, D.A., and Fretz, P.B.: Treatment of equine leg wounds using skin grafts: thirty-five cases, 1975–1988. Can. Vet. J., *31*:761–765.
8. Gelman, C.L., Barroso, E.G., Britton, C.T., et al.: The effects of lasers, electorcautery and sharp dissection on cutaneous flaps. Plast. Reconstr. Surg., *94*:829–833, 1994.
9. Hanselka, D.V.: Use of autogenous mesh grafts in equine wound management. J. Am. Vet. Med. Assoc., *164*:35, 1974.
10. Mackay-Smith, M.P., and Marks, D.: A skin-grafting technique for horses. J. Am. Vet. Med. Assoc., *152*:1633, 1968.
11. Meagher, D.M.: Split-thickness autologous skin transplantation in horses. J. Am. Vet. Med. Assoc., *159*:55, 1971.
12. Stashak, T.S.: Reconstructive surgery in the horse. J. Am. Vet. Med. Assoc., *170*:143, 1977.
13. Stashak, T.S.: Skin grafting in horses. Vet. Clin. North Am. (Large Anim. Pract.), *6*:215, 1984.

Chapter 9

EQUINE ORTHOPEDIC SURGERY

Objective

1. Discuss the indications for, techniques, and complications of commonly used equine orthopedic surgical procedures, including the following:
   - Medial patellar desmotomy
   - Cunean tenectomy
   - Lateral digital extensor tenotomy
   - Inferior check ligament desmotomy
   - Superior check ligament desmotomy (after Bramlage)
   - Superficial digital flexor tenotomy
   - Deep digital flexor tenotomy
   - Sectioning of the palmar annular ligament of the fetlock
   - Palmar digital neurectomy
   - Amputation of the small metacarpal and metatarsal bones
   - Arthrotomy of the midcarpal joint
   - Arthrotomy of the fetlock joint

Medial Patellar Desmotomy

Indications

Upward fixation of the patella occurs when the patellar fibrocartilage and medial patellar ligament fix over the medial trochlear ridge of the femur, inhibiting flexion of the hock and stifle. Some predisposing factors are known, such as poor muscle tone and condition, hindlimb conformation, stifle trauma, and hereditary factors.[4] An increased incidence of upward fixation of the patella is also seen in young horses and ponies, particularly Shetland ponies, and horses with straight hindlimb conformation.[1,4] Good quality radiographs of the stifle joint are necessary to rule out osteochondritis dissecans, especially in young horses. This condition can mimic the signs of intermittent upward fixation of the patella and may be associated with straight limb conformation and distention of the femoropatellar joint as well.

Medial patellar ligament desmotomy should be considered a "last resort" treatment for recurrent upward fixation of the patella. Depending on the duration and severity of the condition, many cases will respond to more conservative therapy. This is especially true in young horses that will improve after appropriate conditioning and development of quadriceps muscle tone through training. Medial patellar desmotomy induces thickening over the entire length of the medial patellar ligament after it heals, which ideally should allow the ligament to disengage from the notch on the medial ridge of the femoral trochlea and prevent locking. Counterirritants injected in and around the medial patellar ligament have also been used to treat more persistent cases with clinical success.[3]

Anesthesia and Surgical Preparation

This surgical procedure is performed with the animal standing. Depending on the temperament of the animal, tranquilization may be indicated. The area of the middle and medial patellar ligaments is clipped and surgically prepared. The tail is wrapped to avoid contamination of the surgical site. Two milliliters of local anesthetic are injected subcutaneously over the medial border of the middle patellar ligament. A 20-gauge, 1-in needle is then inserted through this bleb, and the subcutaneous area around the distal part of the medial patellar ligament is infiltrated with local anesthetic.

Instrumentation

General surgery pack
Blunt-ended bistoury (tenotomy) knife
Curved Kelly forceps

Surgical Technique

A 1-cm incision is made over the medial border of the middle patellar ligament close to the attachment of the ligament to the tibial tuberosity. (The site of the skin inci-sion in relation to the patellar ligaments is illustrated in Figure 9-1A.) Curved Kelly forceps are then forced through the heavy fascia and are passed beneath the medial patellar ligament. This creates a channel for the

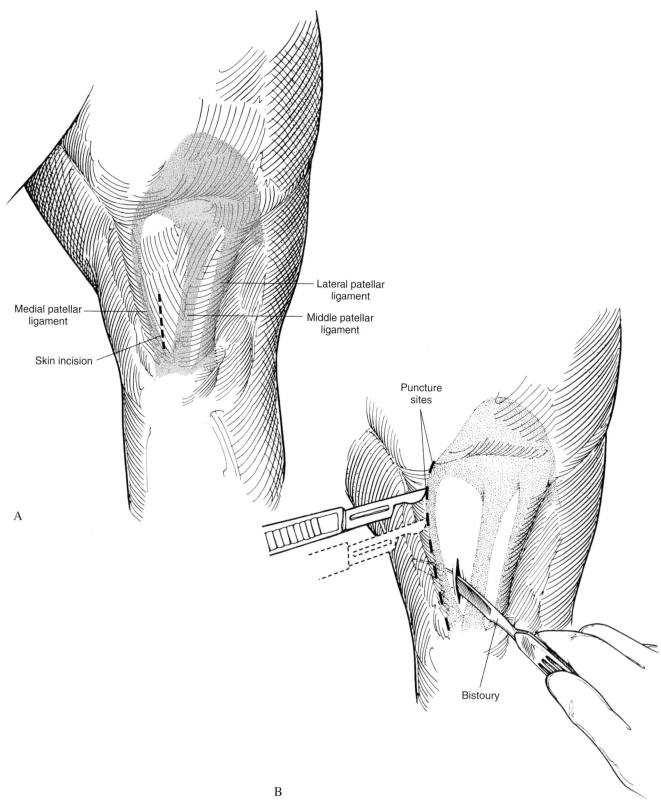

Fig. 9-1. A to D, Medial patellar desmotomy/fenestration.

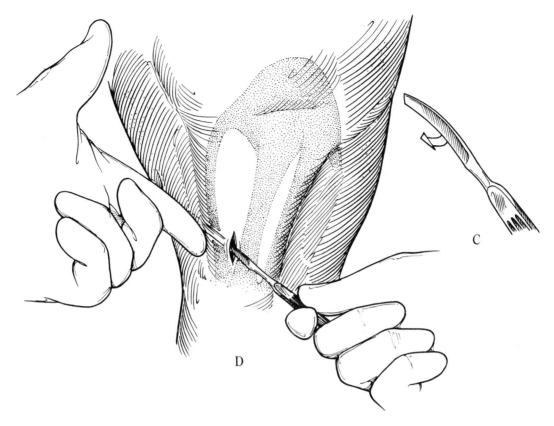

Fig. 9-1. *Continued.*

insertion of a bistoury knife beneath the medial patellar ligament (Figure 9-1*B*). The bistoury knife is inserted so the side of the knife lies flat beneath the patellar ligament. When the knife is positioned, the cutting edge is then turned outward (Figure 9-1*C*). With the left index finger palpating the end of the knife through the skin to ascertain its correct position, the surgeon cuts the ligament with a sawing movement (Figure 9-1*D*). One must ensure that the blade of the bistoury knife completely encloses the medial patellar ligament before it is severed. Once the ligament has been severed, the tendon of the sartorius muscle feels like a tense band medially and may lead the inexperienced operator to believe that the medial patellar ligament has not been completely severed. One or two sutures of nonabsorbable material are placed in the skin incision.

An alternate procedure has been described that achieves the same thickening effect of the medial patellar ligament as desmotomy. Medial patellar ligament splitting involves percutaneous splitting of the medial patellar ligament with a no. 15 blade. The proximal third of the medial patellar ligament is fenestrated, but the parapatellar fibrocartilage is not split (Figure 9-1*B*). The procedure is performed under the guidance of ultrasound and with the patient under general anesthesia and in dorsal recumbency. Medial patellar ligament splitting is described in detail elsewhere.[4] Another approach has been described

where a 16-gauge needle is used to fenestrate the medial patellar ligament.[3] Either of these two approaches is more desirable than cutting the medial patellar ligament.

Postoperative Management

Antibiotics are not used routinely. Hand-walking is useful to control local swelling. The horse should be rested and hand-walked for a minimum of 2 weeks and preferably 4 to 6 weeks. Even with experienced operators, instances of severe swelling and lameness of varying duration are observed occasionally.

Complications and Prognosis

Complications that can arise during surgery include severing of the wrong ligament or inadvertent entrance into the femoropatellar joint with the bistoury (this can potentially occur if the desmotomy is performed too proximad). A complication that can be seen postoperatively is dehiscence of the skin incision and cellulitis (phlegmon) of the limb. These complications can be avoided by careful attention to aseptic technique during the procedure.

When used appropriately, medial patellar ligament desmotomy has a generally favorable prognosis, provided surgery is performed before any secondary gonitis develops. Unfortunately, the procedure is often performed on horses with undiagnosed lameness in which upward fixation of the patella is not the problem. In these cases, the results are less satisfactory.

A condition resembling chondromalacia patellae of man and associated with medial patellar desmotomy has been observed in our clinic.[2] On radiographs, spurring or fragmentation of the distal patella is noted. When viewed arthroscopically, cartilage lesions varying from softening and fibrillation to dissection and fragmentation of the articular cartilage have been seen. It is suggested that the lesions may be caused by maltracking of the patella within the trochlear groove, leading to more lateral positioning of the patella resulting from loss of the medial tensile pull of the medial patellar ligament. That medial patellar desmotomy is the cause of the problem has yet to be proved, however.

References

1. Dugdale, D.: Intermittent upward fixation of the patella and disorders of the patellar ligaments. *In* Current Therapy in Equine Medicine. Edited by N.E. Robinson. Philadelphia, W.B. Saunders, 2006.
2. McIlwraith, C.W.: Osteochondral fragmentation of the distal aspect of the patella in horses. Eq. Vet. J., *22*:157, 1990.
3. Reiners, S.R., May, K., DiGrassie, W., and Moore, T. How to perform a standing medial patellar ligament splitting. *In* 51 Annual Convention of the American Association of Equine Practitioners, AAEP, 2005, Seattle, WA, USA. Ithaca: International Veterinary Information Service (www.ivis.org), 2006; Document No. P2684.1205.
4. Tnibar, M.A.: Medial patellar ligament splitting for the treatment of upward fixation of the patella in 7 equids. Vet. Surg., *31*:462–467, 2002.

Cunean Tenectomy

Relevant Anatomy

The tibialis cranialis muscle originates on the lateral condyle and tuberosity of the tibia and travels distally to just above the hock, where its insertion tendon begins. The tendon passes through the peroneus tertius and then divides into a large dorsal branch and a smaller medial branch. The cunean tendon is the medial branch; it passes obliquely over the distal intertarsal and tarsometatarsal. joints where a small bursa is interposed between the tendon and bone.

Indications

Cunean tenectomy is one of the treatments for bone spavin (degenerative joint disease of the distal intertarsal and tarsometatarsal joints)[3], cunean bursitis (a condition that occurs frequently in Standardbred racehorses), and distal tarsal osteoarthritis. This operation is also used as

a surgical approach to the distal intertarsal and tarsal metatarsal joints as part of surgical arthrodesis of these joints. It is believed that this surgery may benefit horses afflicted with bone spavin by reducing pain caused by pressure exerted by the tendon on the spavin region.[6] In the opinion of those who have performed many cunean tenectomies, this is essentially a "tendon-lengthening" operation. If the surgical site is examined at autopsy months after surgery, the severed ends will have reestablished continuity.

Cunean tenectomy is generally performed only in those cases that are not responsive to more conservative treatment. Other surgical techniques generally have a more favorable prognosis. For example, surgical arthrodesis has been used to treat bone spavin cases refractory to more conservative treatments with a better outcome than cunean tenectomy. Surgical arthrodesis of these joints is beyond the scope of this book, but it is described in the advanced techniques textbook.[4]

The advantages to this procedure are that it usually does not require general anesthesia, it is relatively simple and inexpensive to perform, and it has a rapid recovery. However, the procedure may result in soft tissue enlargement at the surgery site and its clinical benefits are yet to be proven. Although the surgical procedure is described here, it is not used in surgical practice by the author.

Anesthesia and Surgical Preparation

This surgical procedure may be performed with the recumbent animal under general anesthesia or with the standing animal under local anesthesia. For the latter procedure, the limb is clipped, shaved, scrubbed, and prepared for the infusion of local anesthetic. Generally, local anesthetic is infused in an inverted "U" pattern dorsal to the proposed site of the incision. Alternatively, anesthetic can be infused above and below the tendon and into the cunean bursa to distend it. A twitch or tranquilization may be required. The surgical site is prepared for aseptic surgery following infiltration of the local anesthetic.

Instrumentation

General surgery pack

Surgical Technique

The incision for the cunean tenectomy can be either a vertical incision almost perpendicular to the direction of the cunean tendon or an incision that parallels the direction of the fibers of the cunean tendon. If the surgeon is attempting the operation for the first time, we recommend that he/she make a *vertical* incision. This allows the surgeon a certain margin of error if the incision is too distal or too proximal.

If the second method is used and the incision is made in the direction of the fibers, the surgeon must be confident that it is placed directly over the middle of the tendon. To help locate the incision, firm digital palpation is made over the area of the tendon on the medial aspect of the hock; the distal limit of the chestnut is a good landmark (Figure 9-2A). If this incision is too proximal or too distal, it cannot be modified like the vertical incision. The technique described here has the incision following the direction of the cunean tendon.

The incision is made through the skin and subcutaneous tissues and onto the cunean tendon; at this point, the tendon will be visible. A pair of forceps is directed under the cunean tendon and into the cunean bursa, to emerge

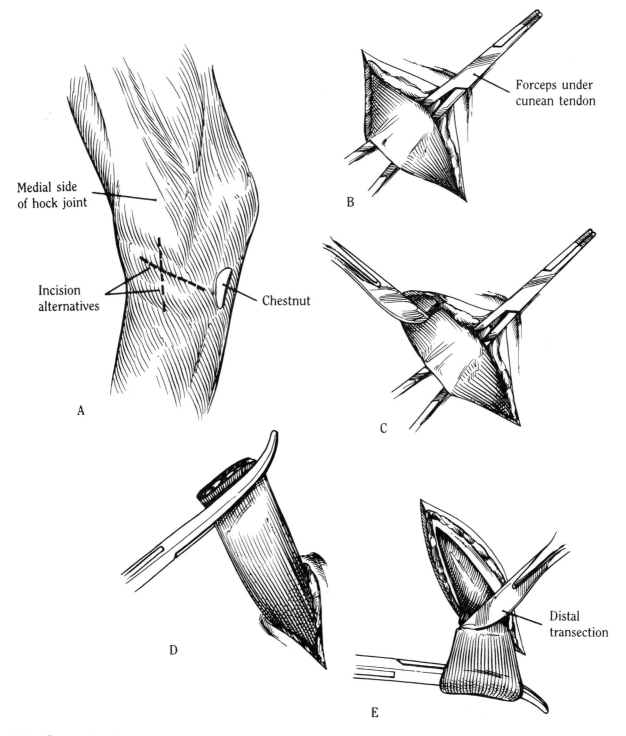

Fig. 9-2. Cunean tenectomy.

from the proximal edge of the tendon (Figure 9-2B). The tendon is then incised at its proximal end (Figure 9-2C), and the distal portion of the tendon is grasped with the forceps (Figure 9-2D). As much of the cunean tendon is removed as possible. The tendon is incised at its distal end near the chestnut (Figure 9-2E).

Following removal of a portion of the tendon, the skin is closed using a synthetic, monofilament, nonabsorbable suture (nylon or polypropylene) in a simple interrupted or vertical mattress pattern. If the animal is under general anesthesia, the surgeon may elect to close the subcutaneous tissues with an absorbable suture before the skin closure. The limb is bandaged using a suitable nonadherent dressing in combination with an elastic adhesive bandage that does not extend above the hock joint.

Postoperative Management

Tetanus prophylaxis is administered, but antibiotics are not used routinely. The bandage is kept in place for approximately 10 days; at the end of this time, the initial bandage and the skin sutures are removed. Exercise generally commences as soon as the skin sutures are removed.

Complications and Prognosis

The efficacy of this procedure in treating the previously mentioned conditions is debatable. Cunean tenectomies have been performed in horses with distal tarsal osteoarthritis with satisfactory results.[1] An owner survey of horses that received cunean tenectomies for treatment of bone spavin reported that 83% of owners felt the procedure improved lameness and that they would have the procedure performed again.[2] Conversely, a statistical analysis of cases treated by this surgical procedure and by other means reported that the operation had limited advantage over conservative methods.[3] The benefit of this operation in returning the horse to performance has also been questioned.[1,5] Soft tissue enlargement at the surgery site is a complication of cunean tenectomy.

References

1. Baxter, G.M.: Review of methods to manage horses with advanced distal tarsal osteoarthritis. In 50th Annual Convention of the American Association of Equine Practitioners, 2004, Denver, CO.
2. Eastman, T.G., Bohanon, T.G., Beeman, G.M., et al.: Owner survey on cunean tenectomy as a treatment for bone spavin in performance horses. In Proceedings of the 43rd Annual American Association for Equine Practitioners Convention 1997, pp. 121–122.
3. Gabel, A.A.: Treatment and prognosis for cunean tendon bursitis-tarsitis of Standardbred horses. J. Am. Vet. Med. Assoc., 175:1086, 1979.
4. McIlwraith, C.W., and Robertson, J.: McIlwraith's and Turner's Equine Surgery: Advanced Techniques, 2nd Ed. Philadelphia, Lippincott Williams & Wilkins, 1998.
5. Platt, D.: Review of current methods available for the treatment of bone spavin. Eq. Vet. Edu., 9:258–264, 1997.
6. Stashak, T.S. (Ed.): Adams' Lameness in Horses, 4th Ed. Philadelphia, Lea & Febiger, 1987.

Lateral Digital Extensor Tenotomy

Relevant Anatomy

The lateral digital extensor muscle originates at the collateral ligament of the stifle, fibula, and lateral tibia; it proceeds distad, lateral to the tibia, and enters the tendon sheath just caudal to the lateral malleolus of the tibia. The tendon sheath is nonpalpable where it is covered by the fascia and extensor retinaculum of the hock. The tendon then continues distad and is palpable as it emerges from the tendon sheath at the level of the proximal third of the metatarsus (Figure 9-3A).

Indications

Lateral digital extensor tenotomy (myotomy) has been used for the treatment of equine stringhalt, a condition characterized by abnormal gait and involuntary hyperflexion of the hindlimb.[7] Stringhalt has been defined as a distal axonopathy.[3] One proposed cause of the exaggerated hyperflexion of the hindlimb is damage to the large, more vulnerable nerve fibers from the muscle spindles in the hindlimb. The etiological agent of stringhalt is unknown; however, two general forms of the disease have been distinguished. Australian stringhalt is associated with ingestion of certain plant toxins, is distinguished by geographical and seasonal patterns of occurrence, and can occur bilaterally. Furthermore, it has been reported to spontaneously resolve itself and may be accompanied by forelimb and laryngeal abnormalties.[4,5] Conventional or "classic" stringhalt is not associated with the ingestion of plant toxin and occurs sporadically. This form of the disease has occurred subsequent to injury to the stifle or hock, particularly trauma that occurs to the dorsum of the metatarsus, upward fixation of the patella, painful foot diseases, and spinal cord disease.[2,4]

Although the exact cause of stringhalt is unknown, resection of the tendon and muscle belly (myotenectomy) has in some cases led to partial or even complete relief of the condition.[6] Benefits of this procedure are that it can be performed in the standing horse with local anesthesia and requires only two incision sites, approximately 2 and 6 cm long each.[1] The following technique involves resection of the tendon plus a large portion of the muscle belly of the lateral digital extensor tendon. This modified technique was designed to improve the surgical success rate.

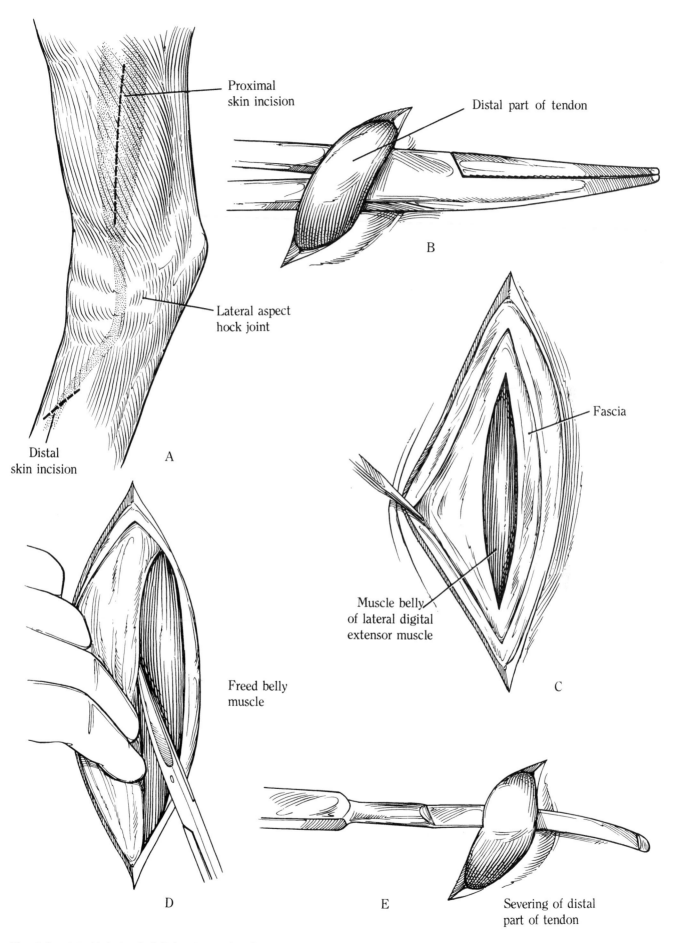

Fig. 9-3. A to H, Lateral digital extensor tenotomy.

Labels within figure:

A
- Proximal skin incision
- Lateral aspect hock joint
- Distal skin incision

B
- Distal part of tendon

C
- Fascia
- Muscle belly of lateral digital extensor muscle

D
- Freed belly muscle

E
- Severing of distal part of tendon

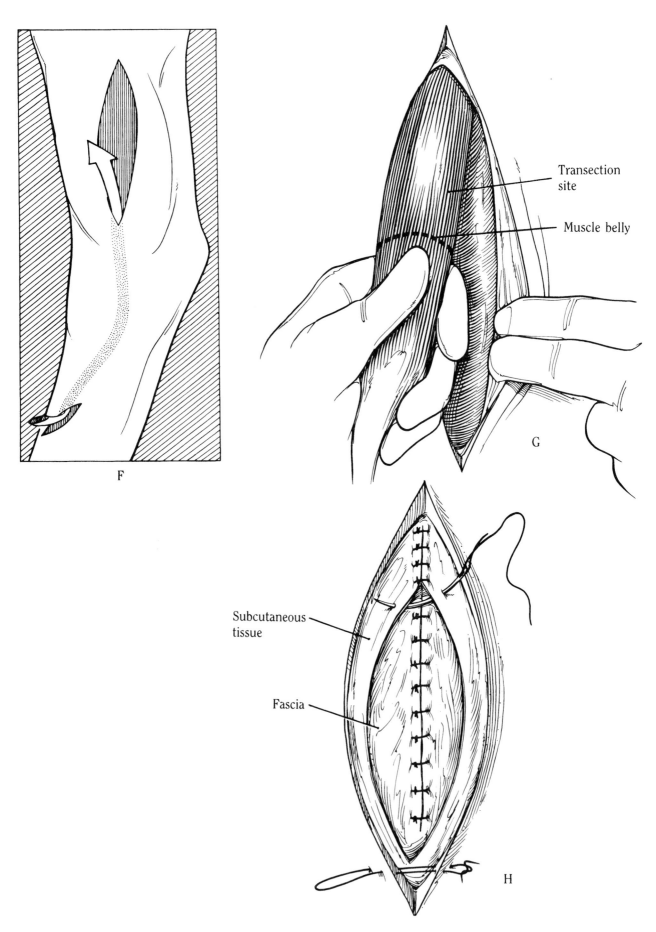

Transection site

Muscle belly

G

Subcutaneous tissue

Fascia

H

Fig. 9-3. *Continued.*

Anesthesia and Surgical Preparation

It is preferable to perform this technique of lateral digital extensor tenotomy with the patient under general anesthesia because more attention can be paid to asepsis and hemostasis. If only a small amount of the muscle is removed, the surgery can be performed under local anesthesia with the animal standing. In this situation, the local anesthetic should be injected about 2 cm above the lateral malleolus of the tibia directly into the muscle belly of the lateral digital extensor. The second injection of local anesthetic should be made in the area below the hock and above the lateral digital extensor tendon, just before it joins the long digital extensor tendon.

The area over the surgical site is clipped and shaved. Two surgical sites are prepared: The first is a large area over the muscle belly, above the hock, and the second is a smaller area over the distal end of the tendon where it merges with the long digital extensor tendon (Figure 9-3A).

Instrumentation

General surgery pack
Blunt-ended bistoury (tenotomy) knife

Surgical Technique

The distal incision is made over the lateral digital extensor tendon immediately proximal to its junction with the long digital extensor tendon. An incision is made directly over the tendon; the tendon is exposed and isolated by dissecting bluntly beneath the tendon and elevating it using either curved Kelly forceps or Ochsner forceps (Fig. 9-3B). Pulling on the tendon at this stage reveals movement of the corresponding muscle belly of the lateral digital extensor tendon; this will assist the surgeon in locating the incision over the muscle belly.

The second incision is made over the muscle belly parallel to the direction of the muscle fibers. The incision should continue through the overlying fascia until the fleshy portion of the muscle belly is visible (Figure 9-3C). The fascia overlying the muscle belly is thick, and the fibers are directed diagonally. Once the muscle belly is freed (Figure 9-3D), the surgeon goes to the first incision over the distal aspect of the lateral digital extensor tendon and severs the tendon (Figure 9-3E). Prior to severing the tendon, one should make sure that the tendon in the distal incision corresponds to the muscle in the proximal incision. Then a pair of Ochsner forceps are placed under the musculotendinous junction; by exerting traction on it, the entire tendon is stripped from its sheath, which overlies the lateral aspect of the hock (Figure 9-3F). The muscle belly is then elevated from the incision and is severed at an oblique angle (Figure 9-3G).

The surgeon should attempt to oversew the muscle stump. This may be difficult because of excess tension, but we believe it reduces postoperative seroma formation. The stump of the muscle is oversewn by grasping the fascia surrounding the muscle belly on the one side and apposing it to the fascia on the opposite side of the muscle belly. Simple horizontal mattress sutures are placed using a synthetic absorbable material. The fascia is closed with simple interrupted or continuous sutures of an absorbable suture material, followed by closure of the subcutaneous tissues with a similar material in a simple interrupted or continuous pattern (Figure 9-3H). The skin is closed with a synthetic, monofilament, nonabsorbable suture material in a simple interrupted pattern. The distal incision is closed in one layer using a similar material in the skin. The wounds are covered with nonadherent dressings, and the entire limb is bandaged.

If the condition is bilateral, the horse is rolled over (if it is under general anesthesia), and the identical procedure is performed on the other pelvic limb.

With the original technique, in which only a small amount of muscle belly is severed, postoperative bandaging is less critical. With this modified muscle-belly severing technique, however, bandaging is essential to minimize seroma formation caused by hemorrhage from the muscle stump. A bandage for this purpose consists of soft cotton and extends from the proximal tibia distad to the pastern.

Postoperative Management

Bandaging is generally required for 2 to 3 weeks, and sutures are removed 2 to 3 weeks postoperatively. Box-stall rest is indicated until the surgical sites are healed. When the sites are healed, hand-walking is commenced for about 2 weeks. After this period of hand-walking, normal training is resumed.

Complications and Prognosis

Dehiscence of the skin sutures sometimes occurs because of the stringhalt nature of the gait, and although it has been suggested that the wounds be resutured,[6] it is preferable to allow healing by secondary intention. Other complications include persistence of clinical signs, seroma formation, and hemorrhage.

The results of this procedure in treating stringhalt have been inconsistent; although many studies show that it is at least beneficial in alleviating some of the hindlimb hyperflexion,[2] flexion of the tarsal cural joint involves other muscles, including the lateral digital extensor, long digital extensor, and cranial tibial muscle.[5] One recent study reported excellent long-term recovery in horses affected with acquired bilateral stringhalt (Australian stringhalt) that received lateral digital myotenectomies.[7] Other treatments for stringhalt vary from rest and removal from pasture, to medical treatments including administration of phenytoin, mephenesin, or baclofen.[7] Clients are advised of these aspects when they present a horse to the clinician for surgery. If the client wants, the surgery is performed; despite the uncertain pathogenesis, the operation offers the only real treatment possibility in horses that do not respond to conservative treatment.

References

1. Adams, S.P., and Fessler, J.F. (Ed.): Atlas of Equine Surgery, Philadelphia, W.B. Saunders, 2000, pp. 381–383.
2. Cahill, J., and Goulden, B.E.: Stringhalt—current thoughts on aetiology and pathogenesis. Eq. Vet. J., 24:161–162, 1992.
3. Cahill, J.I., Goulden, B.E., and Jolly, R.D.: Stringhalt in horses: a distal axonopathy. Neuropathol. Appl. Neurobiol., 12:459, 1986.
4. Crabill, M.R., Honnas, C.H., Taylor, D.S., Schumacher, J., et al.: Stringhalt secondary to the dorsoproximal region of the metatarsus in horses: 10 cases (1986–1991). J. Am. Vet. Med. Assoc., 205:867–869, 1994.
5. Slocombe, R.F., Huntington, P.J., Friend, S.C.E., Jeffcott, L.B., et al.: Pathological aspects of Australian stringhalt. Eq. Vet. J., 24:174–183, 1992.
6. Stashak, T.S. (Ed.): Adams' Lameness in Horses, 4th Ed. Philadelphia, Lea & Febiger, 1987, p. 723.
7. Torre, F.: Clinical diagnosis and results of surgical treatment of 13 cases of acquired bilateral stringhalt (1991–2003). Eq. Vet. J., 37:181–183, 2005.

Inferior (Distal) Check Ligament Desmotomy

Relevant Anatomy

The inferior (distal) check ligament, also known as the *deep digital flexor accessory ligament*, originates from the palmar carpal ligament and joins the deep digital flexor tendon in the metacarpal region. As described previously, the inferior check ligament functions as part of the stay apparatus in the horse to prevent overstretching of the flexor tendon and limit the amount of overextension possible in the metacarpophalangeal joint.

Indications

Inferior check ligament (deep digital flexor accessory ligament) desmotomy has been described as treatment for chronic desmitis of the deep digital flexor accessory ligament and chronic lameness associated with heel pain in horses.[7,8] More commonly, this procedure is indicated as treatment for cases of flexure deformity of the distal interphalangeal (coffin) joint or metacarpophalangeal joint (fetlock) that involve contracture of the deep digital flexor tendon (DDF).[3,4] This includes conditions such as clubfoot and some caudal foot lameness.[8,10] Surgical treatment of flexural deformities is indicated only in cases that have not responded to conservative methods of therapy, which are described in detail in other texts. If after 1 to 2 months of conservative treatment methods are not suc-

cessful, inferior check ligament desmotomy may be indicated.[2]

Flexure deformities may be congenital or acquired at any age in horses. Suggested causative factors for acquired flexure deformities included nutrition, genetics, and pain.[2] Some authors have suggested that excessive feeding in some rapidly growing breeds may result in bone growth that exceeds the elongation rate of the associated tendons. Another potential cause of this disease is speculated to be pain and altered weight bearing associated with orthopedic disease, especially physeal dysplasia.[2]

In terms of function and cosmetics, inferior check desmotomy is a better technique than deep flexor tenotomy for the treatment of distal interphalangeal flexure deformities, except when the dorsal surface of the hoof is beyond vertical.[5]

An ultrasound-guided technique for inferior check desmotomy has been described as well.[10] Suggested advantages to this procedure include selection of the incision site, a smaller incision, no subcutaneous suturing, and decreased tissue swelling after surgery.[10]

Anesthesia and Surgical Preparation

Surgery is performed with the patient under general anesthesia and in lateral recumbency. A lateral or medial approach may be used, but the lateral approach avoids the medial palmar (common digital) artery on the medial side; it is the easiest approach and is recommended for the inexperienced surgeon. A medial approach has one advantage, however, in that, if a blemish develops, it will be on the medial side of the limb and may not be as obvious. If only one leg is affected, the animal is positioned so that the side of the leg to be operated on is uppermost. If both legs are affected, the horse is placed in dorsal recumbency and the legs are suspended from the ceiling. Then the carpometacarpal area is clipped and is surgically prepared.

Instrumentation

General surgery pack

Surgical Technique

A 3–4-cm incision is made over the cranial border of the DDF tendon centered at the junction of the proximal one-third and distal two-thirds of the cannon bone. The position of the incision is illustrated in Figure 9-4A, and the relevant anatomy is illustrated in Figure 9-4B. Following the skin incision, the loose connective tissue over the flexor tendons is dissected bluntly, and the paratenon is incised (Figure 9-4C). The superficial and deep flexor tendons must be identified, but they need not be dissected from each other. Blunt dissection is directed craniad to expose the inferior check ligament, and a cleavage plane is identified between the proximal part of the DDF tendon

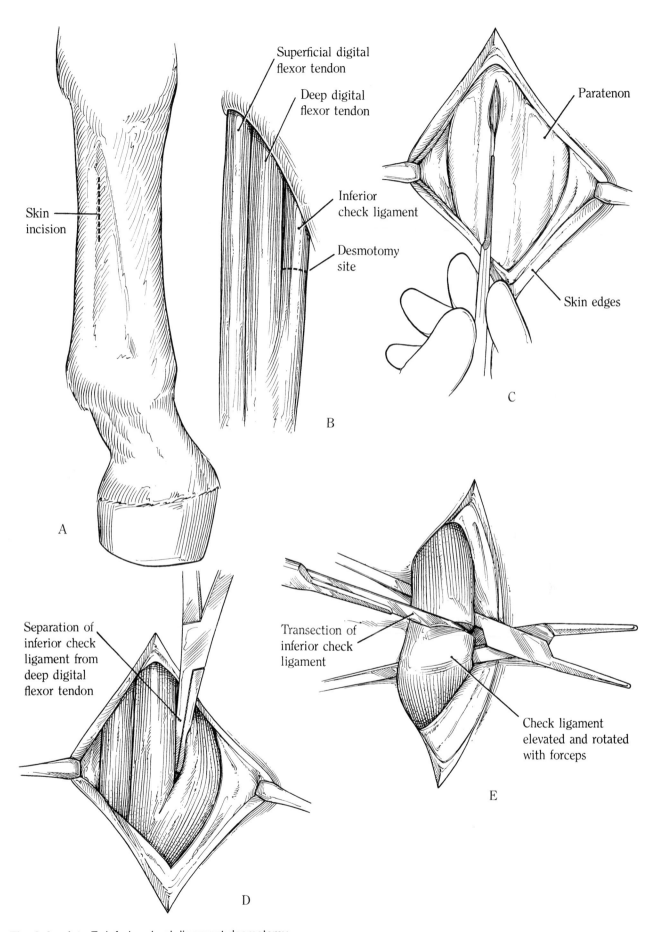

Skin incision

Superficial digital flexor tendon

Deep digital flexor tendon

Inferior check ligament

Desmotomy site

A

B

Paratenon

Skin edges

C

Separation of inferior check ligament from deep digital flexor tendon

D

Transection of inferior check ligament

Check ligament elevated and rotated with forceps

E

Fig. 9-4. A to E, Inferior check ligament desmotomy.

and the inferior check ligament. This cleavage plane is used to separate the check ligament from the DDF tendon (Figure 9-4D). Forceps are inserted between the check ligament and the DDF tendon to separate the structures; then the check ligament is lifted from the incision and is incised with a scalpel (Figure 9-4E). The author prefers to remove a 1-cm segment of the check ligament. This surgical manipulation sometimes disrupts the synovial sheath of the carpal canal, the distal extremity of which extends most of the way down inside the cleavage plane. This event seems to be of little consequence, however. The foot of the patient is then extended manually. The ends of the check ligament become separated, and complete severance of all parts of the check ligament can be ascertained.

The paratenon and superficial fascia are closed in a single layer with simple continuous sutures of synthetic, absorbable material. The skin is closed with nonabsorbable sutures in a suture pattern of the surgeon's choice.

Postoperative Management

A sterile dressing is placed over the incision, and the limb is bandaged from the proximal metacarpus to the coronary band. To apply more pressure over the surgical site (in an attempt to minimize swelling and reduce the potential blemish) a 4-in roll of gauze bandage is placed over the incision and is held in position with pressure from an overlying bandage. The hoof is trimmed to normal conformation. Phenylbutazone (1 to 2 g) is administered intravenously to reduce postoperative pain and to facilitate lowering of the heel. Antibiotics are not administered routinely. Toe extensions may be indicated in more severe cases. Sutures are removed at 12 to 14 days, and bandaging may be discontinued 3 to 4 days later.

Complications and Prognosis

Scarring at the incision site is a common complication of inferior check ligament desmotomies. Proponents of the ultrasound-guided technique for this procedure have reported a reduction in scarring when this method is used.[10] Normal thickening of the check ligament occurs following desmotomy; however, this has not been shown to adversely affect tendon function after healing. Biomechanical studies show that following transection of the accessory ligament, the load is redistributed to the superficial flexor tendon and shifted to the deep digital flexor toward the end of the stance phase.[1] Transfer of the load to the contralateral limb was not observed, and only minor hyperflexion of the metacarpophalangeal joint of the limb that received desmotomy occurred.[1] Overloading of the flexor tendon during locomotion was not considered a concern assuming high-load situations following surgery are avoided, such as jumping.

The results of athletic performance in horses afflicted with flexural deformities after surgery are favorable. A retrospective study of 40 horses treated for distal interphalangeal flexure deformities reported that 9 months to 4 years after surgery, 35 horses were not lame and were used as athletes.[9] Of the other 7 horses, 6 had complications related to the deformity, whereas 1 had complications resulting from surgery.[9] Another study reported that ultrasound-guided inferior check ligament desmotomy corrected 40 of 42 cases of clubfoot and both cases of fetlock deformities (2 horses). The prognosis for the horse returning to athletic function has been suggested to be correlated with the age of the horse receiving surgical treatment; Standardbred foals that received desmotomy at an older age had a decreased chance of racing and training sound.[6]

Generally, the prognosis is poor for horses afflicted with desmitis of the deep digital flexor accessory ligament that is associated with adhesions or tendinitis of the superficial flexor tendon. Desmotomy of the accessory ligament has been shown to restore most of these horses to soundness and even use as a pleasure horse.[7]

References

1. Buchner, H.H.F., Savelberg, H.H.C.M., and Becker, C.K.: Load redistribution after desmotomy of the accessory ligament of the deep digital flexor tendon in adult horses. Vet. Quarterly, *18Suppl*:70–74, 1996.
2. Hunt, R.J.: Flexural limb deformities. *In* Current Techniques in Equine Lameness and Surgery, 2nd Ed. Edited by N.A. White, J.N. Moore. Philadelphia, W.B. Saunders Co., 1998, pp. 326–328.
3. McIlwraith, C.W.: Diseases of joints, tendons, ligaments and related structures. *In* Adams' Lameness in Horses, 4th Ed. Edited by T.S. Stashak. Philadelphia, Lea & Febiger, 1987.
4. McIlwraith, C.W.: Tendon disorders of young horses. In Equine Medicine and Surgery, 3rd Ed. Edited by R.A. Mansmann and E.S. McAllister. Santa Barbara, CA, American Veterinary Publications, 1982.
5. McIlwraith, C.W., and Fessler, J.F.: Evaluation of inferior check ligament desmotomy for treatment of acquired flexor tension contracture. J. Am. Vet. Med. Assoc., *172*:293, 1978.
6. Stick, J.A., Nickels, F.A., and Williams, A.: Long-term effects of desmotomy of the accessory ligament of the deep digital flexor muscle in Standardbreds: 23 cases (1979–1989). J. Am. Vet. Med. Assoc., *8*:1131–1132, 1992.
7. Todhunter, P.G., Schumacher, J., and Finn-Bodner, S.T.: Desmotomy for treatment of chronic desmitis of the accessory ligament of the deep digital flexor tendon in a horse. Can. Vet. J., *38*:637–639, 1997.
8. Turner, T.A., and Rosenstein, D.S.: Inferior check desmotomy as a treatment for caudal hoof lameness. *In* Proceedings of the 88th Annual Meeting of the American Association of Equine Practitioners 1992, pp. 157–163.
9. Wagner, D.C., et al.: Long-term results of desmotomy of the accessory ligament of the deep digital flexor tendon (distal check ligament) in horses. J. Am. Vet. Med. Assoc., *187*:1351, 1985.

10. White, N.: Ultrasound-guided transection of the accessory ligament of the deep digital flexor muscle (distal check ligament desmotomy) in horses. Vet. Surg., 24:373–378, 1995.

Superior Check Ligament Desmotomy (After Bramlage)

Relevant Anatomy

The superficial digital flexor muscle belly is located between the larger deep digital flexor muscle belly and the flexor carpi ulnaris on the caudal aspect of the forelimb. The superior check ligament (the accessory ligament of the superficial digital flexor muscle), which inserts on the caudal surface of the radius, functions in the stay apparatus in the horse.[4] Together with the inferior check ligament (the accessory ligament of the deep digital flexor muscle), it prevents overextension of the fetlock during weight bearing. The cephalic vein runs superficially up the forearm and is used to locate the incision site in this procedure. Branches arising from this vein may require ligation. The brachial artery runs down the medial aspect of the humerus and gives rise to several branches. At the elbow, it becomes the median artery, which runs with the median nerve and courses under the flexor carpi radialis, giving rise to the common interosseous artery.[4] Just proximal to the carpus, the median artery divides into three branches: the palmar branch; the radial artery; and the main branch, which runs through the carpal canal with the flexor tendons and becomes the medial palmar artery. The median nerve also divides proximal to the radiocarpal joint and gives rise to the medial and lateral palmar nerves. There is a nutrient artery that runs near the proximal aspect of the superior check ligament that should, if possible, be avoided.

Indications

Superior check ligament desmotomy was initially described as a surgical treatment for metacarpophalangeal flexural deformities in young horses.[2] Reported results vary,[5,13] however, and it is now recognized that the superficial digital flexor (SDF) tendon is not necessarily the primary unit in metacarpophalangeal flexural deformities.[6] In cases where the SDF appears to be the most involved structure, superior check ligament desmotomy may be indicated.

Superior check ligament desmotomy has been reported as a treatment for superficial digital flexor tendinitis in racehorses.[7] The rationale for the surgery is that it interrupts the transfer of the weight-bearing load on the tendon to the distal radius, bringing the muscle and tendon proximal to the superior check ligament (and therefore enhanced elasticity to the functional unit) into use during weight-bearing.[3]

The technique described is a modification of that previously described.[8] The approach is more caudal, and the limits of the superior check ligament are more easily defined. In addition, the closure of the medial wall of the flexor carpi radialis sheath facilitates elimination of dead space and minimizes the potential for hematoma formation and adhesions.

Anesthesia and Surgical Preparation

Surgery is performed with the patient under general anesthesia and either in lateral recumbency with the affected leg down or in dorsal recumbency with the leg suspended. The latter position is preferable in terms of hemostasis. The leg is clipped from midradius to midmetacarpus. The medial side of the antebrachium is surgically prepared.

Instrumentation

General surgery pack

Surgical Technique

A 10-cm skin incision is made cranial to the cephalic vein, over the flexor carpi radialis tendon and extending from the level of the distal chestnut proximad. The incision is continued through the subcutaneous tissue and antebrachial fascia (Figure 9-5A). A transverse branch of the cephalic vein might require ligation (the incision can often be continued under it). The fascial sheath of the flexor carpi radialis is incised (Figure 9-5B), and Gelpi retractors are placed to expose the medial wall of the sheath, which adheres to the superior check ligament. A stab incision is made through the craniolateral wall of the sheath and superior check ligament (Figure 9-5C). The incision is continued proximad and distad to sever the ligament completely. Complete incision through the check ligament is evidenced by visualizing the muscular portion of the radial head of the deep digital flexor tendon beneath and separation of the superficial digital flexor muscle palmad (Figure 9-5D). An artery (nutrient artery for the superficial digital flexor tendon) may be present at the proximal border of the check ligament. After complete transection of the ligament, the membranous roof of the carpal synovial sheath is seen distally, and the muscle belly of the radial head of the deep digital flexor tendon is seen in central and proximal areas of the incision.

The incision in the flexor carpi radialis sheath is closed with a simple continuous pattern using 2-0 synthetic absorbable material. The antebrachial fascia and subcutaneous tissue is closed with a continuous suture of 2-0 synthetic nonabsorbable material (Figure 9-5E). The skin is closed with interrupted sutures of 2-0 nonabsorbable material.

Postoperative Management

A sterile dressing is placed over the incision, and a pressure bandage is applied. Phenylbutazone is administered

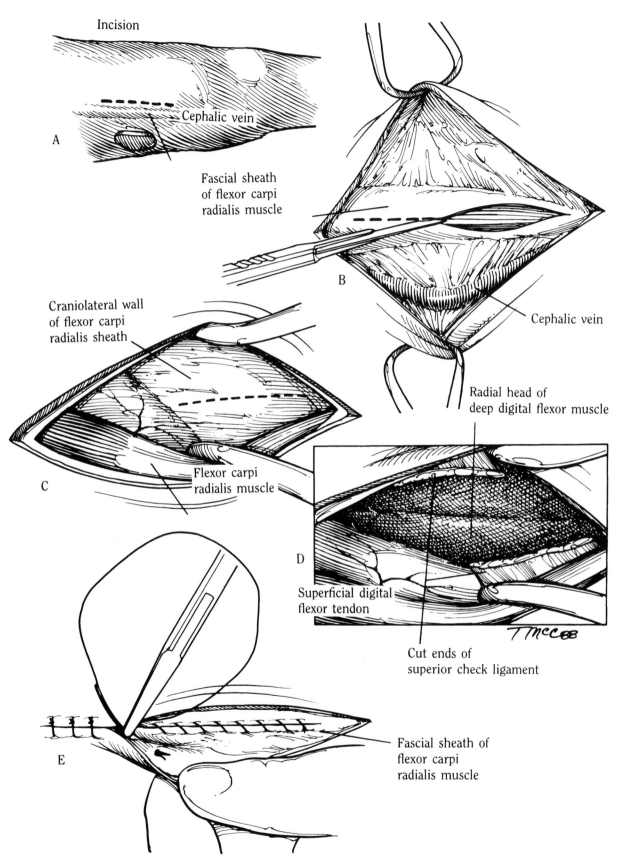

Incision

Cephalic vein

A

Fascial sheath
of flexor carpi
radialis muscle

B

Cephalic vein

Craniolateral wall
of flexor carpi
radialis sheath

C

Flexor carpi
radialis muscle

Radial head of
deep digital flexor muscle

D

Superficial digital
flexor tendon

TMcC88

Cut ends of
superior check ligament

E

Fascial sheath of
flexor carpi
radialis muscle

Fig. 9-5. Superior check ligament desmotomy.

postoperatively, but antibiotics are not used routinely. Sutures are removed at 12 to 14 days, and bandaging may be discontinued 3 to 4 days later.

Complications and Prognosis

Biomechanical studies have suggested that superior check desmotomy used to treat horses with superficial flexor tendinitis may predispose these horses to developing suspensory desmitis. The superior check ligament plays a vital role in maintaining proper metacarpophalangeal and fetlock joint angles in the horse. Following superior check ligament desmotomy, these angles are decreased, which subsequently increases strain on the superficial digital flexure tendon and suspensory ligament and might predispose the horse to other injuries.[1] In one study, Thoroughbred racehorses that received this procedure were shown to be 5.5 times more likely to develop suspensory desmitis than those that were treated nonsurgically.[6]

The efficacy of this procedure in returning racehorses inflicted with tendinitis to full athletic performance is controversial.[11] Most clinical studies of superior check desmotomy have been conducted in Thoroughbred and Standardbred racehorses, despite the fact that superficial flexor tendinitis is common in all sport horses, especially jumpers and 3-day event horses.[11] The prognosis in Standardbred racehorses appears to be slightly better for returning to athletic performance than that for Thoroughbreds, although the results are highly varied. One study showed that 50 of 61 Standardbred racehorses, 83%, returned to racing after treatment for tendinitis.[7] However, only 57% of the 61 horses went on to complete 20 or more starts. Similar results were found in another study, which reported that 35 of 38 (92%) horses returned to racing and 71% of horses started 5 or more races without recurring tendinitis.[11] The prognosis for Thoroughbred racehorses is generally lower in the literature. Reported percentages of horses that returned to racing and completed multiple starts range from 53% to 73%.[10,11] In some studies, these percentages have not substantially exceeded those calculated for Thoroughbred racehorses that are managed with minimal exercise and rehabilitation.[6,11] A minimally invasive technique has been described using an arthroscope and a lateral approach.[12] This technique provides a better cosmetic outcome and less postoperative care than the traditional open approach.

References

1. Alexander, G.R., Gibson, K.T., Day, R.E., and Robertson, I.D.: Effects of superior check desmotomy on flexor tendon and suspensory ligament strain in equine cadaver limbs. Vet. Surg., 30:522–527, 2001.
2. Bramlage, L.R.: Personal communication, 1987.
3. Bramlage, L.R.: Superior check ligament desmotomy as a treatment for superficial digital flexor tendonitis: initial report. In Proceedings of the 32nd Annual Convention of the American Association of Equine Practitioners in 1986:1987, p. 365.
4. Dyce, K.M., Sack, W.O., and Wensing, C.J.G.: Textbook of Veterinary Anatomy, 2nd Ed. Philadelphia, W.B. Saunders, 1996.
5. Fackelman, G.E.: Flexure deformity of the metacarpophalangeal joints in growing horses. Compend. Contin. Educ., 9:51, 1979.
6. Gibson, K.T., Burbidge, H.M., and Pfeiffer, D.U.: Superficial digital flexor tendonitis in Thoroughbred racehorses: outcome following non-surgical treatment and superior check desmotomy. Aust. Vet. J., 75:631–635, 1997.
7. Hogan, P.M., and Bramlage, L.R.: Transection of the accessory ligament of the superficial digital flexor tendon for treatment of tendinitis: long term results in 61 Standardbred racehorses (1985–1992). Eq. Vet. J., 27:221–226, 1995.
8. Jann, H.W., Beroza, G.A., and Fackelman, G.E.: Surgical anatomy for desmotomy of the accessory ligament of the superficial flexor tendon (proximal check ligament) in horses. Vet. Surg., 15:378, 1986.
9. McIlwraith, C.W.: Diseases of joints, tendons, ligaments, and related structures. In Lameness in Horses, 4th Ed. Edited by T.S. Stashak. Lea & Febiger, Philadelphia, 1987, p. 339.
10. Ordidge, R.M.: Comparison of three methods of treating superficial digital flexor tendinitis in the racing Thoroughbred by transection of its accessory ligament alone (proximal check ligament desmotomy) or in combination with either intra-lesional injections of hyaluronidase or tendon splitting. Proceedings of the American Association of Equine Practitioners, 42:164, 1996.
11. Ross, M.W.: Surgical management of superficial flexor tendonitis. In Diagnosis and Management of Lameness in the Horse. Edited by M.W. Ross and S.J. Dyson. Philadelphia, W.B. Saunders, 2003.
12. Southwood, L.L., Stashak, T.S., Kainer, R.A., and Wrigley, R.H.: Desmotomy of the accessory ligament of the superficial digital flexor tendon in the horse with use of a tenoscopic approach to the carpal sheath. Vet. Surg., 28:99–105, 1999.
13. Wagner, P.C., et al.: Management of acquired flexural deformity of the metacarpophalangeal joint in Equidae. J. Am. Vet. Med. Assoc., 187:915, 1985.

Superficial Digital Flexor Tenotomy

Relevant Anatomy

The tendons of the deep and superficial digital flexors share a tendon sheath as they pass through the carpal canal. The tendon of the superficial digital flexor remains superficial up until the fetlock, where it dives deep to insert on the distal tubercles of the first phalanx and the fibrocartilage of the second phalanx.[1] At the level of the first phalanx, the superficial digital flexor tendon forms a sleeve through which the tendon of the deep digital flexor passes to insert on the third phalanx. Local thickenings of deep fascia, the annular ligaments, hold the flexor tendons in place at the fetlock.[1]

The principal vessels and nerves of the distal limb exist on the palmar surface of the distal limb and run superficially between the borders of the suspensory ligament and the flexor tendons. The medial palmar artery, which passes through the carpal canal, is the main blood supply to the distal limb. Smaller metacarpal arteries arising from the median artery run with the suspensory ligament as well. The medial palmar artery branches into the medial and lateral digital arteries, which supply the digit, just proximal to the sesamoids. The medial and lateral nerves (branches of the median nerve) and the palmar and dorsal branches of the ulnar nerve innervate the distal limb. The medial and lateral palmar nerves run superficially in the groove between the suspensory ligament and flexor tendons until midway down the metacarpus, where the medial branch forms an anastomosis with the lateral palmar nerve.[1] Like the arteries, these will continue to the digit as the medial and lateral digital nerves.

Indications

Superficial digital flexor tenotomy is indicated for the treatment of selected cases of flexure deformity of the metacarpophalangeal (fetlock) joint. This condition has been described previously as SDF tendon contracture, but it has become evident that in most cases, more than the SDF tendon is involved.[4] The deep digital flexor tendon is commonly involved, and in a chronic case, the suspensory ligament may be involved as well. In an appropriate patient, however, tenotomy of the superficial flexor tendon may return the fetlock to normal alignment.

The technique of superior check (accessory ligament of the SDF) desmotomy has been advocated as an alternate treatment for flexure deformity of the metacarpophalangeal joint.[2] Effective division of the superior check ligament is more difficult than inferior desmotomy, however, and the value of the operation in treating flexure deformities of the metacarpophalangeal joint is controversial.[2,3,5]

Anesthesia and Surgical Preparation

This technique may be performed with the appropriate patient under local analgesia or in lateral recumbency or dorsal under general anesthesia. The midmetacarpal area is prepared surgically.

Instrumentation

General surgery pack
Blunt-ended tenotomy knife

Surgical Technique

Tenotomy may be performed blindly through a stab incision using a tenotomy knife or under direct visualization through a larger skin incision. The latter technique is illustrated here.

A 2-cm skin incision is made over the junction of the superficial and deep digital flexor tendons at the level of the midmetacarpus (Figure 9-6A). The paratenon is incised, and forceps are used to separate the SDF tendon from the deep digital flexor tendon. A cleavage plane is obvious (Figure 9-6B). When the SDF tendon is separated, it is incised with a scalpel (Figure 9-6C). Following tenotomy, the skin is sutured with nonabsorbable material.

When the surgeon has become familiar with the technique under direct visualization, it is simple to perform the surgery blindly by inserting a tenotomy knife blade through a small skin incision, manipulating it between the superficial and deep digital flexor tendons, rotating it 90°, and then severing the tendon. The stab incision is closed with a single suture.

Postoperative Management

A sterile dressing is placed over the incision, and the leg is bandaged from the proximal metacarpus distad. Phenylbutazone, 1 to 2 g, is administered to facilitate return to function, and the animal is placed on an exercise regimen immediately. The sutures are removed 10 to 12 days after the operation, at which point bandaging is discontinued. If this technique fails to correct the deformity, additional procedures, such as inferior check desmotomy, may need to be performed. In addition, in some cases, inferior check ligament desmotomy is the initial treatment of choice in patients with flexure deformities of the metacarpophalangeal joint.[3,4]

Complications and Prognosis

This procedure is generally recommended for unresponsive cases of metacarpophalangeal joint deformity in an effort to salvage the horse as a pasture pet or for breeding purposes.[4] The prognosis is generally guarded, healing is uncosmetic, and the procedure overall is painful. Arthrodesis of the metacarpholangeal joint can be performed for nonresponsive, severe cases of flexure deformities as well.

References

1. Dyce, K.M., Sack, W.O., and Wensing, C.J.G.: Textbook of Veterinary Anatomy, 2nd ed. Philadelphia, W.B. Saunders, 1996, pp. 585–610.
2. Fackelman, G.E.: Flexure deformity of the metacarpophalangeal joints in growing horses. Compend. Contin. Educ., 1:S1, 1979.
3. McIlwraith, C.W.: Diseases of joints, tendons, ligaments, and related structures. In Adams' Lameness in Horses, 4th Ed.

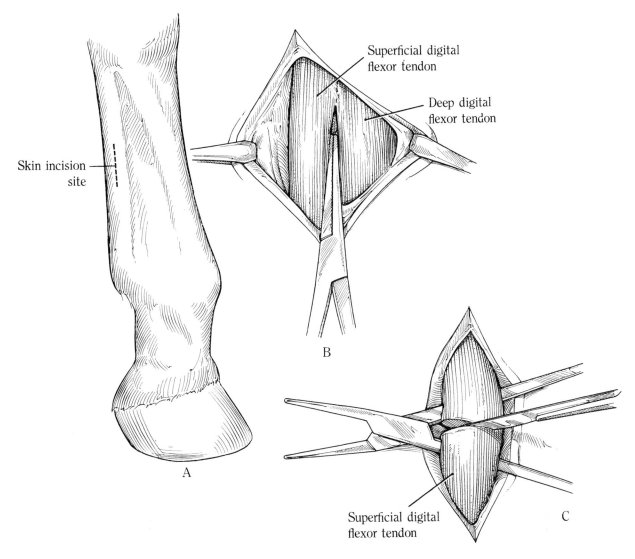

Superficial digital
flexor tendon

Deep digital
flexor tendon

Skin incision
site

B

Superficial digital
flexor tendon

C

Fig. 9-6. A to C, Superficial digital flexor tenotomy.

Edited by T.S. Stashak. Philadelphia, Lea & Febiger, 1987, p. 339.

4. McIlwraith, C.W.: Tendon disorders of young horses. *In* Equine Medicine and Surgery, 3rd Ed. Edited by R.A. Mansmann and E.S. McAllister. Santa Barbara, CA, American Veterinary Publications, 1982.

5. Wagner, P.C., et al.: Management of acquired flexural deformity of the metacarpophalangeal joint in Equidae. J. Am. Vet. Med. Assoc., *187*:915, 1985.

6. Wagner, P.C.: Flexure deformity of the metacarpophalangeal joint (contracture of the superficial digital flexure tendon). *In* Current Practice of Equine Surgery, Edited by N.A. White and J.N. Moore. Philadelphia, J.B. Lippincott Co., 1990, pp. 476–480.

Deep Digital Flexor Tenotomy

Relevant Anatomy

Refer to the previous section on superficial digital flexor tenotomy for a description of structures relevant to this procedure.

Indications

Deep digital flexor (DDF) tenotomy is indicated for the treatment of severe cases of flexural deformity of the distal interphalangeal joint and also as an aid in the

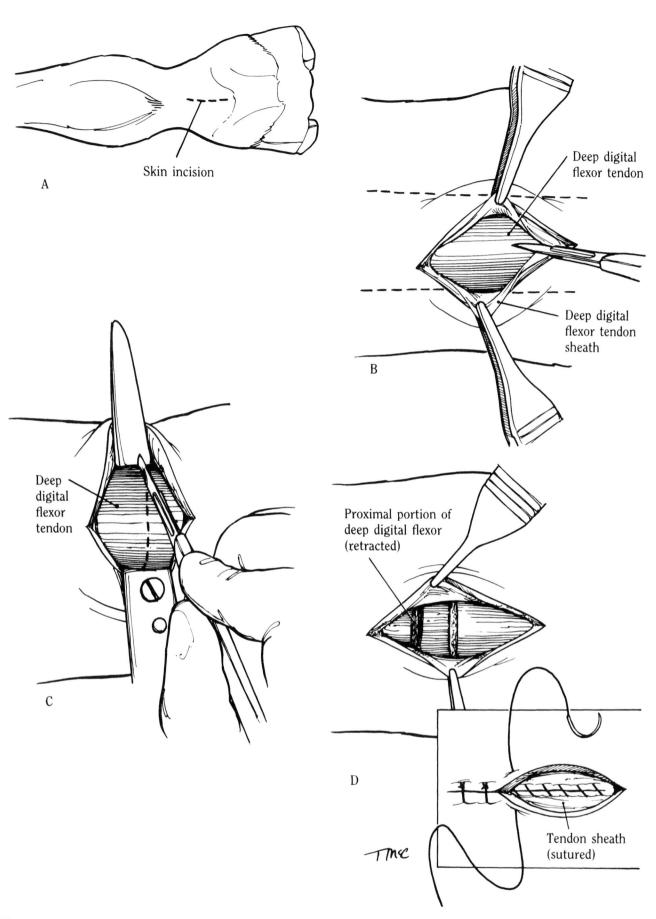

A

Skin incision

B

Deep digital
flexor tendon

Deep digital
flexor tendon
sheath

C

Deep
digital
flexor
tendon

D

Proximal portion of
deep digital flexor
(retracted)

Tendon sheath
(sutured)

TMc

Fig. 9-7. A to D, Deep digital flexor tenotomy.

management of chronic refractory laminitis.[4,6] If a distal interphalangeal joint flexural deformity has progressed to the extent that the dorsal surface of the distal phalanx has passed beyond vertical, secondary contraction of the joint capsule and peritendinous attachments of the distal segment of the deep flexor tendon may lock the digit in its fixed position. In such cases, a good response to inferior check ligament desmotomy cannot be anticipated, but the patient may respond to a DDF tenotomy.

The most common explanation for pedal bone rotation in horses with severe laminitis is separation of the interdigitating sensitive and insensitive laminae at the dorsal aspect of the hoof wall and the continued pull of the DDF tendon on the palmar aspect of the distal phalanx.[2] The rationale for DDF tenotomy in cases of severe laminitis is to reduce the dynamic forces favoring rotation and to reduce the pressure of the distal phalanx on the corium of the sole.[1] Results of a retrospective study support the technique's effectiveness as a salvage procedure in horses with chronic refractory laminitis.[1]

Tenotomy of the DDF tendon can be performed at either the midmetacarpal level or the midpastern region.[4,6] Concerns of distal peritendinous adhesions may guide the surgeon to the midpastern tenotomy.

Anesthesia and Surgical Preparation

Surgery at the midpastern region is performed with the patient under general anesthesia and in lateral recumbency. A pneumatic tourniquet and Esmarch's bandage are advantageous to provide hemostasis. For surgery at the midmetacarpal region, the procedure can be performed standing. The leg is clipped from above the fetlock down to and including the coronary band. The palmar aspect of the pastern is shaved, and the area is surgically prepared.

Instrumentation

General surgery pack
Blunt-ended tenotomy knife

Surgical Technique

For the midpastern approach, a 3-cm skin incision is made on the midline of the palmar aspect of the pastern starting 1 cm proximal to the heel bulbs and extending proximad (Figure 9-7A). Dissection is continued through the subcutaneous tissue to expose the digital flexor tendon sheath. The tendon sheath is incised in the same line and to the same limits of the skin incision to expose the DDF tendon (Figure 9-7B). Curved forceps are placed under the tendon, and it is transected with a scalpel (Figure 9-7C). The tendon ends will retract.

The incision in the tendon sheath is closed with 2-0 absorbable suture in a simple continuous pattern (Figure

9-7D). The subcutaneous tissue may be closed in a simple continuous pattern (optional), and the skin is closed with interrupted sutures using synthetic nonabsorbable material.

Both closure and resection of the synovial sheath have been recommended by different authors.[1,4] We recommend closure of the synovial sheath, based on the finding in one study that closure did not apparently impair tendon healing.[1] The preferred surgical approach at the midmetacarpal region is performed as described for the midmetacarpal superficial digital flexor tenotomy, transecting the deep digital flexor instead. It can easily be performed in the standing horse with the use of sedation and a local block.

Postoperative Management

A sterile dressing is placed over the incision, and the limb is bandaged from the hoof to the carpus. Phenylbutazone is administered as necessary. In cases of flexural deformity, the hoof is trimmed by shortening the heels as much as possible. This may be done gradually. Hand-walking is performed. Corrective shoeing may also be necessary. If postoperative dorsiflexion develops, shoes with caudally extended branches should be applied.

In horses with laminitis, shoeing is an important adjunctive therapy. Reversed, extended heel shoes have been recommended initially, with later substitution with flat shoes and pads.[1]

Complications and Prognosis

Results of a retrospective study support the technique's effectiveness as a salvage procedure in horses with chronic refractory laminitis.[1] Transection of the deep digital flexor tendon will also decrease the pain associated with the acute refractory stage of laminitis, but it does not reverse the pathological changes within the digital lamina.[5] Of horses that received deep digital flexor tenotomies for treatment of chronic laminitis, 77% survived greater than 6 months and 59% survived greater than 2 years.[3]

References

1. Allen, D., et al.: Surgical management of chronic laminitis in horses: 13 cases (1983–1985). J. Am. Vet. Med. Assoc., *189*:1605, 1986.
2. Coffman, J.R.: Biomechanics of pedal rotation in equine laminitis. J. Am. Vet. Med. Assoc., *156*:219, 1970.
3. Eastman, T.G., Honnas, C.M., Hague, B.A., Moyer, W., and von der Rosen, H.D.: Deep digital flexor tenotomy as a treatment for chronic laminitis in horses: 35 cases (1998–1997). J. Am. Vet. Med. Assoc., *214*:517–519, 1999.
4. Fackleman, G.E., et al.: Surgical treatment of severe flexural deformity of the distal interphalangeal joint in young horses. J. Am. Vet. Med. Assoc., *182*:949, 1987.

5. Hunt, R.J., Allen, D., Baxter, G.M., Jackman, B.R., and Parks, A.H.: Mid-metacarpal deep digital flexor tenotomy in the management of refractory laminitis in horses. Vet. Surg., 20:15–20, 1991.

6. McIlwraith, C.W.: Diseases of joints, tendons, ligaments, and related structures. In Adams' Lameness in Horses, 4th Ed. Edited by T.S. Stashak. Philadelphia, Lea & Febiger, 1987, p. 339.

Sectioning of the Palmar (or Plantar) Annular Ligament of the Fetlock

Relevant Anatomy

There are three annular ligaments of the fetlock: the palmar, proximal digital, and distal digital. The palmar annular ligament of the fetlock runs from the abaxial surface of the proximal sesamoid bones and transverses the palmer aspect of the fetlock joint. With the intersesamoidean ligament, it creates a canal through which the superficial and deep digital flexor tendons pass. (Fig 9-8A).

Indications

This surgical procedure is indicated for the treatment of constriction of or by the palmar or plantar annular ligament, tendinitis in the digital sheath, or posttraumatic adhesions of the digital sheath.[1,3] The problem is associated with injury or infection, and the condition may develop in several ways. Direct injury to the annular ligament with subsequent inflammation may cause fibrosis, scarring, and a primary constriction of the ligament; the constricted ligament, in turn, exerts pressure on the superficial and/or deep flexor tendon. A primary injury to the superficial and/or deep flexor tendon with subsequent tendinitis ("bowed tendon") can have the same result because it is associated with swelling of the SDF tendon against the inelastic annular ligament. In some situations, both types of injury may be involved.

The restriction of free tendon movement and tenosynovitis result in pain and persistent lameness. Prolonged permanent damage to the tendon may result. The syndrome can also arise as a primary chronic digital sheath synovitis of unknown cause, with excess production of synovial fluid and fibrous tissue deposition at the proximal reflection of the synovial sheath onto the flexor tendons.[2] Some authors have considered this pathogenesis to be the most common (the cause of the synovitis remains obscure).[2] Fluid distention of the digital flexor tendon sheath above and below the constricted annular ligament causes the characteristic "notched" appearance on the palmar (or plantar) aspect of the fetlock.[1]

Anesthesia and Surgical Preparation

The patient is placed under general anesthesia with the affected leg uppermost. The use of an Esmarch's bandage and a pneumatic tourniquet facilitates the surgery. A routine preparation for aseptic surgery is performed from the proximal metacarpus distad.

Instrumentation

General surgery pack
Blunt-ended tenotomy knife

Surgical Technique

There are many described techniques for performing an annular ligament desmotomy. The open approach has been generally dropped in favor of the other approaches, including the closed approach with scissors, the closed approach with a tenotomy knife, and the tenoscopic guided approach. Only the closed approach will be described here.

This simplified version of the surgery can be performed with the patient under anesthesia (preferred) or standing. Although it does not allow complete visualization of the tendon sheath contents, it does obviate potential problems of wound dehiscence and synovial fistulation that have been experienced with the open technique.

A 2-cm skin incision is made over the proximal outpouching of the digital flexor sheath, and, using Mayo scissors, a subcutaneous tunnel is created distad to the distal extremity of the annular ligament (Figure 9-8B). Mayo scissors are then positioned so that one arm is in the subcutaneous tunnel and one within the sheath and, with appropriate care to avoid the palmar or plantar vessels and nerve, the annular ligament is incised (Figure 9-8C). Attention is also paid not to sever tendinous tissue within the sheath, and one must know the limits of the annular ligament. Conversely, the digital sheath can be distended with saline, and a stab incision can be made through the skin and into the sheath. A blunt tenotomy knife can be inserted into the sheath and turned at a 90° angle to the annular ligament to facilitate transection (Figure 9-8A). The skin alone is closed using 2-0 synthetic nonabsorbable suture material.

Postoperative Management

A sterile dressing is placed over the incision, and a pressure bandage is applied. Antibiotics are not used routinely. Hand-walking is begun in 3 days and is maintained on an increasing plane to preclude the formation of adhesions. The sutures are removed at 14 days, and bandaging is maintained for 3 weeks. With uneventful healing, the main criterion for returning the horse to work is the time necessary for healing of the tendinitis in the superficial flexor tendon.

Complications and Prognosis

Dehiscence of the incision and the development of synovial fistulation are rare complications of the open

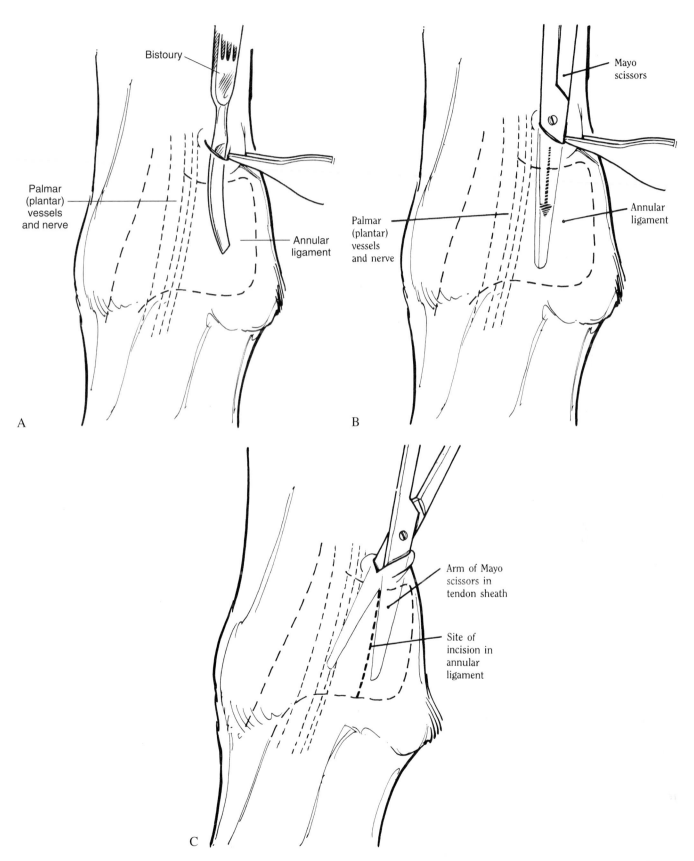

Fig. 9-8.   A, Drawing showing location of palmar/plantar annular ligament transection with blunt tenotomy knife. B and C, Closed technique with scissors.

technique. Such patients are placed on antibiotics, and careful wound management and bandaging are performed. The use of the closed technique virtually obviates this complication.

If extensive changes have not occurred in the superficial or deep flexor tendons, the prognosis is good, but the presence of adhesions or gross pathologic changes decreases the probability for a success. Intrasynovial injections of high molecular weight sodium hyaluronate may be helpful in reducing adhesion formation. Aggressive physical therapy is helpful in reducing pathologic adhesions.

References

1. Adams, O.R.: Constriction of the palmar (volar) or plantar annular ligament in the fetlock in the horse. VM/SAC, 70:327, 1974.
2. Gerring, E.L., and Webbon, P.M.: Fetlock annular ligament desmotomy: a report of 24 cases. Eq. Vet. J., 16:113, 1984.
3. McIlwraith, C.W.: Diseases of joints, tendons, ligaments, and related structures. In Adams' Lameness in Horses, 4th Ed. Edited by T.S. Stashak. Philadelphia, Lea & Febiger, 1987, p. 339.

Palmar Digital Neurectomy

Relevant Anatomy

The lateral and medial palmar digital nerves are continuations of the lateral and medial palmar nerves. The palmar digital nerve is identified just palmar to the digital artery approximately 0.5 cm below the skin surface and deep to the ligament of the ergot. At the fetlock, the medial and lateral palmar nerves each give rise to dorsal branches.

Indications

Palmar, or posterior, digital neurectomy is used to relieve chronic heel pain. The most common indication is navicular disease that is not responsive to corrective shoeing and medical therapy, but it is also used in horses with fracture of the navicular bone, selected lateral-wing fractures of the distal phalanx, and calcification of the collateral cartilages of the distal phalanx.[4,5] This surgical procedure is not benign, and it is not a panacea; a number of potential complications should be explained to the owner prior to surgery. In the hands of a good operator, however, palmar digital neurectomy is a form of long-term relief from the pain of those conditions just listed.

Anesthesia and Surgical Preparation

Neurectomy may be performed under local analgesia with the animal standing or under general anesthesia. If the surgery is performed with the animal standing, it is preferable to inject the local analgesic agent over the palmar nerves at the level of the abaxial surface of the sesamoid bones. The nerves can be palpated in this area, and the infiltration of this area avoids additional trauma and irritation at the surgery site. If neurectomy is performed in a field situation immediately following the use of a diagnostic block of the palmar digital nerve, however, this same block may be used for the surgical procedure. However, the author generally recommends waiting for 10 days after performing a palmar digital nerve block before performing a neurectomy in order to reduce inflammation in the region. General anesthesia is convenient to use, and for the more involved technique of epineural capping, it is certainly indicated.

The area of the surgical incision is clipped, shaved, and prepared for surgery in a routine manner. Plastic adhesive drapes are useful to exclude the hoof as a source of contamination.

Instrumentation

General surgery pack
Iris spatula (epineural capping technique)
CO_2 laser

Surgical Technique

In both the simple guillotine method and the technique of epineural capping, the approach to the nerve is the same. In the simple guillotine technique, an incision 2 cm long is made over the dorsal border of the flexor tendons (Figure 9-9A). If epineural capping is to be performed, the incision is generally 3 to 4 cm long and is continued through the subcutaneous tissue. It is important that the tissues be subjected to minimal trauma. An incision over the dorsal border of the flexor tendons generally brings the operator close to the palmar digital nerve. Variation exists, but the relationship of vein, artery, nerve, and the ligament of the ergot assists the surgeon's orientation (Figure 9-9B). At this stage of the dissection, the surgeon should look for accessory branches of the palmar digital nerve. These branches are commonly found near the ligament of the ergot. If an accessory branch is found, a 2-cm portion is removed using a scalpel.

Guillotine Technique

The nerve is identified and is dissected free of the subcutaneous tissue. The structure can be identified as nerve if it puckers after it is stretched, if scraping its surface reveals the longitudinal strands of the axons, or if a small incision into the nerve body reveals cut transverse sections of bundles of nerve fibers. The nerve is severed at the distal extremity of the incision. Then a hemostat is placed on the nerve, which is stretched while being cut with a scalpel or CO_2 laser at the proximal limit of the incision (Figure 9-9C). This sharp incision is made in such a fashion that the proximal portion of the nerve springs up into the

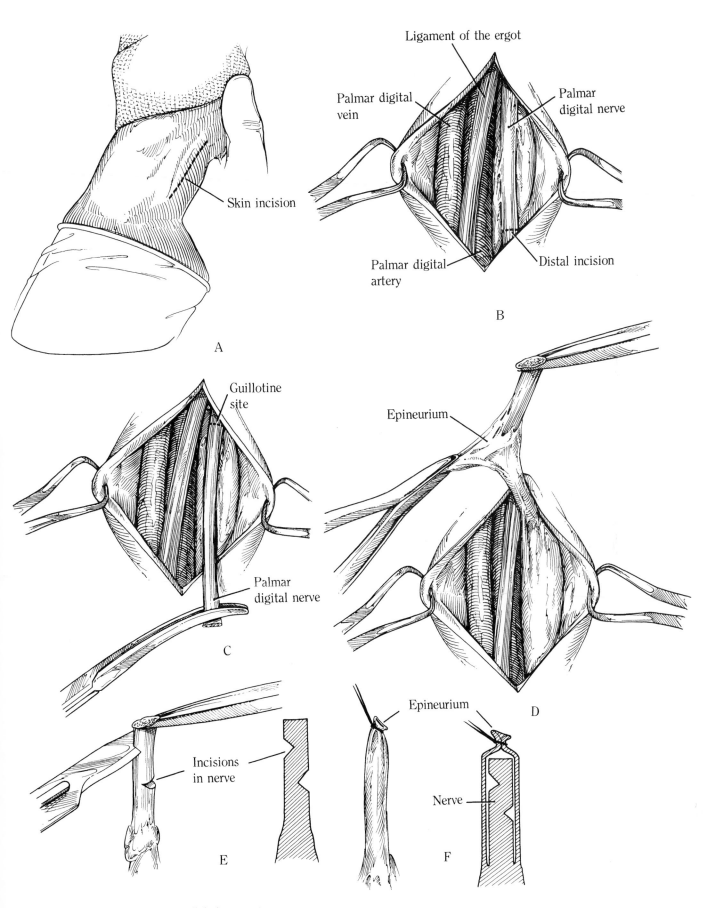

Labels in image:

A — Skin incision

B — Ligament of the ergot; Palmar digital vein; Palmar digital nerve; Palmar digital artery; Distal incision

C — Guillotine site; Palmar digital nerve

D — Epineurium

E — Incisions in nerve

F — Epineurium; Nerve

Fig. 9-9. A to F, Palmar digital neurectomy.

tissue planes and out of sight. It is believed that the severance of untraumatized nerve and its retraction up into the tissue planes helps reduce the problems of painful neuromas. The concept behind using the CO_2 laser is that it seals the nerve ending, even further reducing the possibility of a painful neuroma.

The skin is closed with interrupted sutures of nonabsorbable material.

Epineural Capping

The technique of epineural capping is an additional procedure that is intended to reduce the incidence of painful neuroma,[2] but controlled studies with an adequate number of cases that compare techniques are lacking. Several other procedures that have been described to reduce neuroma formation include electrocoagulation, freezing, capping of the nerve stump with exogenous materials, injection of neurotoxins into the proximal axon stump, and incomplete transection of the proximal nerve stump.[3] However, only the epineural capping technique will be described here. It is important to note also that an inexperienced surgeon's use of epineural capping with undue trauma may well have more complications than the faster guillotine method performed atraumatically.

Surgical dissection and exposure of the nerve are accomplished as in the guillotine technique, except the incision is longer. A section of nerve 3 to 4 cm long is exposed and is freed from all fascia and connective tissue. The nerve is severed as distally as possible and is raised from the incision. The end of the nerve is then held with forceps, and the epineurium is carefully reflected (Figure 9-9D). The epineurium is reflected for 2 to 3 cm, and two incisions are made through half the nerve on each side (Figure 9-9E). The nerve is then severed distal to these cuts, and the epineurium is pulled back over the severed end and is ligated with 2-0 or 3-0 absorbable monofilament (Figure 9-9F). The skin is sutured as described in the guillotine technique.

A modified technique of epineural capping involving cryosurgery has also been developed.[6] Following reflection of the epineurium, a sterile cryoprobe is placed on the proximal portion of the nerve, and the tissue is frozen to -30°C, using a double freeze-thaw cycle. The nerve tissue is then transected, leaving 5 mm of frozen tissue to retract proximally into the epineural sheath. This method is an attempt to minimize neuroma formation.

Postoperative Management

Antibiotics are not used routinely. A sterile dressing is placed on the incision, and a pressure bandage is maintained on the leg for at least 21 days. To minimize postoperative inflammation, 2 g of phenylbutazone are administered daily following surgery for 5–7 days. Sutures are removed 10 days after the operation, and the horse is rested for 60 days.

Complications and Prognosis

Complications of neurectomy include painful neuroma formation, rupture of the deep digital flexor tendon, reinnervation, persistence of sensation because of failure to identify and sever accessory branches of the nerve, and loss of the hoof wall.[5] Neuromas are the most common complication and can arise when the axons in the proximal stump regenerate axon sprouts, which cause pain and hypersensitivity.[1] One retrospective study of 50 horses that received palmar digital neurectomies, the majority by transection and electrocoagulation, reported that 17 horses (34%) had complications, with recurrence of heel pain being the most common.[3] Only 3 of the 17 horses developed neuromas, although this number may have been higher due to undetectable painful neuromas that could not be palpated. In 2 years, 63% of all the horses that received neurectomies were still sound. More recently, a study of 24 horses that received neurectomies using the guillotine technique reported no postoperative complications. The majority of these horses (22 of the 24) were treated for lameness associated with abnormal radiographic findings of the navicular bone and associated structures; the collateral cartilages of the hoof, or in one case, pedal osteitis. Twenty-two of these horses returned to full athletic performance, including jumping, dressage, camp drafting, cutting, and endurance competition.

References

1. Cummings, J.F., Fubini, S.L., and Todhunter, R.J.: Attempts to prevent equine post neurectomy neuroma formation through retrograde transport of two neurotoxins, doxorubicin and ricin. Eq. Vet. J., *20*:451–456, 1988.
2. Evans, L.H.: Procedures used to prevent painful neuromas. *In* Proceedings of the 16th Annual Convention of the American Association of Equine Practitioners in 1970:1971, p. 103.
3. Jackman, B.R., Baxter, G.M., Doran, R.E., Allen, D., and Parks, A.H.: Palmar digital neurectomy in horses: 57 cases (1984–1990). Vet. Surg., *22*:285–288, 1993.
4. Mathews, S., Dart, A.J., and Dowling, B.A.: Palmar digital neurectomy in 24 horses using the guillotine technique. Aust. Vet. J., *81*:402–405, 2003.
5. Stashak, T.S. (Ed.): Adams' Lameness in Horses, 4th Ed. Philadelphia, Lea & Febiger, 1987.
6. Tate, L.P., and Evans, L.H.: Cryoneurectomy in the horse. J. Am. Vet. Med. Assoc., *177*:423, 1980.

Amputation of the Splint (II and IV Metacarpal and Metatarsal) Bones

Relevant Anatomy

The second and fourth metacarpal bones, or splint bones, are attached to the abaxial surface of the medial and lateral proximal sesamoids by fibrous bands.[3] Thus, frequent hyperextension of the fetlock that results in stretching of these bands may be a predisposing factor for fracture of the splint bones.[3] Fracture generally occurs at the most distal third of the splint bone.

Indications

Amputation of the small metacarpal or metatarsal (splint) bones is indicated when these bones are fractured. Horses that race over fences and Standardbreds appear to be most susceptible to this type of injury.[3] Splint bone fractures in Standardbred horses are often associated with suspensory desmitis as well.

The lameness caused by fractures of the splint bone is generally mild and may be an incidental finding in a radiographic examination. If the skin has been broken, osteitis or osteomyelitis at the fracture site may result. These cases are accompanied by more soft-tissue swelling and lameness than are closed fractures of the splint bone.[5]

Occasionally, undisplaced fractures of the splint bone heal following suitable rest, but constant movement at the fracture site generally results in nonunion with an attending callus.[5] The decision to remove the fractured distal end of a splint bone is often controversial. Dealing with the suspensory desmitis alone may be sufficient, and removal of the distal splint bone may be unnecessary.[9]

If infection and accompanying osteomyelitis are present, surgical debridement-curettage or sequestrectomy may be necessary to resolve the infectious process, regardless of the health of the suspensory ligament.

Anesthesia and Surgical Preparation

General anesthesia is recommended for this operation. The horse is placed in either lateral recumbency with the affected splint bone uppermost or dorsal recumbency with the injured leg suspended. The latter method has advantages when more than one splint is to be operated on, and it achieves natural hemostasis during the surgical procedure.

A tourniquet facilitates the surgery if the animal is in lateral recumbency. The surgical site is shaved and prepared for aseptic surgery.

Instrumentation

General surgery pack
Curved osteotome
Chisel
Mallet
Periosteal elevator

Surgical Technique

A variable-length incision is made directly over the splint bone, extending from approximately 1 cm distal to the

distal extremity of the splint bone to approximately 2 cm proximal to the proposed site of amputation (Figure 9-10A). The subcutaneous fascia is incised along the same line as the incision, through the periosteum. The periosteum is elevated off the affected part of the splint bone. The distal end of the splint bone is undermined with the aid of sharp dissection and is freed from surrounding fascia (Figure 9-10B). Then the end is grasped firmly with forceps, such as Ochsner forceps. With further sharp dissection, the splint bone is separated from its attachments to the third metacarpal or metatarsal bone. Some of the attachments to the third metacarpal or metatarsal bone may need to be severed with the aid of a chisel (Figure 9-10C). A curved osteotome can also be used to sever these attachments.

The splint bone should be amputated above the fracture site or the area of infection with the aid of a chisel or osteotome. The splint bone should be removed (a large curette is sometimes necessary to remove diseased bone adequately).[1] The proximal end of the splint bone should be tapered to avoid leaving a sharp edge (Figure 9-10C), and any loose fragments removed or flushed out of the surgical site. The periosteum should be sharply excised to reduce the chances of periosteal proliferation. If infection is present, unhealthy scar tissue must be excised with sharp dissection, and all sequestra removed. Any bleeding should be controlled at this time. When infection is present, generally the region is vascular because of acute and chronic inflammation.

It the fracture is not infected, and is very proximal, the fracture should be repaired by use of a small bone plate with screws only placed into the splint bone (Figure 9-10D). If the fracture is infected and proximal, the distal end should be removed and the proximal segment anchored using a contoured bone plate fixed to the splint bone and cannon bone (Fig 9-10E).[1,8] Bone screws alone may be more likely to cycle and break. If this is not performed, the proximal fragment may become displaced because of the inadequate amount of interosseous ligament holding it in place.

When amputating a lateral splint bone in the pelvic limb, one must be careful to avoid incising the large, dorsal metatarsal artery III (great metatarsal artery), which lies above and between the third and fourth metatarsal bones in the interosseous space.[6] If large amounts of fibrous tissue are present because of an infectious process, the artery may be difficult to dissect from the soft tissue component. If the artery is inadvertently severed, it can be ligated without causing problems associated with loss of blood supply to the distal limb.

Following removal of the splint bone, the subcutaneous tissue should be closed with a synthetic absorbable suture. Considerable dead space may result from removal of the bone, especially if much bony and fibrous tissue reaction was present. Some patients with a severe infectious process or significant dead space may require a Penrose drain for a few days (see Chapter 7, "Principles

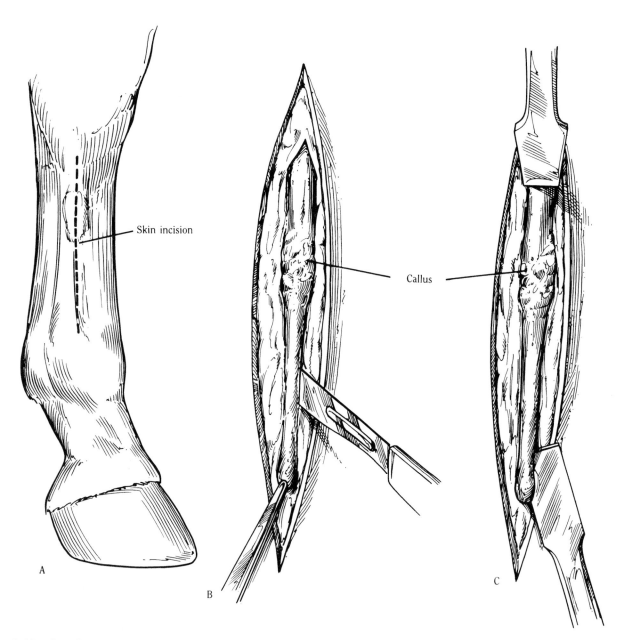

Fig. 9-10. A to C, Amputation of the small metacarpal and metatarsal (splint) bones. D and E, Bone plate fixation of proximal splint bone fractures.

of Wound Management and the Use of Drains"). However, a good pressure bandage is often adequate to reduce dead space. Only in rare instances is an ingress-egress system of flushing indicated. The skin should be closed with a monofilament nonabsorbable suture using a simple interrupted pattern. The incision is covered with an antimicrobial dressing and is placed under a pressure bandage.

Postoperative Management

Tetanus prophylaxis is administered. Antibiotics are used in cases of acute (active) osteitis or osteomyelitis, although

with appropriate preoperative wound management and thorough wound debridement, the infection usually resolves without the need for preoperative antimicrobial therapy.[1] The limb should be kept under a pressure bandage for 3 to 4 weeks. Despite careful hemostasis, the surgical procedure is generally accompanied by some hemorrhage. It is therefore wise to change the bandage in the first 1 to 2 days postoperatively. After that time, pressure bandages are changed every 5 to 7 days, or sooner if needed. If drains are in place, they should generally be removed the second or third postoperative day. Skin sutures should be removed 10 to 14 days after surgery.

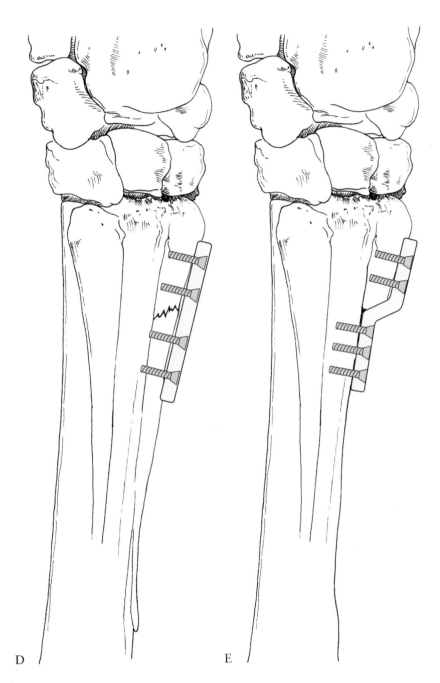

D   E

Fig. 9-10. *Continued.*

Complications and Prognosis

In Standardbred horses, suspensory desmitis rather than the fractured splint bone may limit the prognosis for return to athletic soundness.[2,9]

References

1. Allen, D., and White, N.A.: Management of fractures and exostosis of the metacarpals II and IV in 25 horses. Eq. Vet. J., *19:*326, 1987.
2. Bowman, K.F., Evans, L.H., and Herring, M.E.: Evaluation of surgical removal of fractured distal splint bones in the horse. Vet. Surg., *11:*116, 1982.
3. Dyson, S.J.: The metacarpal region. *In* Diagnosis and Management of Lameness in the Horse. Edited by M.W. Ross and S.J. Dyson, Philadelphia, W.B. Saunders, 2003, pp. 362–375.
4. Harrison, L.J., May, S.A., and Edwards, G.B.: Surgical treatment of open splint bone fractures in 26 horses. Vet. Rec., *128:*606–610, 1991.
5. Haynes, P.F.: Diseases of the metacarpophalangeal joint and the metacarpus. *In* Symposium on Equine Lameness. Vet. Clin. North Am. (Large Anim. Pract.), *2:*33, 1980.
6. Milne, D.W., and Turner, A.S.: An Atlas of Surgical Approaches to the Bones of the Horse. Philadelphia, W.B. Saunders, 1979.
7. Peterson, P.R., Pascoe, J.R., and Wheat, J.D.: Surgical management of proximal splint bone fractures in the horse. Vet. Surg., *16:*367–372, 1987.

8. Stashak, T.S. (Ed.): Adams' Lameness in Horses, 4th Ed. Philadelphia, Lea & Febiger, 1987.

9. Verschooten, F., Gasthuys, F., and De Moor, A.: Distal splint bone fractures in the horse: an experimental and clinical study. Equine Vet. J., *16*:532, 1984.

Arthrotomy of the Midcarpal Joint

Relevant Anatomy

There are three main articulations within the carpal joint: the radiocarpal, midcarpal, and carpometacarpal articulations. The radiocarpal articulation is fairly mobile and provides 90 to 100° of flexion, and the midcarpal joint allows approximately 45° of flexion.[2] The carpometacarpal and intercarpal articulations have no significant movement. All articulations share a common fibrous capsule, but the synovial layer is distinct for each articulation, with the exception of the metacarpal and midcarpal joint cavities, which communicate with each other.[2]

Indications

Arthrotomy of the intercarpal joint is indicated for surgical excision of osteochondral fragments and osteophytes. The use of arthrotomy to remove osteochondral fragments from the carpus has generally been replaced by the technique of arthroscopic surgery, and various advantages of arthroscopy have been identified.[4] Arthroscopy requires specialized equipment and considerable learning and experience; however, we believe that arthrotomy is still a valid technique—but only when the foregoing resources are unavailable.

The technique described here details one of five possible approaches to the various bones of the carpal joint.[5] This approach is most common because of the higher incidence of injuries to the distal radial and proximal carpal bones in fast-gaited horses, particularly racehorses.[7] During high-speed exercise, these bones are especially prone to injury due to the repetitive loading of one bone against the other, which is attributed to in part by the negligible amount of weight-bearing forces the intraarticular ligaments support.[1,10] This arthrotomy approach is also used for the repair of slab fractures of the third carpal bone, which is presented in *Equine Surgery: Advanced Techniques.*[3]

The exact location of the lesion should be ascertained with preoperative radiographs of the affected limb. As with all elective surgical procedures on horses' limbs, the presence of any other problems should be ascertained prior to surgery.

Anesthesia and Surgical Preparation

The surgery is performed under general anesthesia with the horse placed in lateral recumbency and the affected limb down. Some surgeons prefer to operate with the horse in dorsal recumbency and the limb elevated to take advantage of natural hemostasis. Prior to anesthetic induction, the patient's leg is clipped from the coronary band to midradius all the way around the leg. Following anesthetic induction, the area of surgical excision is shaved, and routine surgical preparation is performed. By preparing the limb before surgery, the anesthetic time can be reduced.

Instrumentation

General surgery pack
Curettes
Retractors
Periosteal elevators
Bulb syringe

Surgical Technique

After draping (the use of sterile plastic adherent drapes is recommended for this procedure), the following structures should be identified: the tendinous insertion of the extensor carpi radialis muscle, the tendon of the extensor carpi obliquus muscle, the antebrachial joint, and the midcarpal joint. Identification of these structures is facilitated by flexing and extending the carpal joint. A straight 3-cm skin incision extending from the middle of the face of the radial carpal bone to the middle of the face of the third carpal bone and 5 to 8 mm medial to the extensor carpi radialis tendon is made (Figure 9-11A).

The incision is continued through the subcutaneous fascia, carpal extensor retinaculum, and joint capsule. Synovial fluid will flow from the incision when the joint is entered (Figure 9-11B). Any blood vessels or their visible lumens should be cauterized at this point. Using suitable retractors, the surgeon carefully retracts the edges of the incision in the carpal extensor retinaculum and joint capsule; this will expose the proximal surface of the third carpal bone and the distal surface of the radial carpal bone.

If the osteochondral chip fragments are not visible immediately, a pair of curved forceps can be used to gently probe the articular margins of the third carpal and radial carpal bones. Any movement or instability along these edges should be investigated further because they are usually the location of the offending chip fractures.

Chip fractures may be difficult to identify because they may be embedded in fibrous tissue. Rarely are they completely loose and detached. To remove the fractures from their attachments, the chip can be grasped with forceps and dissected free with a no. 15 scalpel blade. Another method is to take a small, sharp, periosteal elevator and pry the fragment loose (Figure 9-11C). The resultant defect is then curetted down to the subchondral bone (Figure 9-11D). This curettage has been recommended to ensure filling the defect with fibrocartilage. Curettage has been reported to decrease the likelihood of exostosis

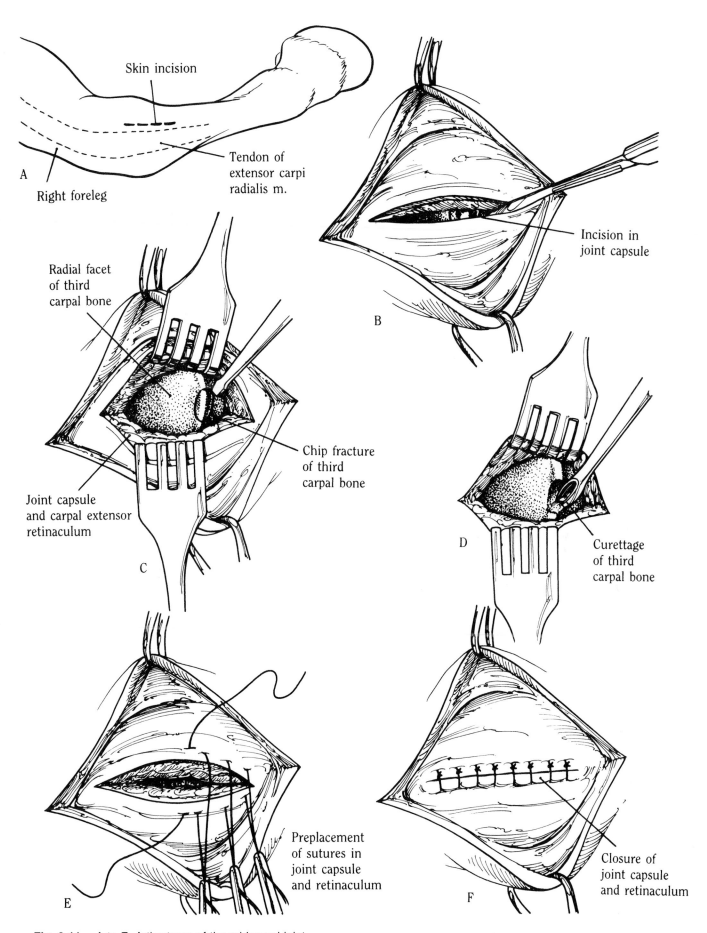

A — Right foreleg — Skin incision — Tendon of extensor carpi radialis m.

B — Incision in joint capsule

C — Radial facet of third carpal bone — Chip fracture of third carpal bone — Joint capsule and carpal extensor retinaculum

D — Curettage of third carpal bone

E — Preplacement of sutures in joint capsule and retinaculum

F — Closure of joint capsule and retinaculum

Fig. 9-11. A to F, Arthrotomy of the midcarpal joint.

141

formation postoperatively. Intraoperative radiographs should be taken to confirm complete removal. Copious lavage should be performed to remove only small fragments of bone.

Closure is performed in three layers. The joint capsule and retinaculum are closed with a layer of simple continuous or interrupted sutures of synthetic absorbable material. The sutures should not penetrate the synovial membrane. Preplacement of the sutures in the joint capsule and extensor retinaculum ensures an accurate apposition and a tight seal (Figure 9-11E and F), but is not required if a continuous pattern is used.

Following joint capsule closure, 4 to 5 ml of Ringer's solution with 1 million units of potassium penicillin are flushed into the joint using a 20-gauge needle. The subcutaneous fascia is closed with a simple continuous pattern using synthetic absorbable sutures. The skin is closed with a simple interrupted, cruciate, or near-far-far-near pattern using synthetic monofilament sutures, and the limb is wrapped with a tight pressure bandage. Control of minute capillary ooze will be possible if the tourniquet is released when the pressure wrap has been applied.

Postoperative Management

The limb is wrapped in a firm pressure bandage for 3 weeks, during which time the bandage is changed several times. Skin sutures are removed at 10 to 12 days. Care must be taken when bandaging the carpal joint to prevent formation of a pressure sore on the accessory carpal bone. During convalescence, the horse is kept in a box stall. The convalescence and aftercare depend on the individual case and the severity of the injury to the carpal bone. Generally, it is 3 to 6 months before the horse should return to its athletic activities.

Complications and Prognosis

In a retrospective study of Thoroughbred racehorses, horses treated surgically for carpal injury (81% of which involved the midcarpal joint) had a significantly better prognosis for returning to racing and performed better than those horses that did not receive surgical treatment.[7] Of the horses that received surgery, 76% raced subsequently and 48% won at least one race. Studies also show that early diagnosis and surgical treatment of midcarpal joint injuries greatly increases the horse's chance of returning to racing by preventing the progression of the defect to a third carpal slab fracture, which exacerbates articular damage even further.[6,10]

References

1. Bramlage, L.R., Schneider, R.K., and Gabel, A.A.: A clinical prospective on lameness originates in the carpus. Eq. Vet. J., 6Suppl:12–18, 1988.
2. Budras, K.D., Sack, W.O., and Rock, S.: Anatomy of the Horse, 3rd Ed. Hannover, Germany, Schlutersche, 2001, pp. 12–13.
3. McIlwraith, C.W., and Robertson, J.: McIlwraith's and Turner's Equine Surgery: Advanced Techniques, 2nd Ed. Philadelphia, Lippincott Williams & Wilkins, 1998.
4. McIlwraith, C.W., Yovich, J.V., and Martin, G.S.: Arthroscopic surgery for the treatment of osteochondral chip fractures in the equine carpus. J. Am. Vet. Med. Assoc., 191:531, 1987.
5. Milne, D.W., and Turner, A.S.: An Atlas of Surgical Approaches to the Bones of the Horse. Philadelphia, W.B. Saunders, 1979.
6. Pool, R.R.: Joint disease in the athletic horse: a review of pathological findings and pathogenesis. In Proceedings of the 41st Annual AAEP Convention. 1995, pp. 20–34.
7. Raidal, S.L., and Wright, J.D.: A retrospective evaluation of the surgical management of equine carpal therapy. Aust. Vet. J., 74:198–202, 1996.
8. Raker, C.W., Baker, R.H., and Wheat, J.D.: Pathophysiology of equine degenerative joint disease and lameness. In Proceedings of the 12th Annual Convention of the American Association of Equine Practitioners in 1965:1966, p. 229.
9. Riddle, W.E.: Healing of articular cartilage in the horse. J. Am. Vet. Med. Assoc., 157:1471, 1970.
10. Scheider, R.K.: Diagnostic arthroscopy in occult carpal lesions. In Current Techniques in Equine Surgery and Lameness, 2nd Ed. Edited by N.A. White and J.N. Moore. Philadelphia, W.B. Saunders, 1998

Arthrotomy of the Fetlock Joint and Removal of an Apical Sesamoid Chip Fracture

Relevant Anatomy

The suspensory apparatus in the horse—which includes the proximal sesamoid bones, distal sesamoidean ligaments, and the suspensory ligament—has two important functions: to prevent hyperextension of the fetlock joint and to store and redistribute some of the weight-bearing force from the joint to the limb. Injury to the suspensory apparatus is common in horses, particularly in performance breeds such as Thoroughbreds and Standardbreds. Often, it manifests as a fracture in the proximal sesamoid bones, of which apical fractures are usually the most common.[1,5]

Indications

Arthrotomy and removal of the fractured fragment comprise the treatment of choice for an apical chip fracture of the proximal sesamoid bone.[2] This can be performed via arthroscopy or arthrotomy. If left unoperated, the result will be either a fibrous union or displacement of the fragment proximad, which, in turn, can lead to exostosis formation and joint-surface irregularity.[6]

Anesthesia and Surgical Preparation

This surgical procedure is performed with the horse under general anesthesia and, depending on the surgeon's preference, the horse may be placed in lateral or dorsal recumbency. With dorsal recumbency and the leg suspended, natural hemostasis is achieved. If surgery is performed in lateral recumbency, Esmarch's bandage and a tourniquet are generally used. Prior to anesthetic induction, the patient's leg is clipped from proximal cannon to coronary band all the way around the leg. Following anesthetic induction, the area of the surgical incision is shaved, and routine surgical preparation is performed. Draping may include the use of a plastic adhesive drape.

Instrumentation

General surgery pack
Weitlaner retractor
Bone curette
Rongeurs
Periosteal elevator

Surgical Technique

The limb is maintained in an extended position while surgical entry into the joint is made. With the leg in this position, it is easier to identify the branch of the suspensory ligament. An incision approximately 5 cm long is made over the palmar or plantar recess (volar pouch) of the metacarpo- (metatarso-) phalangeal joint immediately dorsal and parallel to the branch of the suspensory ligament and palmar or plantar to the distal aspect of the metacarpus or metatarsus (Figure 9-12A). The incision extends from approximately 1 cm below the distal extremity of the splint bone to the proximal border of the collateral sesamoidean ligament. The incision is continued through the thin subcutaneous areolar connective tissue in the same line, and Weitlaner retractors are placed to facilitate exposure of the joint capsule. It may be easier to identify the joint capsule if the joint has been distended with saline prior to making the incision. A 3-cm incision is made through the joint capsule (fibrous joint capsule plus synovial membrane) to enter the joint (Figure 9-12B). Care is taken to avoid the collateral sesamoidean ligament distally and the vascular plexus on the palmar (plantar) aspect of the distal metacarpus or metatarsus proximally. Following entry into the joint, the fetlock is flexed, and the edges of the joint capsule are retracted to expose the palmar articular surface of the third metacarpus and the articular surface of the proximal sesamoid bone.[3]

The apical fragment to be removed is identified, and it is incised from the suspensory ligament using a no. 15 scalpel blade or periosteal elevator (Figure 9-12C).

Trauma to the suspensory ligament is minimized by careful, sharp dissection. As the soft tissue attachments are severed, the chip is removed using Ochsner forceps or small rongeurs (Figure 9-12D). The fracture site is curetted smooth, and the joint is vigorously flushed with sterile Ringer's solution. Intraoperative radiographs should be taken to confirm complete removal. The hypertrophic synovial membrane is also removed.

The fibrous joint capsule is closed with a layer of simple interrupted or continuous sutures of synthetic absorbable suture material. The sutures in the fibrous joint capsule should not penetrate the synovial membrane. Preplacement of the sutures in the joint capsule facilitates accurate apposition and a tight seal, but is not necessary when using a simple continuous pattern. Following closure of the joint capsule, 8 to 10 ml of Ringer's solution (to which 1 million U of potassium penicillin may be added) are flushed into the joint using a 20-gauge needle (Figure 9-12E). The subcutaneous fascia is closed with a simple continuous pattern using synthetic absorbable material, and the skin is closed with simple interrupted or near-far-far-near sutures of monofilament nonabsorbable material. The tourniquet is removed, a sterile dressing is placed over the incision, and a firm bandage is placed on the leg.

Postoperative Management

The use of antibiotics is optional. The skin sutures are removed in 10 to 12 days, and the bandage is maintained on the leg for another 10 days. Convalescent time after removal of an apical sesamoid chip should be at least 4 months, but it varies, depending on the degree of concurrent injury in the suspensory ligament and other soft tissues.

Complications and Prognosis

The prognosis depends largely on the size of the fracture fragment and the presence and degree of suspensory desmitis.[4] Sport horses with large apical fragments accompanied by suspensory branch injury may require 6 to 12 months of recovery and have a poor prognosis. Nonsport horses without preexisting injury generally have a very favorable prognosis. Surgical removal carries the best prognosis for horses with proven speed when they are operated on within 30 days of injury and have no evidence of suspensory desmitis or osteoarthritis; the prognosis for return to racing was 65% for those horses that had raced previous to injury.[6] In Standardbreds, conservative therapy dramatically reduced the racing performance when preinjury values were compared to postinjury values.[6]

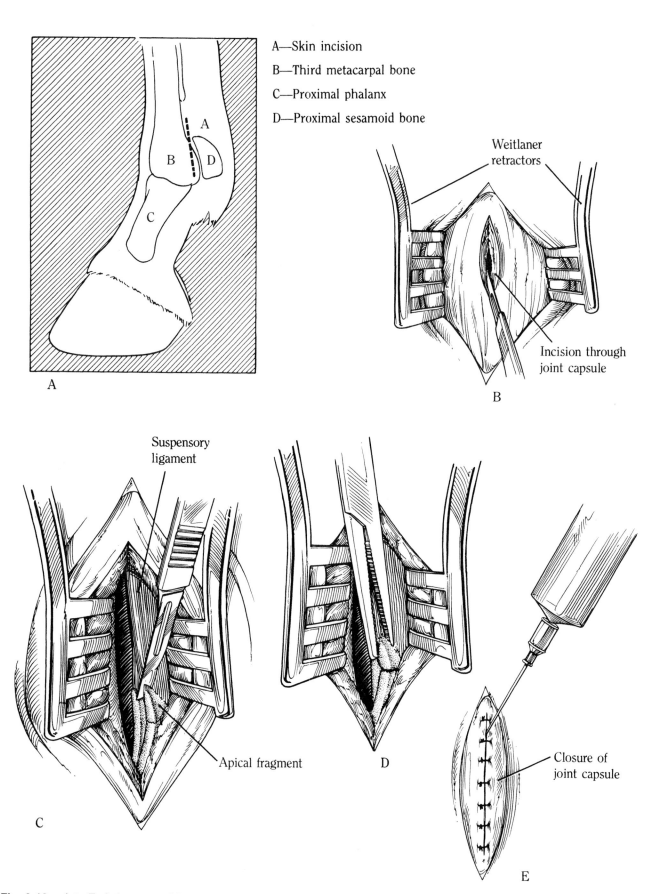

A—Skin incision

B—Third metacarpal bone

C—Proximal phalanx

D—Proximal sesamoid bone

Weitlaner
retractors

Incision through
joint capsule

Suspensory
ligament

Apical fragment

Closure of
joint capsule

Fig. 9-12. A to E, Arthrotomy of fetlock joint for removal of apical sesamoid fracture.

References

1. Bukowiecki, C.F., Bramlage, L.R., and Gabel, A.A.: In vitro strength of the suspensory apparatus in training and resting horses. Vet. Surg., *16:*126–130, 1987.

2. Churchill, E.A.: Surgical removal of fractured fragments of the proximal sesamoid bone. J. Am. Vet. Med. Assoc., *128:*581, 1956.

3. Milne, D.W., and Turner, A.S.: An Atlas of Surgical Approaches to the Bones of the Horse. Philadelphia, W.B. Saunders, 1979.

4. Richardson, D.W.: The metacarpophalangeal joint. *In* Diagnosis and Management of Lameness in the Horse. Edited by M.W. Ross and S.J. Dyson. Philadelphia, W.B. Saunders Co., 2003, pp. 348–362.

5. Ruggles, A.J., and Gabel, A.A.: Injuries of the proximal sesamoid bones. *In* Current Techniques in Equine Surgery and Lameness. Edited by N.A. White and J.N. Moore. Philadelphia, W.B. Saunders Co., 1998, pp. 403–408.

6. Spurlock, G.H., and Gabel, A.A.: Apical fractures of the proximal sesamoid bones in 109 Standardbred horses. J. Am. Vet. Med. Assoc., *183:*76, 1983.

Chapter 10

EQUINE UROGENITAL SURGERY

Objectives

1. Describe a technique for routine castration and discuss potential serious complications.
2. Discuss several approaches for performing a cryptorchidectomy.
3. Describe common urogenital surgical techniques in the mare, including Caslick's operation for pneumovagina, urethroplasty, cesarean section, and repair of third-degree perineal lacerations.
4. Describe techniques for performing circumcision and penile amputation in the male.

Castration

Relevant Anatomy

In the male horse, the scrotum is located high between the hindlimbs on the ventral portion of the caudal abdomen. The left testicle in the horse is commonly larger and more caudad than the right.[6] Externally, the median or scrotal raphe divides the scrotum into roughly equal left and right halves.

The scrotum contains the testicles, the distal components of the spermatic cord, the cremaster muscles, and the epididymis. There are four primary layers of the scrotum: the outermost skin and associated connective tissue, the smooth muscle fibers of the tunica dartos, the loose connective tissue of the scrotal fascia, and the innermost parietal vaginal tunic.[6] The testes are comprised of parenchyma encapsulated by a fibrous layer, the tunica albuginea. Most of the parenchyma consists of seminiferous tubules.[6] The remaining interstitial tissues are comprised of Leydig cells, blood vessels, lymphatic vessels, and immune cells.[6] The head of the epididymis is attached to the dorsolateral surface of the testicle and terminates in a coiled tail at the posterior end. The ductus deferens continues from the epididymis with the spermatic cord, which runs from the testicles to the vaginal rings. The spermatic cords contain the ductus deferens, testicular artery, pampiniform plexus, lymph vessels, nerves, and smooth muscle, which are all enclosed by the parietal layer of the vaginal tunic.

Indications

Castration is usually performed to facilitate the management of a particular animal when it is in the company of females or other males. Castration can be performed at any time; however, the colt is often left intact for 12 to 18 months to allow for development of certain desirable physical characteristics. Other animals may be castrated at a later age when it is no longer desirable to maintain them as stallions. Prior to castration, it should be ascertained that the animal is healthy and that both testes are descended. If a horse is anesthetized and only one testis is descended, the surgery should be aborted unless the surgeon is comfortable with cryptorchid castration.

Many methods of castration are available. This section describes a two-phase emasculation preceded by separate dissection of the common tunic because the authors believe it is the optimal technique for the prevention of untoward sequelae. In the technique of "closed" castration, the common vaginal tunic is dissected, but not opened, and emasculation of the entire cord within the tunic is performed as a single procedure. Because several structures are enclosed within the jaws of the emasculator, there is a greater chance that a vessel will be emasculated inadequately. This technique should be restricted to patients with small testes. In a modified-closed technique, the vaginal tunic is sharply incised over the spermatic cord, the vascular structures exteriorized and emasculated, followed by emasculation of the entire cord.

In the "open" technique, the common tunic is opened with the initial skin incision, and prior dissection of the tunic from the subcutaneous tissue is not performed. This method is commonly used without any problems, but the chances of inadequate tunic removal with consequent hydrocele are increased.

A technique of primary closure in multiple layers with ablation of the scrotum has been described.[1] In this technique, the ventral scrotum is ablated. The testicles are removed by emasculation combined with transfixation ligatures. Additional skin may have to be removed, so the scrotum is completely ablated when the skin edges are apposed. Closure of the subcutaneous and subcuticular tissues is performed in three or four layers. This method is certainly more time consuming than other procedures, but postoperative scrotal swelling is usually eliminated.[1]

Anesthesia and Surgical Preparation

Castration may be performed on the standing animal under local analgesia or with the animal in recumbency under general anesthesia. The technique depends on the temperament of the animal, the experience of the surgeon, and in some situations, the tradition and environment in which the horse is castrated.

For castration of the standing animal, a tranquilizer or sedative may be administered to the horse, and local infiltration analgesia is performed. A combination of detomidine hydrochloride (20 to 40 µg/kg) or xylazine hydrochloride (0.3 to 0.5 mg/kg) and butorphanol tartate (0.01 to 0.05 mg/kg) is commonly used and provides reliable sedation.[8,9] Following surgical preparation of the area, the skin is infiltrated on a line 1 cm from the median raphe with 10 ml of local analgesic solution; this infiltration is continued into the subcutaneous tissue. Local analgesia can be injected directly into the testis. It is also important to infiltrate the spermatic cord in the region of emasculation with a long 18- to 20-gauge needle.

For castration of the recumbent animal, several anesthetic regimens are available and suitable. Anesthesia may be induced by intravenous administration of a xylazine (1.0 mg/kg) and ketamine hydrochloride (2.2 mg/kg) mixture.[12] If the procedure is prolonged, a second dose may be given intravenously according to the desired time of anesthesia. Alternatively, guaifenesin in combination with thiamylal sodium may be used, or if rapid induction is desired, thiamylal sodium or thiopental sodium alone is suitable.

For a right-handed operator, the horse is cast with the left side down. The upper hindleg is tied craniad, and the surgical site is prepared; clipping or shaving is not necessary. It can be easier to position the horse in dorsal recumbency using bales to hold the horse in place.

Instrumentation

General surgery pack
Emasculators
LDS stapler (US Surgical)

Surgical Technique

This castration technique is illustrated here in the recumbent animal. Prior to making the first incision it is helpful to inject local anesthetic into the testis and spermatic cord. This will reduce the movements during the procedure and lengthen the effective time of the general anesthetics. Castration is performed through separate incisions for each testis, with incisions located approximately 1 cm from the median raphe (Figure 10-1A). The lower testis is grasped between thumb and forefingers, and the first skin incision is made for the length of the testis (Figure 10-1B). The incision is continued through the tunica dartos and scrotal fascia, leaving the common tunic (tunica vaginalis parietalis) intact. At the same time, pressure exerted by the thumb and forefingers causes the testis, which is still contained within the common tunic, to be extruded (Figure 10-1C). The testis is then grasped in the left hand (for a right-handed operator), and the subcutaneous tissue is stripped from the common vaginal tunic as far proximally as possible (Figure 10-1D). The use of a gauze sponge can facilitate the stripping of the subcutaneous tissue from the common tunic. At this point, a closed, modified closed or an open technique can be performed. For the open technique, the surgeon incises the common tunic over the cranial pole of the testis (Figure 10-1E) and, hooking a finger within the tunic to maintain tension, continues the incision proximad (Figure 10-1F).

The testis is now released from within the common tunic. The mesorchium is penetrated digitally to separate the vascular spermatic cord from the ductus deferens, common tunic, and external cremaster muscle (Figure 10-1G). The latter structures are severed, with attention to removing as much of the common tunic as possible (Figure 10-1G). The severance of this musculofibrous portion of the spermatic cord may be performed conveniently with emasculators, and the crush need only be applied for a short period of time. The testis is then grasped, and the spermatic vessels are emasculated (Figure 10-1H).

Care must always be taken to apply the emasculator correctly without incorporating skin between its jaws and to prevent stretch on the spermatic cord at the time of emasculation. An optional preliminary to emasculation is to place forceps proximally on the cord as a safeguard against loss if a failure occurs during emasculation. The emasculator remains in position for 1 to 2 minutes, depending on the size of the cord, and is then released.

Another technique that can minimize the amount of hemorrhage following castration is to use an LDS stapling

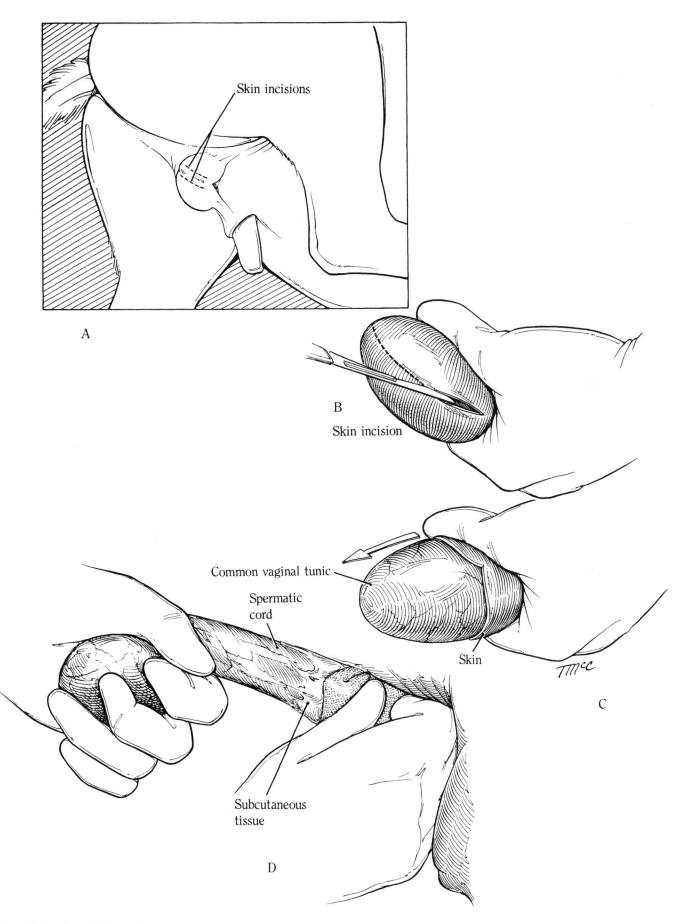

Skin incisions

A

Skin incision

B

Common vaginal tunic

Spermatic cord

Skin

C

Subcutaneous tissue

D

Fig. 10-1. A to L, Castration.

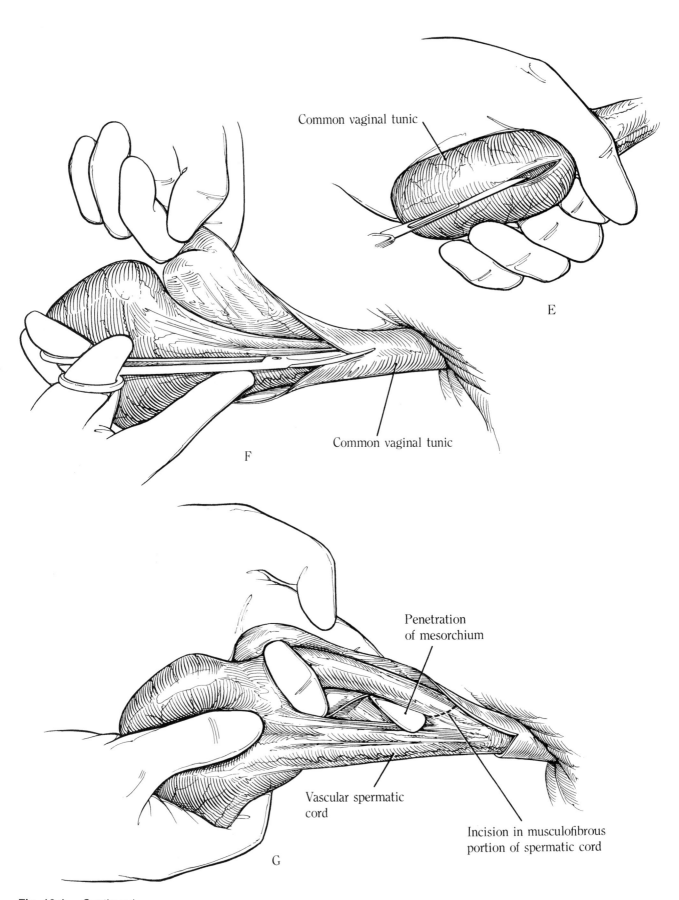

Common vaginal tunic

E

Common vaginal tunic

F

Penetration
of mesorchium

Vascular spermatic
cord

Incision in musculofibrous
portion of spermatic cord

G

Fig. 10-1. *Continued.*

Emasculation of spermatic cord

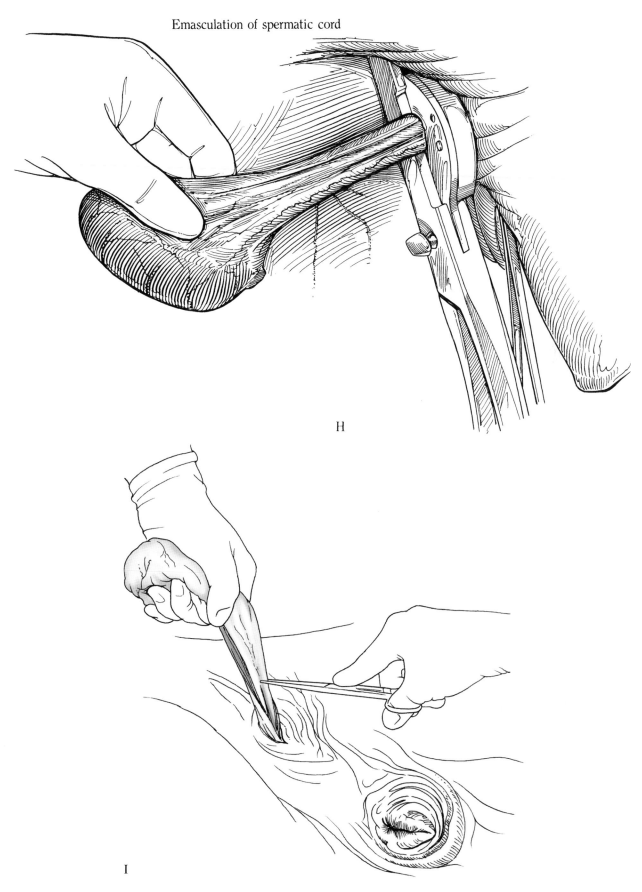

H

I

Fig. 10-1. *Continued.*

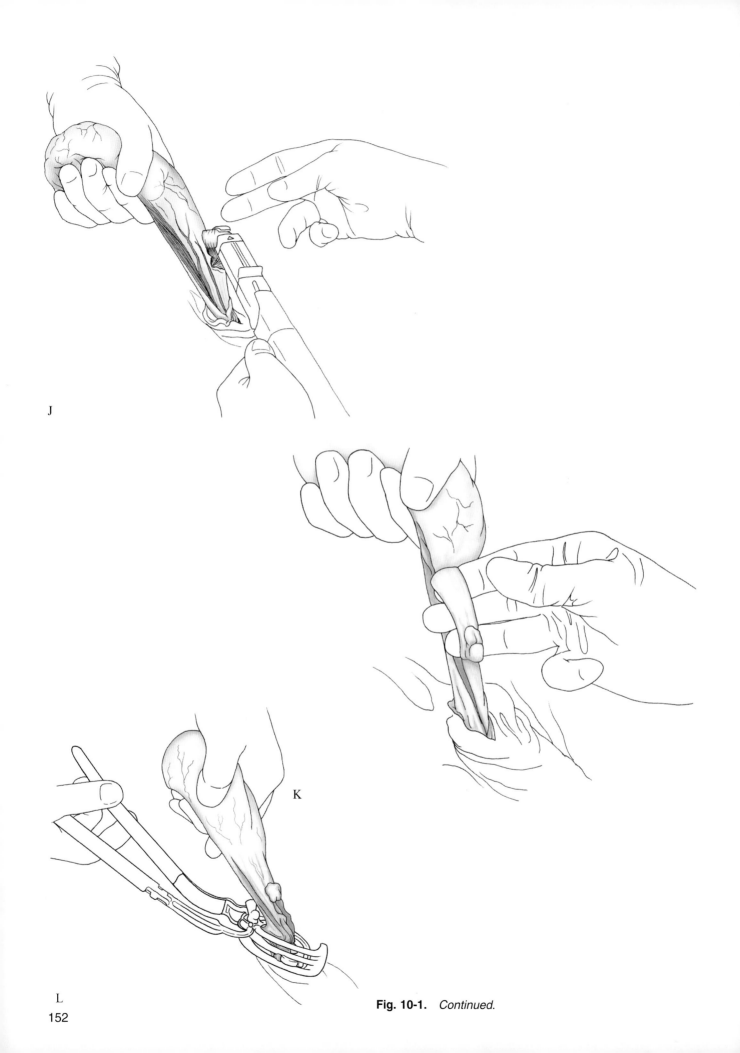

J

K

L

Fig. 10-1. *Continued.*

device to ligate the spermatic vasculature. The testis is approached as previously described, up to the point just following stripping of the subcutaneous fascia (Figure 10-2A to D). At this point a small incision is made into the vaginal tunic over the spermatic cord (Figure 10-1I). The vascular portion of the spermatic cord is exteriorized. An LDS stapling device (US Surgical/Tyco Healthcare) with the dividing blade removed is used to place two ligating staples around the vasculature (Figure 10-1J). The vasculature is transected distal to the staples (Figure 10-1K) and the emasculator placed over the tunic and the testis removed (Figure 10-1L).

The skin incisions are enlarged by pulling them apart with the fingers until a 10-cm opening is obtained. The median raphe may also be removed to further facilitate drainage. However, this may cause more hemorrhage. Any redundant adipose tissue or fascia is also removed.

Postoperative Management

Tetanus immunization is administered, and antibiotics usually are not indicated. The horse should be kept under close observation for several hours after castration to make sure that it is not hemorrhaging, and under general observation for the first 24 hours for other complications and periodically during the first week following surgery. During the first 24 hours the horse should be confined with limited exercise. Uneventful healing is the usual result with good drainage and satisfactory exercise. The animal should be forcibly exercised twice daily from the day following surgery until healing is complete. The new gelding should be separated from mares for a week at least to ensure that no pregnancies will occur.[11] It has been suggested that a gelding can impregnate a mare up to 60 days after castration.

Complications and Prognosis

Complications of equine castration are uncommon, but they can be life threatening to the horse and of great concern to the surgeon. To minimize postoperative complications, good communication with the client is required.

A number of possible complications may arise following castration: (1) severe hemorrhage is usually associated with inadequate emasculation of the testicular artery of the spermatic cord, but considerable hemorrhage can occur from one of the branches of the external pudendal vein in the scrotal wall or septum, if accidentally ruptured[15] or in the transected external cremaster muscle; (2) excessive swelling of the surgical site can arise because of inadequate drainage or inadequate exercise, or a hydrocele may form because of collection of fluid in a common tunic that has been inadequately resected; (3) evisceration may occur through an inguinal hernia; (4) acute wound infection and septicemia may occur; scirrhous cord formation is due to chronic infection and generally can be related to poor technique and inadequate exercise or

drainage; and (5) persistent masculine behavior can occur following removal of two normal testes; and/or (6) penile paralysis.

Hemorrhage

Minor hemorrhage may occur for several hours, but significant hemorrhage beyond approximately 12 hours may require surgical intervention. If the source of hemorrhage is the testicular artery, ligation using a synthetic absorbable suture material may be required. This procedure may warrant general anesthesia if the horse is difficult to manage. Curved forceps, such as Mixter curved hemostatic forceps, are helpful. Standing laparoscopy can be used to look for intraabdominal bleeding.

Edema

Edema of the scrotum and prepuce, a more common complication of castration, usually begins on the third or fourth postoperative day and is often associated with inadequate exercise. Simply turning the gelding out to pasture without forced exercise is often inadequate because of postoperative pain. Horses with excessive edema of the scrotum and prepuce should be checked for a temperature rise because it may indicate impending infection. To help reestablish drainage, a sterile surgical glove is donned, and the scrotal incision is opened cautiously. Parenteral antibiotics, such as procaine penicillin G, may be indicated, as well as a conscientious program of forced exercise. Phenylbutazone may be indicated to reduce soreness and to encourage pain-free movement. Long-standing chronic infections with abscess formation in the inguinal canal may need surgical exploration and abscess drainage.

Visceral Prolapse

Visceral prolapse through the inguinal canal and open scrotum is the most serious potential complication of castration. Eventration of the intestine or omentum may occur within the first few hours after castration before swelling has closed the inguinal canal, but it has been observed up to 6 days after surgery.[2] The incidence of herniation following routine castration is fairly low; one study reported evisceration of the small intestine in 4.8% of the 568 colts that were castrated.[12] Furthermore, there was no association found between open and closed techniques of castration and the incidence of herniation or evisceration in these horses.[12] Some authors believe a half-closed castration technique, which involves opening of the vaginal cavity and ligation of both the parietal vaginal tunic and spermatic cord, minimizes the risk of herniation and evisceration.[14] It has been suggested that breeds such as draft horses, Standardbred horses, warm-bloods, and some mustangs have a higher incidence of eventration and should have a ligature placed around the spermatic cord when being castrated.

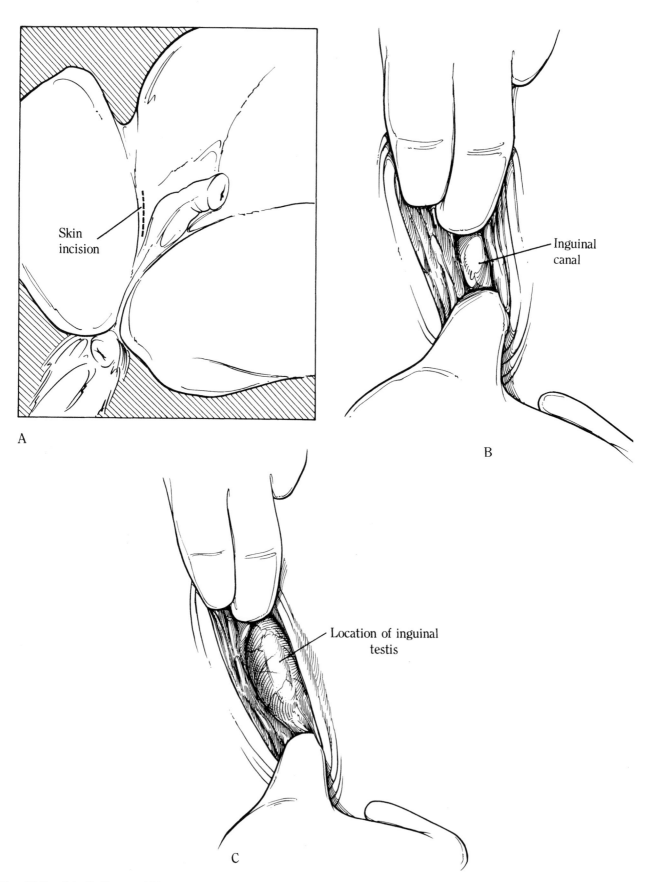

Fig. 10-2. A to S, Cryptorchidectomy.

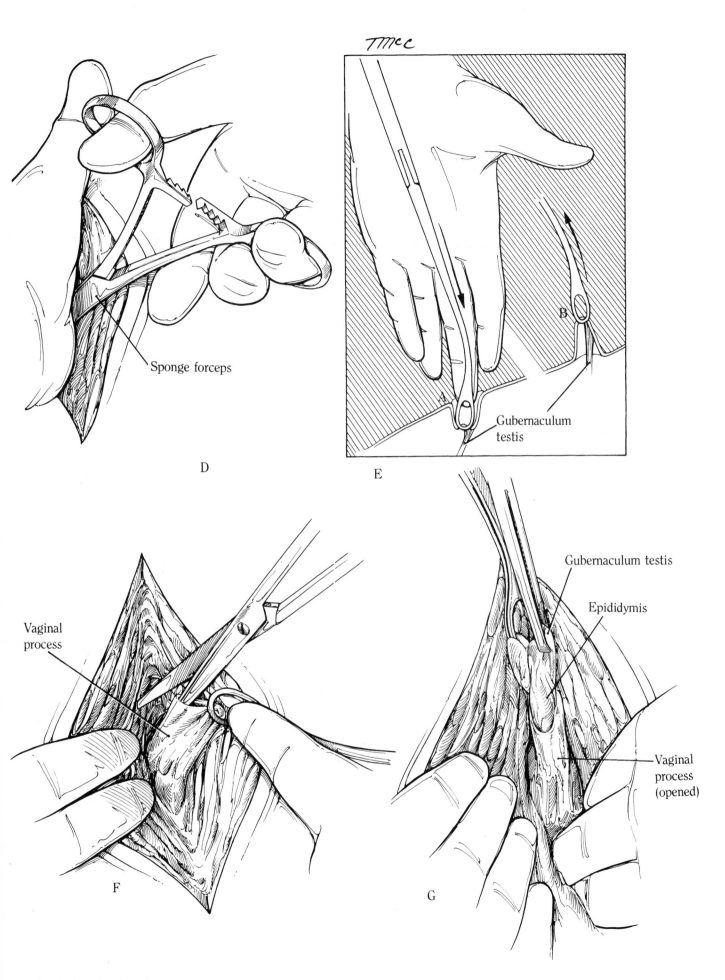

TMcc

Sponge forceps

D

Gubernaculum
testis

E

Vaginal
process

F

Gubernaculum testis

Epididymis

Vaginal
process
(opened)

G

Fig. 10-2. *Continued.*

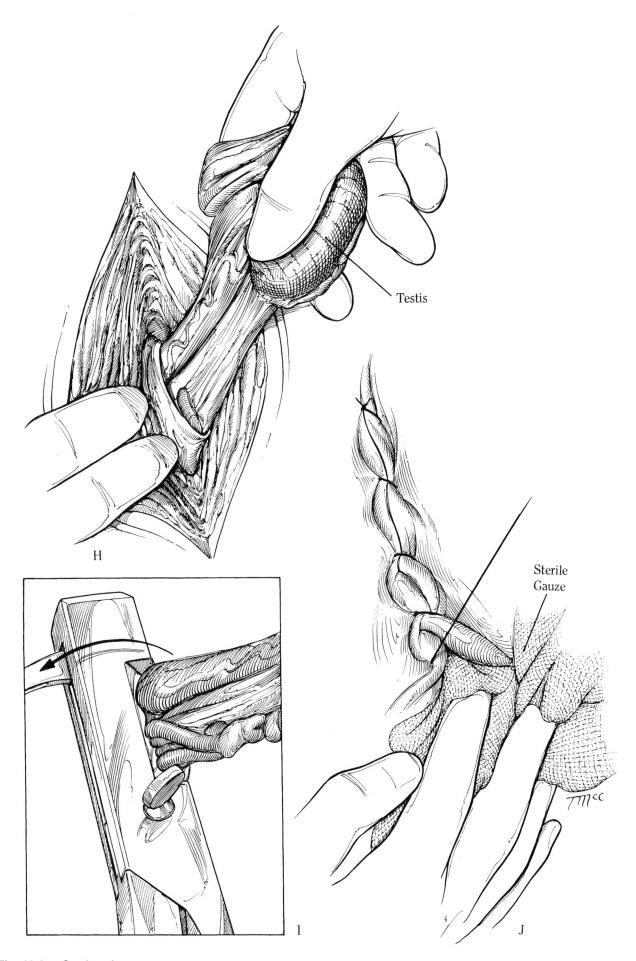

Testis

Sterile
Gauze

H

I

J

Fig. 10-2. *Continued.*

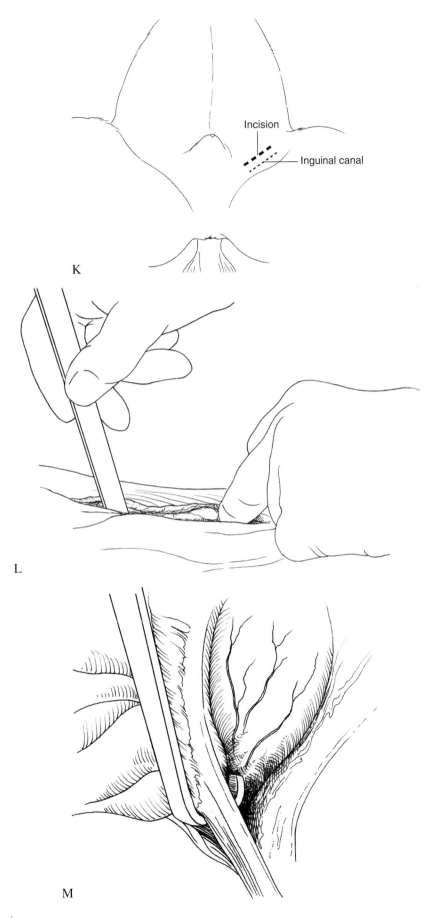

K

L

M

Fig. 10-2. *Continued.*

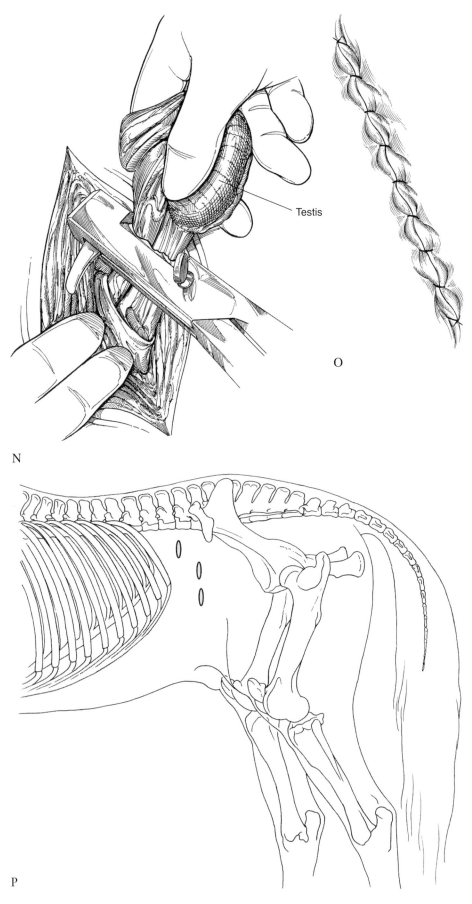

Testis

O

N

P

Fig. 10-2. *Continued.*

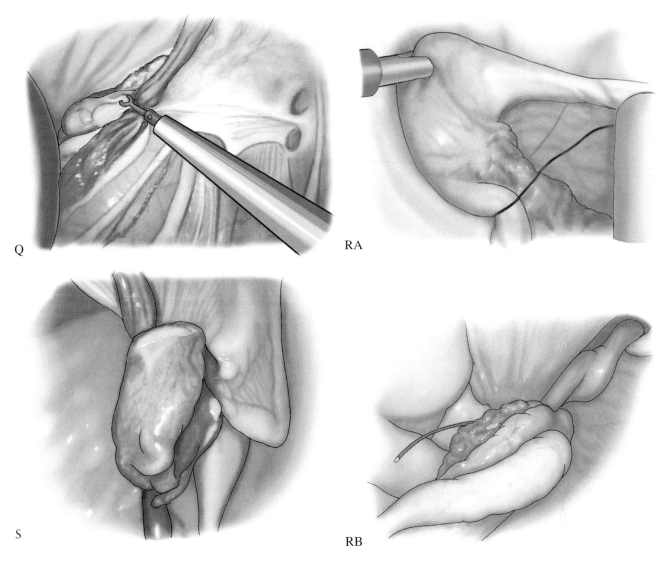

Q RA S RB

Fig. 10-2. *Continued.*

The postoperative complication rate is high for repair of intestinal prolapse, and the condition requires immediate attention.[12] If management of the eventration is beyond the capabilities of the surgeon, the offending viscera, unless it is extensive, can be replaced in the scrotum; the scrotum can be packed with sterile gauzes and temporarily closed with several simple interrupted sutures; and, following the appropriate fluid therapy and parenteral antibiotics, the animal can be referred to an equine surgical facility.

If the eventration is to be managed where the horse was gelded because referral is out of the question, preoperative planning is essential. The appropriate instruments, drapes, and isotonic solutions for lavage must be obtained, and preoperative broad-spectrum antibiotic therapy should commence. Plans for balanced, movement-free general anesthesia must also be made.

With the animal under general anesthesia and in dorsal recumbency, the offending viscera is cleaned by lavage of balanced electrolyte solutions. The incision and scrotal area are prepared for aseptic surgery as thoroughly as possible. Debris, such as straw or blood clots, may have to be manually removed from the bowel in the earlier stages of preparation for surgery. Small segments of bowel, if viable and relatively uncontaminated, can be replaced in the abdomen. Some enlargement of the inguinal ring may be required if the bowel has become congested and edematous. Greater lengths of intestine may be sufficiently contaminated or devitalized that resection and anastomosis will be required. The internal ring may have to be enlarged, a portion of normal bowel exteriorized, and then anastomosis performed. If a portion of omentum is the only abdominal content involved, it can be excised, and remaining healthy omentum can be replaced in the abdomen.

Closure of the internal ring is usually impossible, but closure of the external ring using preplaced simple interrupted synthetic absorbable suture material is necessary, as described in the next section of this chapter on cryptorchidectomy.

Packing of the external canal, as shown in Figure 10-2*J*, is then performed. Fluid therapy should be instituted, as well as other adjunctive therapy for shock, such as flunixin meglumine. The prognosis following eventration is always guarded. A long-term complication may be adhesion of bowel to the inguinal ring (discussed later in this section).

Persistent Masculine Behavior

Many practitioners and horsemen believe that if a stallion is "cut-proud" (a small quantity of epididymis was not removed during surgery), he will continue to show stallionlike behavior. That removal of identifiable epididymal tissue or another piece of a long spermatic cord has resolved the problem in some instances and lends some support to this idea.[15] Testicular or adrenal tissue has not been demonstrated in these removed segments, however, and the problem has been proposed to be psychological.[5] If one suspects that testicular tissue is still present in a gelding, we suggest measuring testosterone levels 30 to 100 min after injecting 6,000 to 12,000 IU of human chorionic gonadotropin (HCG).[4]

Wound Infection

Wound infection may be either acute or chronic. Acute infection can be treated by enlarging the scrotal incisions to allow drainage and by increasing exercise. Antibiotics may be useful. Chronic infection, or scirrhous cord formation, generally requires a second surgery to remove the abnormal tissue. This procedure generally requires more surgical time and plans should be made accordingly.

Penile Paralysis

Penile paralysis (paraphimosis), a rare complication, is usually seen when phenothiazine tranquilizers have been used. If the penis is flaccid and does not retract in 4 to 8 hours, mechanical support of the penis is indicated. *Priapism* is an abnormally prolonged erection of the penis, not associated with sexual desire.[7] It also has been associated with the use of phenothiazine tranquilizers, but fortunately, it is an even rarer complication of castration. Priapism has been treated medically using an anticholinergic agent, benztropine mesylate.[10] The condition has also been treated by drainage and irrigation of the corpus cavernosum penis, along with creation of a vascular shunt between that structure and the corpus spongiosum penis.[5] Description of this procedure is beyond the scope of this book, and the references should be consulted for further details.[7]

Adhesions

Other long-term complications of castration are uncommon, but they are serious and require surgical management. Adhesions of small intestine may occur following ascending infection.[3] We have seen this condition cause a chronic low-grade colic because of incomplete obstruction of the lumen of the small intestine. Muscular hypertrophy, fibrosis, and thickening of the bowel wall aboral to the adhesion usually result. A ventral midline celiotomy, in combination with an inguinal approach, may be required to treat an adhesion in this region. Following identification of the offending bowel and the extent of the adhesion, the adhesion is broken down by carefully separating the bowel from the inguinal region. If the adhesion is of long duration, blind transection of the adhesion with scissors may be required. Standing laparoscopy may be helpful in diagnosing and treating adhesions. With either method, the risk of tearing the intestinal wall and contaminating the abdominal cavity with intestinal contents is real and may be fatal. Peeling the bowel off the adhesion has been successful, but it leaves a raw, bleeding edge that itself is prone to future adhesion formation. Daily rectal examinations, if the horse's size and temperament permit, allow the surgeon carefully to "wipe away" any potentially adhering bowel from these raw surfaces.

References

1. Barber, S.M.: Castration of horses with primary closure and scrotal ablation. Vet. Surg., *14:*2, 1985.
2. Boussauw, B., and Wilderjans, H.: Inguinal herniation 12 days after a unilateral castration with primary wound closure. Eq. Vet. Educ., *8:*248–250, 1996.
3. Crouch, G.M., Snyder, J.R., and Harmon, B.G.: Adhesion of the ileum to the inguinal ring in a gelding. Eq. Pract., *5:*32, 1983.
4. Cox, J.E.: Experiences with a diagnostic test for equine cryptorchidism. Eq. Vet. J., *7:*179, 1975.
5. Pickett, B.W., et al.: Factors affecting sexual behavior of the equine male. *In* Proceedings of the 25th Annual Convention of the American Association of Equine Practitioners in 1979:1980, p. 61.
6. Riegel, R.J., and Hakola, S.E.: Illustrated atlas of equine anatomy and common disorders of the horse, volume II. Marysville, Equistar Publications, 2000.
7. Schumacher, J., and Hardin, D.K.: Surgical treatment of priapism in a stallion. Vet. Surg., *16:*193, 1987.
8. Schumacher, J.: Testis. *In* Equine Surgery. Edited by J.A. Auer and J.A. Stick. St. Louis, Saunders, pp. 775–810, 2006.
9. Searle, D., Dart, A.J., Dart, C.M., and Hodgson, D.R.: Equine castration: review of anatomy, approaches, techniques and complications in normal, cryptorchid and monorchid testes. Aust. Vet. J., *77:*428–434, 1999.
10. Sharrock, A.G.: Reversal of drug induced priapism in a gelding by medication. Aust. Vet. J., *58:*39, 1982.
11. Shideler, R.K., Squires, E.L., and Pickett, B.W.: Disappearance of spermatozoa from the ejaculate of geldings. J. Reprod. Fertil., *27(Suppl.):*25, 1979.
12. Shoemaker, R., Bailey, J., Janzen, E., and Wilson, D.G.: Routine castration in 568 draught colts: incidence of evisceration and omental herniation. Eq. Vet. J., *36:*336–340, 2004.

13. Thomas, H.L., Zaruby, J.F., Smith, C.L., and Livesey, M.A.: Postcastration eventration in 18 horses: the prognostic indicators for long-term survival (1985–1995). Can. Vet. J., 39:764–768, 1998.
14. Van Der Velden, M.A., and Rutgers, L.J.E.: Visceral prolapse after castration in the horse: a review of 18 cases. Eq. Vet. J., 22:9–12, 1990.
15. Walker, D.F., and Vaughan, J.T.: Bovine and Equine Urogenital Surgery. Philadelphia, Lea & Febiger, 1980.

Cryptorchidectomy by the Inguinal and Parainguinal Approach

Relevant Anatomy

In the fetal colt, the testes descend from the abdominal cavity through the inguinal canal to the scrotum just prior to birth or within 2 weeks after.[4] The entrance of the canal from the abdominal cavity, the deep inguinal ring, is located at the caudal border of the internal abdominal oblique muscle. The canal terminates externally at an opening in the aponeurosis of the external abdominal oblique muscle, called the *superficial inguinal ring*. If one or both testes fails to reach the scrotum, it may remain within the abdomen or the canal itself resulting in cryptorchidism. If the testis has traversed the vaginal ring but has not reached the scrotum, the horse is considered an inguinal cryptorchid ("high flanker"). If the testis has not traversed the vaginal ring and has not descended into the inguinal canal, the horse is considered an abdominal cryptorchid. In this case, the vaginal process with the attached gubernaculum will usually be developed and it may be inverted into the abdominal cavity or descended into the canal.[4] Cryptorchidism may be unilateral or bilateral and, in cases of inguinal cryptorchids, may spontaneously resolve itself after a year or more following birth. Horses with abdominal testis(es) will not spontaneously resolve. If the condition does not resolve, then surgical removal of the retained testis(es) is necessary.

The previous section contains additional pertinent anatomy for this technique. For both the inguinal and parainguinal approaches, a thorough understanding of the orientation of the gonadal structures is crucial to successfully locating the testis. In particular, the surgeon relies on the attachment between the tail of the epididymis and the vaginal process to do so.

Indications

There are multiple techniques used for cryptorchidectomy. They can be used to remove both abdominally retained and inguinally retained testis. The most commonly used techniques are the inguinal, parainguinal, and standing laparoscopic techniques. Each will be described.

A rectal examination performed on a cryptorchid patient may enable one to ascertain whether the cryptorchid testis(es) is abdominal or inguinal. Inguinal testes may be nonpalpable on external examination of the inguinal canal. The rectal palpation of the ductus deferens through the vaginal ring indicates that the testis is in the inguinal canal.[1,3] If the ductus deferens cannot be palpated passing through the vaginal ring, the testis is considered to be within the abdomen.[6] We do not routinely perform a rectal examination prior to cryptorchidectomy. Because of altered behavior frequently seen in these cases, the horses are usually fractious and are therefore at an increased risk for rectal perforation. Unlike the broodmare, these animals have not usually been subjected to routine rectal palpation, and this further increases the risk. Arabians, because of a smaller anus and rectum, may be particularly predisposed to this problem.[2] Transrectal ultrasound can be used to diagnose an intraabdominal testis; however, it is not always possible to find the testis.

Anesthesia and Surgical Preparation

The horse is placed under general anesthesia in dorsal recumbency. General anesthesia can be induced with xylazine and ketamine and maintained using "triple drip" (see Chapter 2, "Anesthesia and Fluid Therapy"). The inguinal area is prepared for aseptic surgery in a routine manner and draped.

Instrumentation

General surgery pack
Sponge forceps
Emasculator
Spay hook (parainguinal approach)

Surgical Technique

Inguinal Approach

A 12- to 15-cm skin incision is made over the external inguinal ring and is continued through the superficial fascia (the site of the incision is illustrated in Figure 10-2A). Sharp dissection is then abandoned in favor of blunt dissection with fingertips to separate the subcutaneous inguinal fascia and to expose the external inguinal ring. Large branches of the external pudendal vein are in this region, and trauma to these vessels should be avoided. Dissection is continued beyond the external inguinal ring and through the inguinal canal until the vaginal ring is located with the finger (Figure 10-2B). With an inguinal cryptorchid, the testis contained within the common vaginal tunic would be located in the canal at this time (Figure 10-2C). The common tunic is isolated, and the testis is removed as previously described for normal castration. A closed castration technique is generally used.

With an abdominal cryptorchid, however, the testis will not be obvious. In this situation, the vaginal ring is located, and curved sponge forceps are carefully introduced through the inguinal canal so that the jaws are placed through the vaginal ring into the vaginal process (Figure 10-2D). The partially opened jaws of the forceps are pressed against the vaginal process and are closed (Figure 10-2E). The forceps grasp the vaginal process and associated gubernaculum testis, and the forceps are then withdrawn (Figure 10-2E). This is the critical part of the technique and the most difficult part for the inexperienced surgeon, because excessive force ruptures the vaginal process. The cordlike gubernaculum may then be palpated within the everted vaginal process by rolling it between the thumb and forefinger. When the gubernaculum is identified, the vaginal process is opened with Metzenbaum scissors (Figure 10-2F), and the gubernaculum is grasped with Ochsner forceps. Traction on the gubernaculum causes the tail of the epididymis to be presented (Figure 10-2G). Generally, gentle traction on the epididymis pulls the testis through the vaginal ring. Pushing around the vaginal ring with the fingers at the same time usually is sufficient to deliver the testis, but manual dilation of the vaginal ring is necessary in some cases.

At this point, the testis is positively identified (Figure 10-2H) and is emasculated (Figure 10-2I). In some instances, the testis cannot be retracted sufficiently to enable emasculation, so the cord is ligated and the testis sharply amputated. If the opening made in the vaginal process to deliver the testicle is considerable and if intestinal herniation is a possibility, the external inguinal ring is closed using a large-diameter synthetic absorbable suture material in either a preplaced interrupted pattern or a simple continuous pattern. The strong aponeurosis of the external abdominal oblique muscle is opposed to the fascia on the opposite side of the ring. The dead space is then closed using a no. 2-0 synthetic absorbable suture material. Conversely, a sterile gauze bandage may be packed over the external inguinal ring (Figure 10-2J); this protects against herniation while normal swelling obliterates the inguinal canal. Finally, the skin is sutured with a synthetic absorbable suture, either in a continuous pattern or with simple interrupted sutures with long ends (Figure 10-2J). If the opening in the vaginal process is small (barely enough to squeeze the testicle through), packing will usually be unnecessary. Surgical judgment and some experience will decide whether to pack the external ring or not.

The foregoing technique cannot be used in certain instances, such as when accidental rupture of the vaginal process, vaginal ring, or medial wall of the inguinal canal results in the loss of vital landmarks or when the horse has been subjected to a previous, unsuccessful attempt at surgery. In these situations, the first alternative is digital exploration of the boundaries of the vaginal ring to locate the gubernaculum and the ductus deferens or epididymis. Occasionally, the testes are encountered during the digital exploration. If these methods fail to locate the testis, manual exploration of the abdomen with the entire hand may be necessary. The hand may be admitted through a dilated (ruptured) vaginal ring or through the internal abdominal oblique muscle. The internal abdominal oblique muscle forms the medial wall of the inguinal canal and is thin and easily penetrated in this location. If the testis or ductus deferens is not found immediately, the ampullae should be located at the dorsal aspect of the bladder and traced craniad to the ductus deferens and testis. Termination of the ductus deferens with no epididymis or testis suggests the absence of a testis.

Parainguinal Approach

To perform the parainguinal approach, the horse is anesthetized and placed in dorsal recumbency as described for the inguinal approach. The ventral abdomen is aseptically prepared and draped to allow access to the inguinal areas. A 10-cm incision is made to allow access to the inguinal areas. A 10-cm incision is made through the skin parallel to and 4 cm axial to the inguinal canal (Figure 10-2K). The inguinal canal is explored as for the inguinal approach (Figure 10-2B) to assess the presence of an inguinal testis. If there is an inguinal testis, it is removed as previously described. If no inguinal testis is present, an incision of similar length is made into the external rectus sheath using a scalpel blade. It is important to not make the incision any deeper than the sheath. The rectus abdominus muscle is bluntly divided, and the internal rectus sheath is bluntly penetrated along with the peritoneum. A spay hook is placed through the incision into the peritoneal space. The tip of the spay hook is swept through the region of the vaginal ring to pick up the gubernaculum (Figure 10-2L and M). The gubernaculum is removed from the abdomen and traction is placed until the testis is removed from the abdomen. The testis is emasculated (Figure 10-2N). The external rectus sheath is closed in a simple continuous pattern using no. 1 polyglyconate (Figure 10-2O). The subcutaneous tissue and skin are closed respectively using a no. 2-0 synthetic absorbable suture material using a simple continuous pattern.

Postoperative Management

Tetanus immunization is administered. If gauze packing is placed, it is removed at 24 hours postoperatively. Sutures and gauze pack are removed, the horse is discharged, and the owner is given instructions for routine postcastration management. If suture closure of the inguinal canal is performed, we prefer to hospitalize the horse for 72 hours. Horses can begin exercise in 2 weeks.

Complications and Prognosis

The potential postoperative complications following cryptorchid surgery are the same as described previously for routine castration. Management of the complications is the same for both procedures, and the reader is referred to "Complications and Prognosis" in the section earlier in this chapter titled "Castration." The noninvasive approaches described here are considered superior to the invasive technique. Complications of the invasive technique may be severe, whereas the most common reported complication of the noninvasive technique is failure to identify the vaginal process or ring. Nonetheless, there are inherent risks associated with the noninvasive approach, such as trauma to abdominal structures or inadvertently clamping bowel instead of the vaginal process. Severe swelling may occur but it can be resolved with hydrotherapy. The prognosis is very favorable with either technique. The author prefers the parainguinal approach because it is easier to close the external rectus sheath than the external inguinal ring. Scrotal ablation and primary closure techniques have been described with apparently fewer complications, better cosmetic results (less postoperative swelling), and less postoperative discomfort. Further details of these methods are available.[3,5]

References

1. Adams, O.R.: An improved method of diagnosis and castration of cryptorchid horses. J. Am. Vet. Med. Assoc., *145*:439, 1964.
2. Arnold, J.S., Meagher, D.M., and Loshe, C.L.: Rectal tears in the horse. J. Eq. Med. Surg., *2*:55, 1978.
3. Barber, S.M.: Castration of horses with primary closure and scrotal ablation. Vet. Surg., *14*:2, 1985.
4. Dyce, K.M., Sack, W.O., and Wensing, C.J.G.: Textbook of Veterinary Anatomy, 2nd Ed., Philadelphia, W.B. Saunders, 1996, pp. 565–567.
5. Palmer, S.E., and Passmore, J.L.: Midline scrotal ablation for unilateral cryptorchid castration in horses. J. Am. Vet. Med. Assoc., *190*:283, 1987.
6. Stickle, R.L., and Fessler, J.F.: Retrospective study of 350 cases of equine cryptorchidism. J. Am. Vet. Med. Assoc., *172*:343, 1978.

Laparoscopic Cryptorchidectomy

Relevant Anatomy

The anatomical structures relevant to this procedure are the same as discussed in the previous sections. The perspective is different, however, due to the flank approach. The testis will hang from the dorsal body wall at the mesorchial attachment and is very easy to locate and identify even if previous surgical attempts have been made.

Indications

This technique is an effective, less invasive, method for removal of cryptorchid testes than a flank or inguinal

approach. The benefits of laparoscopy in horses include a shorter convalescence time, better visualization, and more complete exploration of the abdominal cavity. This technique describes the use of hand-tied or pretied ligatures to facilitate intraabdominal amputation of cryptorchid testes in the standing horse.

Anesthesia and Surgical Preparation

For standing laparoscopic procedures in the horse, fasting should begin prior to surgery to prevent intestinal contents from interfering with visualization in the abdomen. The surgery is performed in stocks, generally, with the tail wrapped and secured either to the horse or stocks. The appropriate flank or flanks are aseptically prepared for surgery depending on the location of the abdominally retained testes. Both flanks should always be prepared on bilateral cryptorchids or where the castration history is unclear. Sedation is achieved intravenously with xylazine (0.5 mg/kg) combined with butorphanol (0.05 mg/kg). Further sedation is achieved with either continuous IV infusion of detomidine (20 mg detomidine in 1 liter polyionic replacement fluids) through a jugular catheter or with detomidine injected into the epidural space (40 g/kg detomidine brought to a total volume of 10–12 ml with sterile saline). The skin and musculature of the left flank is desensitized with local portals site blocks (Figure 10-2P) or with an inverted L block using local anesthetic, such as 2% Lidocaine or 2% Mepivacaine (see Chapter 2).

Instrumentation

General surgery pack
3 to 4 surgical drapes
Additional towel clamps
Telescope (see Chapter 3, "Surgical Instruments")
Light source with attached light cord
Mare urinary catheter
Veress needle, teat cannula, or trochar catheter
Sharp and blunt trochars
3–6 cannulas, 10 mm in diameter and 15 to 20 cm long
10-mm serrated laparoscopic scissors
1–2 10-mm acute claw graspers
Laparoscopic injection needle
Knot pusher
Endoscopic suture materials
Laparoscopic video camera (optional)

Surgical Technique

After draping, a 1-cm incision is made in the appropriate flank (left for left-sided of bilateral cryptorchids, right for right-sided cryptorchids) at the base of the tuber coxae, midway between the tuber coxae and the last rib. The incision should include the skin and the fascia of the external abdominal oblique muscle. A mare urinary catheter or a 10-mm diameter, 20-cm long cannula with a blunt trochar is placed through the incision, directed upward toward the opposite stifle, and inserted through the body wall in one continuous motion.[4] Presence in the peritoneal space is confirmed by listening for air being drawn into the abdomen. Insufflation tubing is attached to the cannula and insufflation with CO_2 begun. If a laparoscopic cannula is used, the laparoscope can be inserted to confirm presence in the peritoneal space. The abdomen is insufflated to a pressure of 12–15 mm Hg.[2] Second and third portals are placed 10 cm dorsal and slightly rostral and 10 cm ventral, respectively, to the first portal (Figure 10-2P). The laparoscope is placed in the dorsal most portal, and the abdomen explored. Instruments can be placed in the middle or ventral portals to lift the small colon to observe the opposite inguinal area and determine the location of the testes. The ipsilateral testis is identified (Figure 10-2Q), and grasped and the mesorchium infiltrated with 2% lidocaine using a laparoscopic injection needle. A laparoscopic slipknot (4–5 modified roeder using size no. 1 polyglyconate) in a knot pusher is placed into a 5-mm reducing cannula and inserted in the middle cannula.[1,3] The loop is advanced into the abdomen, and an acute claw grasper is placed into the ventral cannula, through the loop, and the testis grasped. The loop is placed over the testis onto the mesorchium and tightened (Figure 10-2R). The long end of the suture is cut and the mesorchium transected distal to the knot. The pedicle is assessed for bleeding (Figure 10-2S).

A single ligature is generally sufficient; however, a second one can be placed if necessary. In cases of bilateral cryptorchids, the right testis can generally be removed from the left side after placing a 4th cannula in the left flank and lifting the small colon.[4] After the testis has been amputated, the ventralmost incision is enlarged and the testis removed. The external abdominal oblique fascia is closed in the enlarged incision using a no. 0 polygloconate in a simple continuous pattern. The skin is closed with a synthetic, nonabsorbable suture material.

Postoperative Management

Generally, the convalescence time for laparoscopic procedures is shorter than other approaches. The horse should be kept in confinement for 3 days and then can return to full exercise. If only one testis was abdominal and the other was removed through standard castration, the horse should begin hand-walking at 24 hours postsurgery.

Complications and Prognosis

The complications that have been encountered in this procedure include peritonitis, wound infection, intestinal perforation, and hemorrhage. In the hands of a skilled surgeon, the prognosis for laparoscopic cryptorchidectomy is very good because this technique is generally considered less invasive than other approaches. The recovery time and contamination is reduced with this technique,

and abdominal testes may be viewed and extracted more easily.

References

1. Carpenter, E.M., Hendrickson, D.A., James, S., Franke, C., Frisbie, D., Trostle, S., and Wilson, D.: A mechanical study of ligature security of commercially available pre-tied ligatures versus hand tied ligatures for use in equine laparoscopy. Vet. Surg., 35:55–59, 2006.
2. Fischer, A.T.: Equine Diagnostic & Surgical Laparoscopy. Philadelphia, W.B. Saunders, 2001.
3. Shettko, D.L, Frisbie, D.D., and Henrickson, D.A.: A comparison of knot security of commonly used hand-tied laparoscopic slipknots. Vet. Surg., 33:521–524, 2004.
4. Trumble, T., and Hendrickson, D.A.: Standing male equine urogenital endoscopic surgery. Vet. Clin. North Am.: Eq. Pract., 16:269–284, 2000.

Caslick's Operation for Pneumovagina in the Mare

Relevant Anatomy

The external genitalia of the mare is comprised of the perineum and the vulva. The perineum describes the area extending from the base of the tail to the ventral commissure of the vulva.[3] Between the anus and vulva is the perineal body, formed by muscle fibers of the external anal sphincter and constrictor vulvae muscles.[3] The vulva consists of two labia, which meet at the ventral and dorsal commissures, and the clitoris. The labia are normally held together at the vulvar cleft by paired constrictor vulvae muscles. In most mares, the majority of the vulva is located ventral to the pelvic floor. Some mares, Thoroughbreds in particular, will have a slightly more dorsally orientated vulva, which can interfere with closure at the vulvar cleft and result in aspiration of air, endometritis, and sterility.

The vestibule is the termination of the internal genital tract and connects the vulva to the vagina. Normally, the vestibule slopes dorsally in the cranial direction and extends up to the transverse fold, which is the remnant of the hymen at the vaginovestibular junction.[5] The transverse fold of mucosa is identified approximately 5 to 10 cm cranial to the brim of the pelvis on the floor of the vagina (Figure 10-4B). The urethral orifice opens just caudal to and underneath the transverse fold. Cranial to the transverse fold, the vagina continues to the fornix at the cervix. Most of the vagina is retroperitoneal, with the exception of the cranial portion that is covered with peritoneum.

Indications

The operation for pneumovagina in the mare is to prevent the involuntary aspiration of air into the vagina.

Pneumovagina is caused by faulty closure of the lips of the vulva as a result of poor conformation or injury. Mares in which the lips of the vulva are tilted toward the anus are prone to vaginitis, cervicitis, metritis, and infertility due to contamination from material aspirated through the vulva. Old, thin, debilitated mares with sunken ani usually are more prone to pneumovagina. At least 80% of the vulval labia should be located ventral to the pelvic floor, and the vulval seal should be at least 2.5 cm deep and resistant to parting. In addition, the labia should be at an angle of at least 80° or nearly perpendicular to the horizontal.[1] Breeding or foaling injuries may also result in pneumovagina because the skin and mucosa of the labia become misshapen, resulting in a faulty seal. Some mares, especially in racing, may aspirate air even though they have good vulvar conformation, whereas others may have overlapping vulvar lips with relatively good conformation. These mares are also candidates for Caslick's operation. This operation is also performed in combination with other surgery of the mare's perineum, such as repair of first-, second-, and third-degree perineal lacerations.[4]

Anesthesia and Surgical Preparation

Caslick's operation is performed with the animal under local anesthesia by direct infiltration of the vulvar labial margin. The surgery is best performed in a set of stocks, where dangers to the mare and operator are minimal; some mares require a twitch and, occasionally, tranquilization. Prior to the surgery, the feces should be manually removed from the rectum, and the tail should be bandaged and secured out of the surgical field. A thorough cleansing of the perineal region should be performed using a mild disinfectant solution, and all traces of the disinfectant solution should be removed by rinsing with water. Cotton or paper towels are recommended, rather than a scrub brush. Approximately 5 ml of local anesthetic are used for local infiltration into each side (Figure 10-3A and B).

Following desensitization of the required length of mucocutaneous junction of the vulva and labia, a final preparation of the surgical site is performed using a suitable, nonirritating antiseptic applied with cotton or gauze sponges.

Instrumentation

General surgery pack

Surgical Technique

Using tissue scissors, the surgeon removes a ribbon of mucosa approximately 3 mm wide from each vulvar labium (Figure 10-3C). To facilitate trimming the tissue, thumb forceps are used to grasp the ribbon of tissue and to apply downward pressure to stretch the area. A common mistake is to remove too much tissue. Conse-

quently, many practitioners now just use a scalpel blade to incise into the local anesthetic bleb to create a fresh edge (Figure 10-3E). Most mares require that this operation be performed on successive years, and if excessive tissue is removed, subsequent repairs will be more difficult. The length of the vulva and labia to be sutured will vary, depending on the conformation of the individual mare. This length may vary from the upper half of the vulva to as much as 70% of its length. Once the ribbon of tissue is removed with scissors, or the scalpel incision made, the raw surface is generally much wider than one would anticipate because tissue edges under tension retract (Figure 10-3D). This tension is due to swelling caused by the local analgesic infiltration. Bleeding from the edges usually is minimal.

When the ribbon of tissue has been removed with either scissors or a scalpel blade, the raw edges are apposed using a simple continuous suture pattern (Figure 10-3F). A nonabsorbable, noncapillary suture material such as no. 2-0 nylon or no. 2-0 polypropylene is preferred. Vertical mattress, simple interrupted, and continuous interlocking patterns, and Michel clips, have also been used successfully. The suture pattern depends on individual preference, but the raw edges should be in good apposition no matter what pattern is used (Figure 10-3G). Skin staples have also been used successfully without prior removal of mucosa.[2]

To avoid excessive stress on the suture line at its ventral end during breeding or speculum examination, a "breeder's stitch" may be inserted ventral to Caslick's closure.

The area where the stitch is placed is desensitized and is infiltrated 2 cm in all directions from where the suture is to be placed (Figure 10-3G). Using sterile umbilical tape, the surgeon places a single interrupted suture at the most ventral part of Caslick's operation (Figure 10-3H). The stitch should not be so ventral that it interferes with breeding, nor should it be so loose that it may lacerate the stallion's penis (Figure 10-3I). Excessive penetration of the stallion's penis during natural cover in mares with Caslick's operation can be avoided with the use of a stallion/breeding roll.[1]

Postoperative Management

Generally, postoperative topical or systemic antibiotics are not indicated. The sutures can be removed 7 to 10 days postoperatively.

To prevent unnecessary damage at parturition, the vulvar labia should be surgically separated (episiotomy), and the Caslick's operation should be performed 1 or 2 days after foaling. It may also be necessary to separate the labia during natural mating or during manipulations of the reproductive tract for examination or therapy. If the labia become separated for any reason, the Caslick's surgery should be redone at the earliest opportunity to prevent pneumovagina.

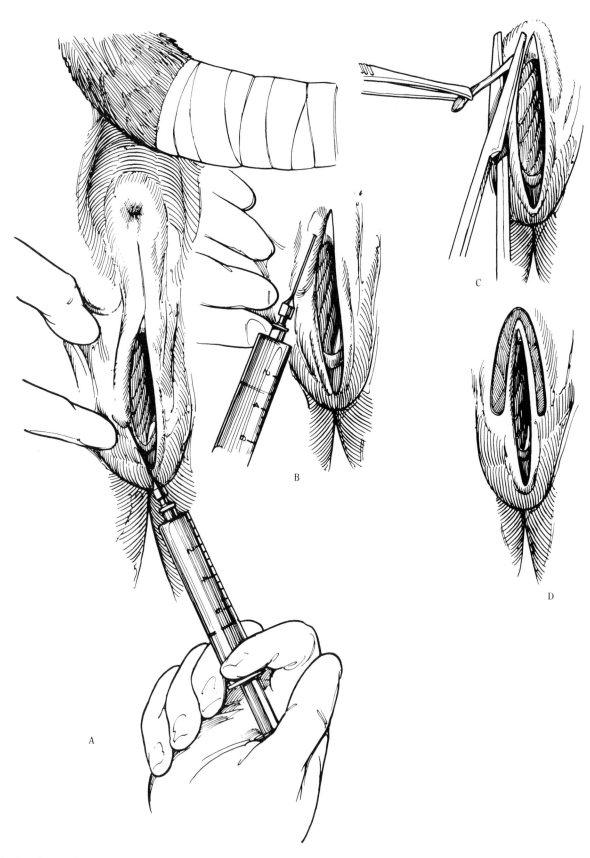

Fig. 10-3. A to I, Caslick's operation.

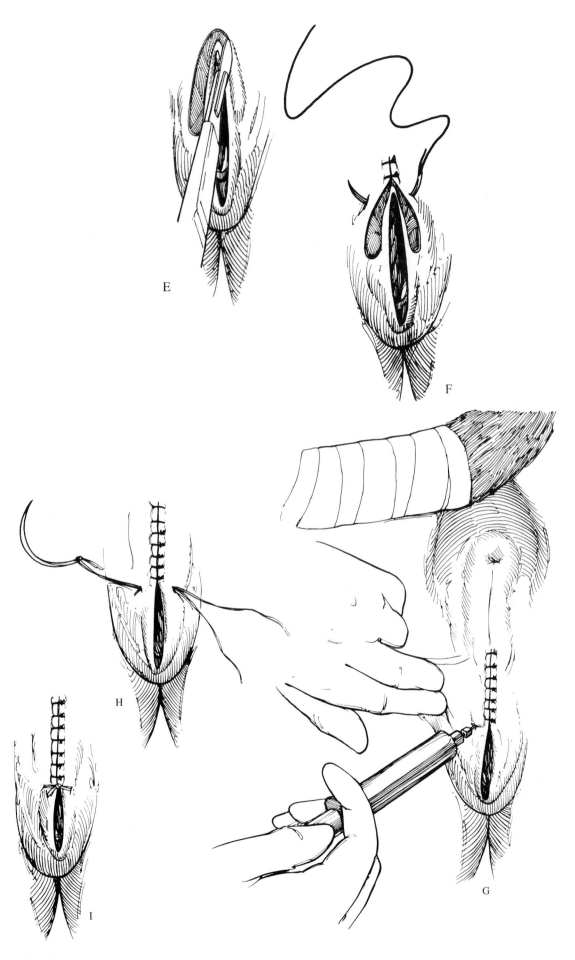

Fig. 10-3. *Continued.*

167

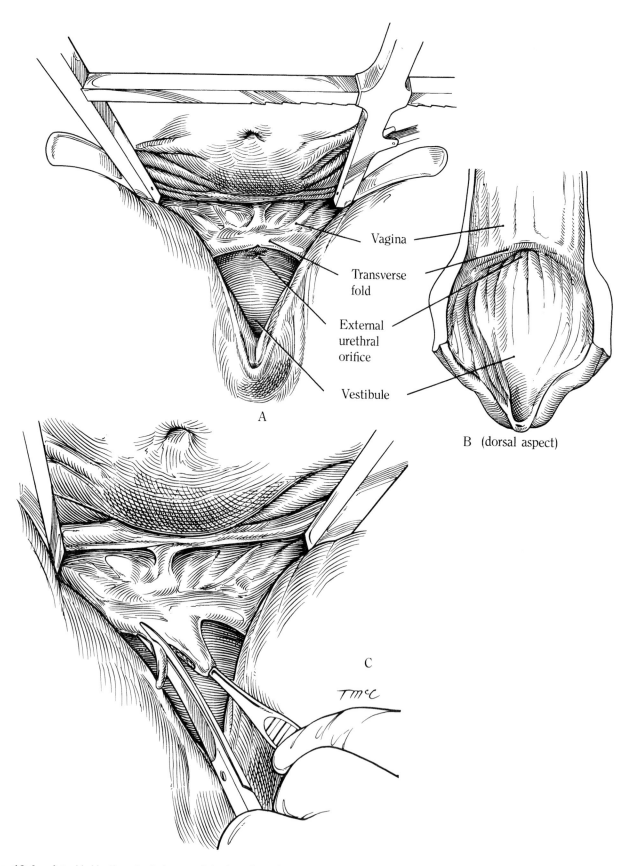

Vagina

Transverse fold

External urethral orifice

Vestibule

A

B (dorsal aspect)

C

TMcC

Fig. 10-4. A to H, Urethroplasty by caudal relocation of the transverse fold.

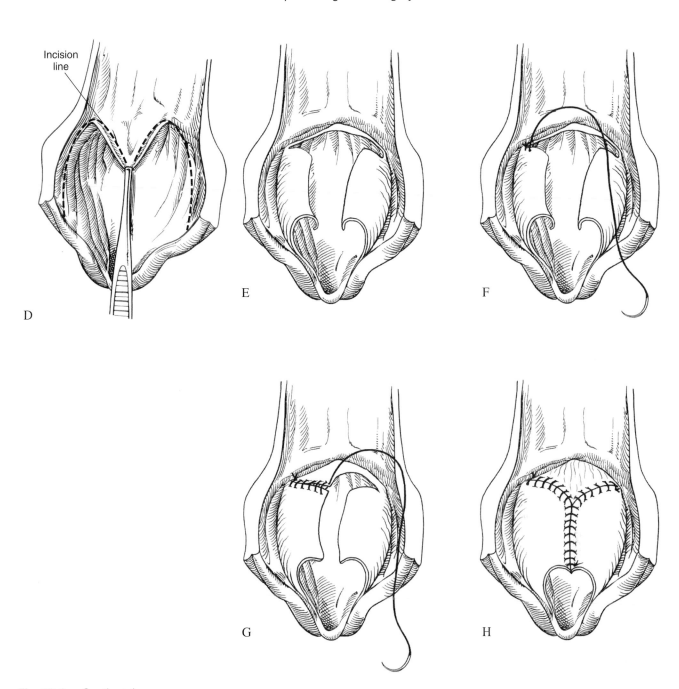

Fig. 10-4. *Continued.*

Complications and Prognosis

Complications of this procedure include recurrence of pneumovagina and wound dehiscence. Certain mares may be candidates for other procedures, such as episioplasty and urine-pooling surgery, to achieve optimal fertility.[4] A mare that still has vaginal aerophagia following Caslick's operation should be considered a candidate for additional surgery. Animals in which the perineal region is sunken beneath both tuber ischii and in which the dorsal commissure of the vulva becomes horizontal, with rostral displacement of the anus, may not respond to Caslick's operation alone. Older, multiparous mares seem

to be more prone to this condition, especially if they are unthrifty.

References

1. Ansari, M.M.: The Caslick operation in mares. Compend. Contin. Educ. Pract. Vet., 5:107, 1983.
2. Candle, A.B., et al.: Skin staples for non-scarified Caslick procedures. Vet. Med., 78:782, 1983.
3. Dyce, K.M., Sack, W.O., and Wensing, C.J.G.: Textbook of Veterinary Anatomy, 2nd Ed. Philadelphia, W.B. Saunders, 1996, pp. 551–572.

4. McIlwraith, C.W., and Turner, A.S.: Equine Surgery: Advanced Techniques, 2nd Ed. Baltimore, Williams & Wilkins, 1998.
5. Woodie, B.: Vulva, vestibule, vagina, and cervix. *In* Equine Surgery, 3rd Edition. Edited by J.A. Auer and J.A. Stick. St. Louis, Saunders, 2006, p. 835.

Urethroplasty by Caudal Relocation of the Transverse Fold

Relevant Anatomy

The urethral orifice opens just caudal to and underneath the transverse fold (the remnant of the hymen at the vaginovestibular junction). The transverse fold of mucosa is identified approximately 5 to 10 cm cranial to the brim of the pelvis on the floor of the vagina (Figure 10-4B). Other relevant anatomy is discussed in previous sections of this chapter.

Indications

This reconstructive technique is indicated for treatment of urine pooling in the vagina, also known as *vesicovaginal reflux*. Urine pooling is more common in older, multiparous mares when sunken vaginas develop. The ventral floor of the vagina slopes cranioventrad, and uterine fluid and urine accumulate in the fornix of the vagina around the cervix. Vaginitis, cervicitis, endometritis, and temporary or permanent sterility may result. The aim of this operation is to promote caudal evacuation of urine and to prevent its pooling in the vagina.

Anesthesia and Surgical Preparation

The surgery is performed on the standing mare restrained in stocks. Tranquilization and epidural anesthesia are used. If the epidural anesthetic is ineffective, local infiltration of the surgical site can be performed. The tail is wrapped and is tied away from the surgical field. The vestibule and vagina are flushed with dilute povidone-iodine solution (not performed routinely by all surgeons), and the perineal area is prepared for aseptic surgery. The bladder should be emptied using a Foley catheter. The surgeon may elect to leave the catheter in place during surgery to help identify the incision and ensure that adequate tissue is available for closure.

Instrumentation

Long-handled surgical instruments
Self-retaining retractor (Glasser retractor)
Foley catheter

Surgical Technique

A self-retaining retractor (Glasser retractor) is placed in the vulva to expose the surgical area (Figure 10-4A).

Long-handled instruments facilitate the performance of this procedure. The transverse fold is grasped at the center with a pair of thumb forceps and is retracted caudad approximately 5 cm using moderate tension (Figure 10-4C and D). The dotted line in the figure indicates the line of mucosal resection. Using curved scissors or scalpel, the surgeon removes the lateral edge or transects, respectively, the retracted transverse fold from the point of attachment of the thumb forceps to the junction of the fold with the vestibular wall (Figure 10-4C and D).[1] A scalpel blade is then used to carry the incision from the junction of the fold and the vestibular wall in a horizontal line to the vulvar lips. The incision must be dorsal enough so that the two lateral flaps can be sutured together without tension. A similar incision is made on the right side (Figure 10-4E). The suture line is started at the left lateral corner of the incision (Figure 10-4F). The mucosa is inverted to the midpoint of the urethral fold. A second suture line is started at the right lateral wall and closed similarly to the left. When the second suture line meets the first suture line, it is carried through to the end of the dissected folds to form a "Y" shaped closure (Figure 10-4H).[1]

It is important to have minimal tension on the transverse fold when it is sutured into this new position; otherwise, the surgery will fail because of pressure necrosis at the sutures. In addition, the transverse fold should not be sutured more than 2 cm from the floor of the vestibule or the fold could be torn during copulation. It is also important that the new urethral aperture be of sufficient size so that normal urine flow is not restricted.

Postoperative Management

Tetanus prophylaxis is provided, and a course of systemic antibiotics is instituted. Caslick's operation is performed at the same time as the urethroplasty. The vagina is not interfered with for 2 weeks. After surgery, mares should not be sexually active for 30 to 60 days; during this time, any uterine infection should be treated. Artificial insemination should be used when possible.

Complications and Prognosis

Complications of this procedure include failure to resolve urine pooling secondary to suture line failure.

This technique is usually effective in eliminating urine pooling in mares with a vaginal slope of 5 to 30°.[2] Mares with a greater slope have a less-favorable prognosis.

References

1. McKinnon, A.O., and Beldon, J.O.: A urethral extension technique to correct urine pooling (vesicovaginal reflux) in mares. J. Am. Vet. Med. Assoc., *192*:647–650, 1988.

2. Monin, T.: Vaginoplasty: A surgical treatment for urine pooling in the mare. *In* Proceedings of the 18th Annual Convention of the American Association of Equine Practitioners in 1972:1973, p. 99.

Cesarean Section in the Mare

Relevant Anatomy

The uterine body in the mare ranges from 18 to 20 cm in length and occupies both retroperitoneal and peritoneal spaces.[15] The cervix, ranging from 5 to 8 cm in length, is within the pelvic cavity dorsal to the bladder and urethra. The lumen of the cervical canal is lined by longitudinal mucosal folds that merge with the endometrial folds in the body.[15] The uterine horns are approximately 20 to 25 cm in length and are suspended by the mesometrium, or broad ligament. The equine placenta has a diffuse attachment, and the cut edge of the uterus is felt to be prone to bleeding.

There are three primary layers to the uterine wall: the tunicae mucosa, muscularis, and serosa, referred to as the *endometrium, myometrium,* and *perimetrium,* respectively.[15] The innermost endometrium lines the lumen and consists mostly of epithelial and glandular tissue. The myometrium contains a highly vascularized layer and a thin, longitudinal layer of smooth muscle. The serosa is the outermost layer, which is composed of visceral peritoneum and two peritoneal sheets of the mesometrium.

The uterine artery, the uterine branch of the ovarian artery, and the uterine branch of the vaginal artery supply blood to the uterus and are contained within the broad ligament.

Indications

This operation is indicated for treatment of various types of dystocia in the mare; the most common indications are transverse presentation,[12,13] some instances of uterine torsion,[11,13] instances of uterine rupture,[3] and the production of gnotobiotic foals.[1] Although uterine torsion is best managed by a standing flank laparotomy and manual repositioning of the gravid uterus, a ventral midline celiotomy is indicated if the mare is intractable, if the uterus is ruptured, or if the torsion cannot be corrected with the animal in the standing position. In such cases, hysterotomy is performed first, making untwisting of the torsion easier.[11]

Fetal manipulation with the animal under general anesthesia or fetotomy, if the fetus is deemed nonviable, are also used in many instances of dystocia. The particular method used to handle a problem commonly depends on the experience and preference of the clinician. Repeated manipulations and attempts at fetotomy can damage the sensitive mucosal lining of the vagina and cervix, result in lacerations of the genital tract, and compromise the mare's future reproductive health.[4] If the surgeon lacks the equipment, is not familiar with the correct fetotomy technique, or lacks anesthetic assistance, a cesarean section may be the best option. Cesarean section should not be considered as a last resort in the mare.

Anesthesia and Surgical Preparation

Various anesthetic regimens have been advocated, in an effort to minimize fetal depression. Epidural anesthesia combined with chloral hydrate and guaifenesin and a low oblique flank surgical approach have been used successfully in Europe.[12,13] We prefer a ventral midline approach to the abdomen performed with the mare under general anesthesia. Although a flank incision is adequate to correct torsion of the uterus, the small paralumbar fossa makes it a poor choice for cesarean section.

Induction of anesthesia with guaifenesin, with or without thiamylal sodium, is preferred to induction with a bolus of thiobarbiturate. Methohexital sodium as an induction agent is superior to thiopental sodium for obtaining live gnotobiotic foals by cesarean section.[1] Induction with xylazine (0.8 mg/kg i.v.) followed by an injection of a ketamine (2.2 mg/kg i.v.)-diazepam (0.04 mg/kg i.v.) solution and maintenance with halothane and oxygen has yielded consistent, satisfactory results.[1,8] The level of halothane required for maintenance of anesthesia can be minimized by performing local infiltration of the ventral midline incision line. In many situations, the foal is already dead because of the protracted dystocia and advanced involution of the uterus by the time cesarean section is performed, and whatever anesthetic regimen is considered best for the mare is appropriate.

The use of halothane as an anesthetic agent has been associated with increased bleeding of the uterine incision. This bleeding is associated with congestion of the myometrial vessels and is more significant in species that have diffuse placentation. In an experimental study of cesarean section in mares, mares anesthetized with halothane had increased bleeding from the uterine incision than mares anesthetized with methoxyflurane.[7] If an encircling suture of the incision edge is used, however, bleeding problems are avoided, and halothane remains a safe anesthetic.

If the ventral midline approach is used, the mare is placed in dorsal recumbency and is clipped and prepared for aseptic surgery in a routine manner. According to the systemic status of the patient, appropriate fluid therapy and medication are administered.

Instrumentation

General surgery pack

Surgical Technique

The abdomen is entered through a ventral midline incision, which is used for the ventral midline laparotomy described in Chapter 12, "Equine Dental and Gastrointestinal Surgery." The uterus enclosing the fetus is located, and an incision site over a limb is chosen, just as in bovine cesarean section. This area is exteriorized as much as possible to minimize contamination of the peritoneal cavity. A more cranial limb should be chosen; otherwise, it may be difficult to close the hysterotomy incision because of caudal retraction of the uterus once the fetus is removed. The uterus is incised using a scalpel, and the foal is removed. Unless the allantochorion has already separated or will lift off easily, it should be left in the uterus.

Before closing the uterus when equine cesarean section is performed, any large bleeding vessels should be ligated. The allantochorion is separated for a distance of 2 to 5 cm from the margin of the uterine incision, and a continuous suture of rapidly absorbing synthetic suture material (Caprosyn) is placed around the entire margin of the uterine incision for hemostasis (Figure 10-5, inset).[8] The technique consists of a simple continuous pattern penetrating all layers of the uterus; it is necessary because the equine endometrium is only loosely attached to the myometrium, and there is little natural hemostasis for the

large subendometrial veins. In addition, halothane may cause congestion of these veins. Bleeding is virtually impossible to control by clamping and ligation. If the uterus has been ruptured, a continuous suture to stop bleeding may not be necessary because hemorrhage may have ceased.[3] The uterus is closed with a double inverting layer of sutures using no. 1 polyglyconate (Maxon) or no. 2 lactomer 9-1 (Polysorb) (Figure 10-5). Although hemostatic sutures have been advocated in the past to reduce hemorrhage from hysterotomy sites, recent studies suggest that this practice does not decrease the incidence of anemia, and the time to place these sutures may outweigh any benefits.[2,5] However, the author continues to use these sutures.

The abdomen is closed as for ventral laparotomy in the horse, which is described in Chapter 12. Great care should be exercised when separating the allantochorion at the margin of the uterine incision and avoiding its inclusion in the suture lines. If rupture has occurred, copious lavage of the abdomen with warm physiologic solutions during surgery is indicated because of the increased risk of contamination from uterine contents.[3]

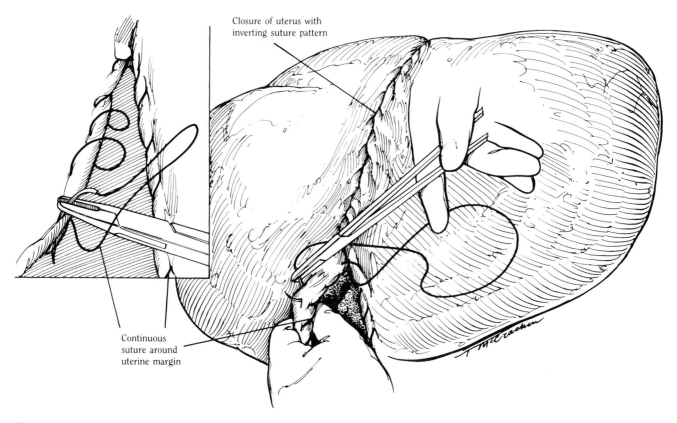

Closure of uterus with inverting suture pattern

Continuous suture around uterine margin

Fig. 10-5. Cesarean section in the mare and uterine closure.

Postoperative Management

Tetanus prophylaxis, antibiotics, and oxytocin are administered. Appropriate fluid therapy is continued or is instituted if the patient is compromised systemically.

As soon as the mare is standing and it is safe to milk her, colostrum should be obtained and given to the foal. The foal should be introduced to the mare as soon as the mare is stable enough on her feet not to be a danger to the foal. For the next 5 to 7 days, rectal or vaginal examination is indicated to assess uterine size.

Prolonged retention of the placenta is of significant concern in the horse, and the mare should be monitored and treated for retention of fetal membranes if necessary. Immediate forced traction of the placenta should be avoided in case the uterus is torn, especially in mares that have had uterine rupture. The placenta will usually pass on its own. If not, gentle manual removal with careful separation of the placenta from the uterine wall may eventually be indicated.[3]

Complications and Prognosis

In women, postoperative infection can be reduced by prophylactic antibiotics, even when these drugs are administered in the immediate postoperative period, rather than preoperatively.[9] Although undesirable transfer of antibiotics is of concern in infants, we see no reason not to commence antibiotics preoperatively in mares. Anemia and bleeding from the hysterotomy site is a common and serious complication following cesarean sections. One study showed a 22% prevalence rate of this complication.[6] Although not as common, bleeding from uterine arteries can also occur and be fatal. Retained placenta, metritis, uterine tears, vaginal or cervical tears, colitis, peritonitis, decreased fertility, and incisional dehiscence are among some of the other reported complications that can occur following cesarean section.[5,14] Of these, retained placenta and decreased fertility are probably the most common.

The prognosis for survival of the mare after elective cesarean section is very good and nears 100% in the literature.[5,14] An 85% survival rate has been reported for mares receiving cesarean sections for correction of dystocia. The survival rates of foals delivered via cesarean section for correction of dystocia is less promising; most of the literature reports an approximate 30% survival rate. This number is greatly influenced by the duration and severity of the dystocia. Premature separation of the placenta can cause fetal asphyxia and death.[14] This is evidenced by the much higher survival rate of foals delivered by elective cesarean sections.[14]

Although an oblique low flank laparotomy approach has been used successfully in Europe,[12,13] we believe that the ventral midline approach offers the best exposure and fewer complications during healing of the incision. As discussed in the section of Chapter 12 on ventral midline laparotomy, fears regarding dehiscence or herniation following the use of this approach are unfounded.

References

1. Edwards, G.B., Allen, W.D., and Newcomb, J.R.: Elective caesarean section in the mare for the production of gnotobiotic foals. Eq. Vet. J., 6:122, 1974.
2. Embertoson, R.M.: The indications and surgical techniques for cesarean section in the mare. Eq. Vet. Educ., 4:31–39, 1992.
3. Fischer, A.T., and Phillips, T.N.: Surgical repair of a ruptured uterus in five mares. Eq. Vet. J., 18:153, 1986.
4. Frazor, G.S.: Fetotomy technique in the mare. Eq. Vet. Educ., 13:151–159, 2001.
5. Freeman, D.E., Hungerford, L.L., Schaeffer, D., Lock, T.F., et al.: Caesarean section and other methods for assisted delivery: comparison of effects on mare mortality and complications. Eq. Vet. J., 31:203–207, 1999.
6. Freeman, D.E., Johnston, J.K., Baker, G.J., Hungerford, L.L., and Lock, T.F.: An evaluation of the haemostatic suture in hysterotomy closure in the mare. Eq. Vet. J., 31:208–211, 1999.
7. Heath, R.B.: Personal communication, 1980.
8. Hopper, S.A.: Equine cesarean section for acute dystocia. In Proceedings of the 11th Annual American College of Veterinary Surgeons in 2001, pp. 183–188.
9. Itskovitz, J., Paldi, E., and Katz, M.: The effect of prophylactic antibiotics on febrile morbidity following cesarean section. Obstet. Gynecol., 53:162, 1979.
10. Juzwiak, J.S., Slone, D.E., Santschi, E.M., and Moll, H.D.: Cesarean section in 19 mares: results and postoperative fertility. Vet. Surg., 19:50–52, 1990.
11. Pascoe, J.R., Meagher, D.M., and Wheat, J.D.: Surgical management of uterine torsion in the mare: a review of 26 cases. J. Am. Vet. Med. Assoc., 179:351, 1981.
12. Vandeplassche, M., et al.: Caesarean section in the mare. In Proceedings of the 23rd Annual Convention of the American Association of Equine Practitioners in 1977:1978, p. 75.
13. Vandeplassche, M., et al.: Some aspects of equine obstetrics. Eq. Vet. J., 4:105, 1972.
14. Watkins, J.P., Taylor, T.S., Day, W.C., and Varner, D.D.: Elective cesarean section in mares: eight cases (1980–1989). J. Am. Vet. Med. Assoc., 197:1639–1645, 1990.
15. Wenzel, J.G.W.: Anatomy of the uterus, ovaries, and adnexa. In Large Animal Urogenital Surgery, 2nd Ed. Edited by D.F. Wolfe and D.H. Moll. Baltimore, Williams & Wilkins, 1999.

Circumcision of the Penis (Reefing)

Relevant Anatomy

The penis of the horse is musculocavernous and can increase in size by up to three times during erection. There are two cavernous spaces of the shaft; the corpus cavernosum, formed by the union of the two crura, and the corpus spongiosum, which gives rise to the glans cranially. These erectile bodies are encapsulated in a thick, fibroelastic layer called the *tunica albuginea*.

The penis is attached caudally to the ischial arch of the pelvis through the paired crura. The urethral process is located at the fossa glandis, the ventral depression of the cranial aspect of the glans. The entrance to the inner sleeve of the prepuce, or sheath, is called the *preputial ring*. The preputial ring is the cranial border of the preputial fold.

Indications

This operation is indicated for the removal of neoplasms, granulomas (including those associated with repeated habronema infestation), and scar tissue or chronic thickening of the preputial membrane that prevents retraction of the penis.[1,2] Circumscribed lesions of the preputial ring may require only simple surgical removal and suturing of the skin edges. More extensive lesions cause deformity, and consequently, a complete ring of tissue is removed.

Anesthesia and Surgical Preparation

The horse is positioned in dorsal recumbency under general anesthesia, the penis is held in extension with towel clamps or a gauze loop around the neck of the glans, and the surgical area is prepared and draped for aseptic surgery. Catheterization of the urethra and the use of a tourniquet are optional.

Instrumentation

General surgery pack
Stallion catheter
Tourniquet

Surgical Technique

Figure 10-6A shows a lesion on the internal preputial membrane with the lines of excision demarcated. If the lesion involves the cranial rim of the inner prepuce, retraction of the inner lining will be essential before the incisions are made. The placement of a tourniquet proximally will improve visualization at the time of surgery. Two circumferential skin incisions are made cranial and caudal to the lesion (Figure 10-6B), and the preputial membrane is tensed by the use of towel forceps. A plane of dissection superficial to the deep fascia of the penis is found, and the tissue between the two circumferential incisions is removed. A third longitudinal incision connecting the two circumferential incisions facilitates the ease of dissection. One should be careful not to cut the large subcutaneous vessels around the penis during the blunt dissection. It is necessary to ligate one subcutaneous vein on each side of the penis. Once the tissue between the two circumferential incisions is removed, two healthy skin margins are left proximally and distally, ready for reapposition (Figure 10-6C). The edges are brought together and are closed with a layer of simple interrupted sutures

of no. 2-0 glycomer 631 (Biosyn) (Figure 10-6D). If a subcutaneous layer is used, no attempt is made to secure this to the underlying tunica albuginea.

Postoperative Management

Tetanus prophylaxis is administered, and the use of postoperative antibiotics is recommended. The horse is hand-walked to help minimize preputial swelling, and sutures can be removed in 14 days. If this surgery is performed on a stallion, the animal should be isolated from mares for 3 to 4 weeks.[2]

Complications and Prognosis

The primary complication that may occur during this procedure is mild hemorrhage. This can generally be avoided by ligation of larger vessels and cautery of smaller vessels. Infection and suture dehiscence may occur if the stallion is not prohibited from sexual activity in the postoperative period. Overall, the prognosis for this procedure is good provided that the underlying tunics are not involved in the lesion.

References

1. Walker, D.F., and Vaughan, J.T.: Bovine and Equine Urogenital Surgery. Philadelphia, Lea & Febiger, 1980.
2. Vaughan, J.T.: Surgery of the male equine reproductive system. *In* The Practice of Large Animal Surgery. Edited by P. Jennings. Philadelphia, W.B. Saunders, 1984, p. 1088.

Amputation of the Penis

Relevant Anatomy

Relevant anatomy for this procedure is described in the previous section.

Indications

The indications for penis amputation in the horse are invasive neoplastic lesions, granulomas associated with habronemiasis, and intractable paralysis or priapism of the penis. The procedure is illustrated as it would be performed for a squamous cell carcinoma of the glans of the penis. In this situation, the penis is amputated at a point distal to that required for penile paralysis, and the operation is therefore easier. The proximal amputations are more difficult because of the greater diameter of the penis and the reflections of the prepuce.[3] En bloc amputation, penile amputation with sheath ablation, and penile retroversion involve extensive resection and have been described for treatment of neoplasia that extends to subcutaneous tissues or regional lymph nodes.[1,2]

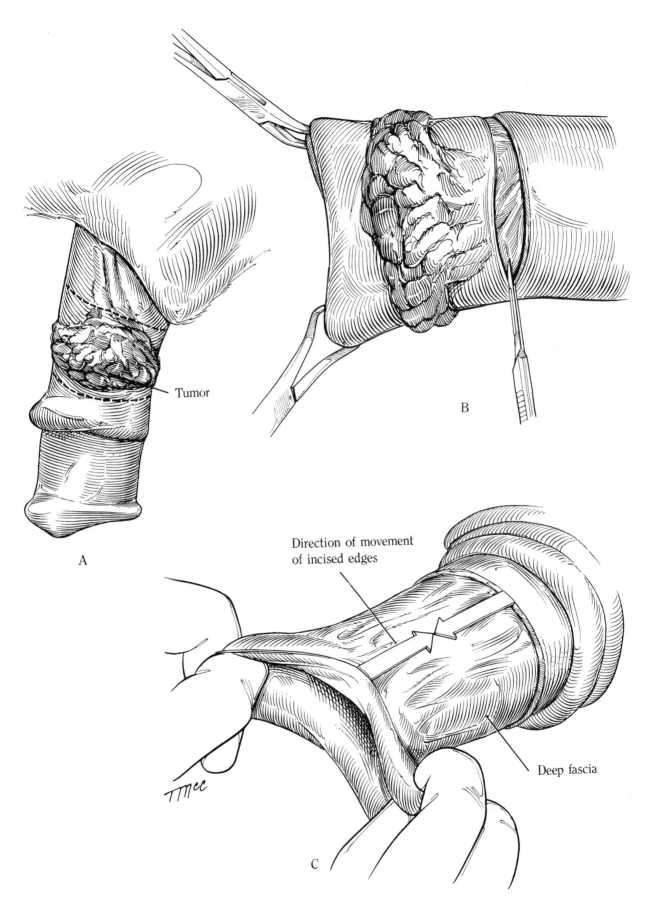

Tumor

**Direction of movement
of incised edges**

Deep fascia

A

B

C

Fig. 10-6. A to D, Circumcision of the penis (reefing).

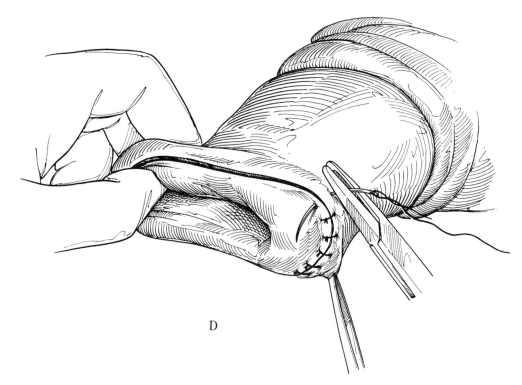

D

Fig. 10-6. *Continued.*

Anesthesia and Surgical Preparation

The horse is positioned in dorsal recumbency under general anesthesia. The penis is prepared for aseptic surgery in a routine manner, and a sterile catheter is passed to identify the urethra. A tourniquet of rubber tubing is applied proximal to the site of amputation (Figure 10-7A). The penis is also extended and stabilized using a gauze loop around the neck of the glans (not illustrated).

Instrumentation

General surgery pack

Surgical Technique

A triangular skin incision is made on the ventral aspect of the penis, and the incision is continued through the fascia and corpus spongiosum (Figure 10-7B). The apex of the triangle is located on the midline in a caudal direction. The triangle has a 3-cm base with sides approximately 4 cm in length. These incisions should extend down to the urethral mucosa, and the connective tissue within the triangle is removed and discarded. With the catheter as a guide, the urethral mucosa is split longitudinally on the midline from the base to the apex of the triangular defect. Then the catheter is removed.

The edges of the urethra are sutured to the skin edges along the sides of the triangular defect using simple interrupted sutures of no. 2-0 glycomer 631 (Caprosyn) (Figure 10-7C). The urethra and penis are then transected. The incision extends from the base of the triangle at a slightly oblique angle craniad toward the dorsal surface of the penis (Figure 10-7D). The principal blood vessels encountered are the branches of the dorsal arteries and veins of the penis that lie between the deep fascia and the tunica albuginea. Other vessels lying in the loose connective tissue beneath the superficial fascia may require ligation.

The tunica albuginea is closed over the transected corpus cavernosum penis using simple interrupted sutures of no. 0 polyglyconate (Maxon) (Figure 10-7E). The first suture is placed in the midline, and the next two sutures bisect these halves. Generally, seven sutures are used, and preplacement of the sutures to minimize excess tension on a single suture is preferable. The transected base of the urethral mucosa is then sutured to the skin using simple interrupted sutures of no. 2-0 glycomer 631 (Caprosyn); these sutures should pass through the underlying stump (Figure 10-7F). Alternatively, the closure can be made in one layer using simple interrupted sutures, with four bites taken through urethral mucosa, ventral and dorsal tunica albuginea, and skin. At this point, the tourniquet is removed.

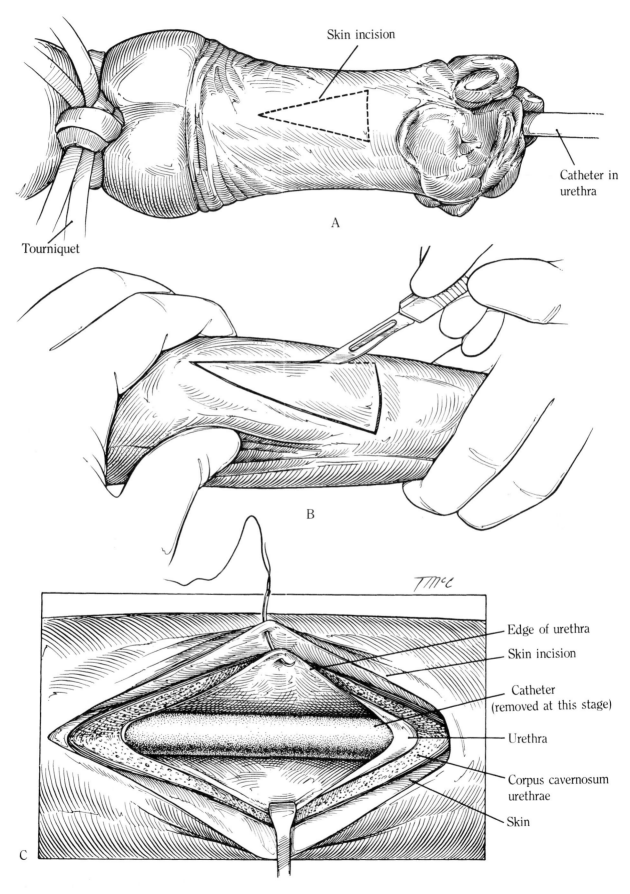

Skin incision

Catheter in
urethra

Tourniquet

A

B

Edge of urethra

Skin incision

Catheter
(removed at this stage)

Urethra

Corpus cavernosum
urethrae

Skin

C

Fig. 10-7. A to F, Amputation of the penis.

177

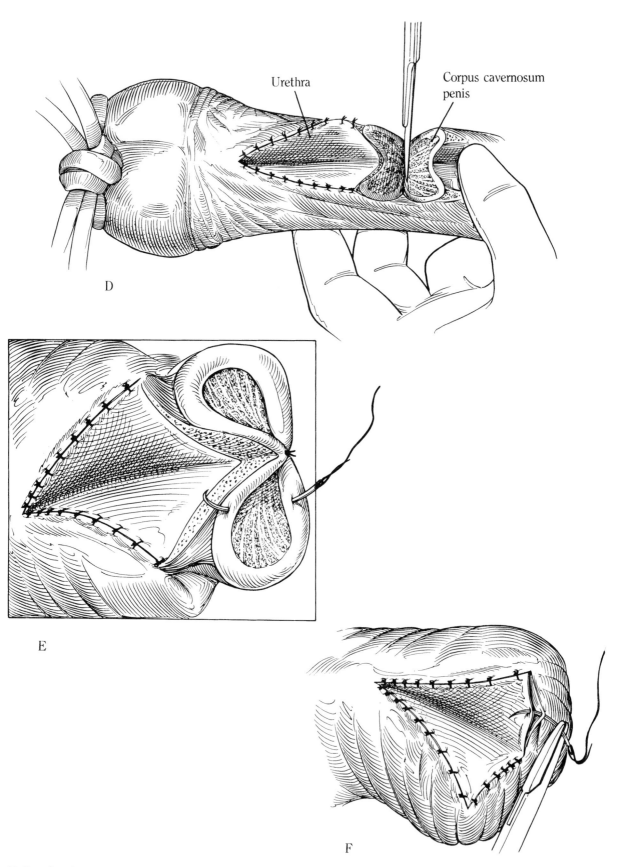

Urethra

Corpus cavernosum penis

D

E

F

Fig. 10-7. *Continued.*

Postoperative Management

Tetanus prophylaxis is administered, and systemic antibiotics may be used for 4 to 5 days. Sutures should be removed in 14 days. A stallion should not be exposed to mares for 4 weeks.

Complications and Prognosis

Complications include edema of the prepuce, hemorrhage, dehiscence, granuloma formation, recurrence of neoplasia, and urethral stenosis.[1,2] Some hemorrhage will be observed following removal of the tourniquet, but excessive hemorrhage can cause a dissecting hematoma and wound breakdown. Minor dehiscence of the suture line, if it occurs, will not cause a significant problem; granulation and epithelialization will occur. Urethral stenosis should not be a problem if the triangulation technique is used. If wound dehiscence is extensive, however, stenosis secondary to fibrosis may result.

Horses treated with penile amputation for squamous cell carcinoma have a favorable prognosis. One study reported a 17% mortality rate due to recurrence.[2]

References

1. Doles, J., Williams, J.W., and Yarbrough, T.B.: Penile amputation and sheath ablation in the horse. Vet. Surg., *30*:327–331, 2001.
2. Mair, T.S., Walmsley, J.P., and Phillips, T.J.: Surgical treatment of 45 horses affected by squamous cell carcinoma of the penis and prepuce. Eq. Vet. J., *32*:406–410, 2000.
3. Walker, D.F., and Vaughan, J.T.: Bovine and Equine Urogenital Surgery. Philadelphia, Lea & Febiger, 1980.

Aanes' Method of Repair of Third-Degree Perineal Laceration

Relevant Anatomy

The relevant anatomy for this procedure was discussed in previous sections of this chapter.

Indications

Perineal lacerations in the mare occur during parturition when the foal's limb(s) or head are forced caudad and dorsad.

The injury is seen predominantly in primiparous mares and is usually due to violent expulsive efforts by the mare in combination with some degree of malposition of the fetus, such as dorsopubic position or footnape posture. The injury is also seen following forced extraction of a large fetus or extraction before full dilation of the birth canal.[4]

First-degree lacerations occur when only the mucosa of the vagina and vulva are involved. Second-degree lacerations occur when the submucosa and muscularis of the vulva, anal sphincter, and the perineal body are involved, but there is no damage to the rectal mucosa. Third-degree perineal lacerations occur when there is tearing through the rectovaginal septum, musculature of the rectum and vagina, and the perineal body (Figure 10-8A).[2] Reconstruction of third-degree perineal lacerations is necessary to return the mare to breeding soundness. The communication between the rectum and vagina results in the constant presence of fecal material in the vagina. Reconstruction is performed occasionally in riding horses to eliminate the unpleasant sound made by air aspirated into the vagina.

Generally, surgery is not performed on an emergency basis. The torn tissues are edematous, necrotic, and grossly contaminated, and it is advisable to wait a minimum of 4 to 6 weeks before attempting repair. Repairs attempted earlier than this are usually unsuccessful. While waiting for repair, the mare should remain under close observation. The excessive straining caused by the injury can lead to prolapse of the viscera, including eversion of the urinary bladder.[5]

The cervix should also be examined for lacerations prior to repair because lacerations of the cervix result in a poor prognosis for return to breeding soundness. Mares with lacerations of the cervix are more susceptible to endometritis and early abortion.[1] Upon discovery of the injury, tetanus immunization should be administered. Some cases may require a course of antibiotics. A preoperative diet of grass hay and alfalfa hay should be commenced to maintain proper fecal consistency. Diets consisting of a low-bulk, highly digestible complete feed, such as Buckeyer Maturity Senior, can reduce the bulk of the feces to minimize stress on the repair.

The following technique is performed in two stages: in the first operation, a shelf is constructed between the rectum and vagina; the second operation involves reconstruction of the perineal body. The aim of two-stage repair is reduction of the incidence of straining and subsequent tearing of sutures. Delaying reconstruction of the perineal body avoids reduction in the size of the rectal lumen, minimizes the accumulation of feces, and reduces the number of muscular contractions necessary to void feces. Moreover, suturing of rectal mucous membrane is avoided in this technique, which decreases straining because of suture irritation.[3] However, many surgeons will choose to complete the reconstruction in one stage, using the same techniques. If the feces are appropriately soft, this can be very successful.

Anesthesia and Surgical Preparation

The mare is tranquilized, is placed in stocks, and an epidural anesthetic is administered (refer to Chapter 2 for details of epidural anesthesia in the horse). The tail is wrapped and tied in a cranial direction to avoid interference during surgery. Feces in the rectum and vagina

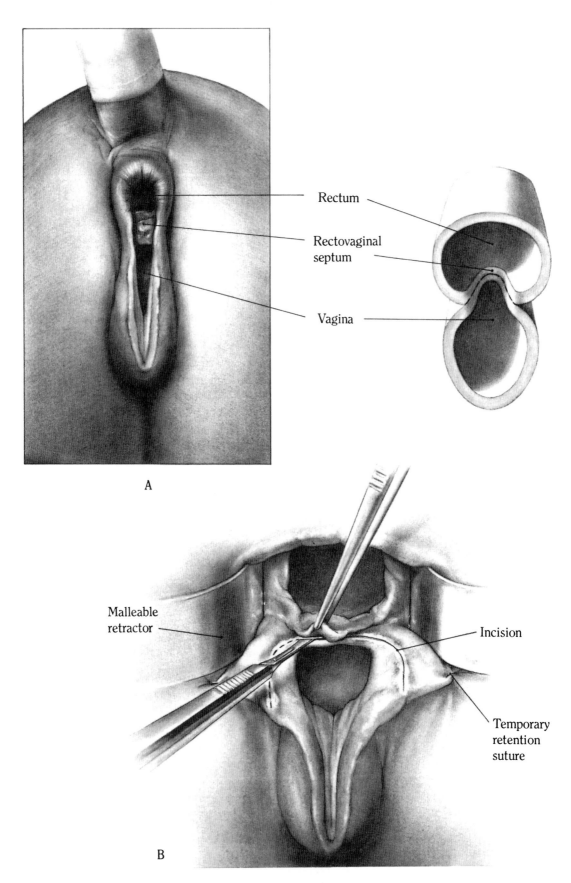

Rectum

Rectovaginal septum

Vagina

A

Malleable retractor

Incision

Temporary retention suture

B

Fig. 10-8. A to H, Aanes' method of repair of third-degree perineal laceration.

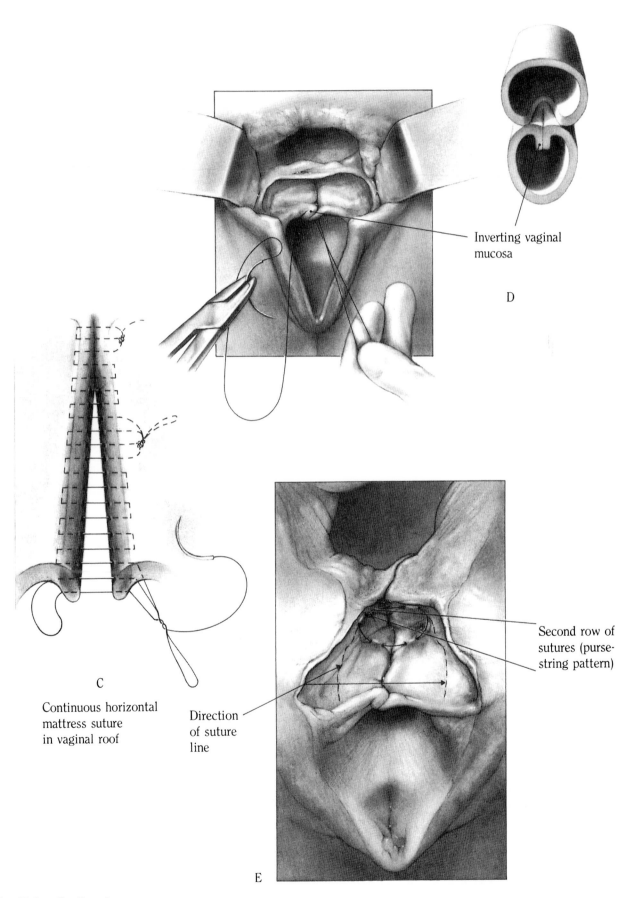

Inverting vaginal
mucosa

D

C

Continuous horizontal
mattress suture
in vaginal roof

Direction
of suture
line

Second row of
sutures (purse-
string pattern)

E

Fig. 10-8. *Continued.*

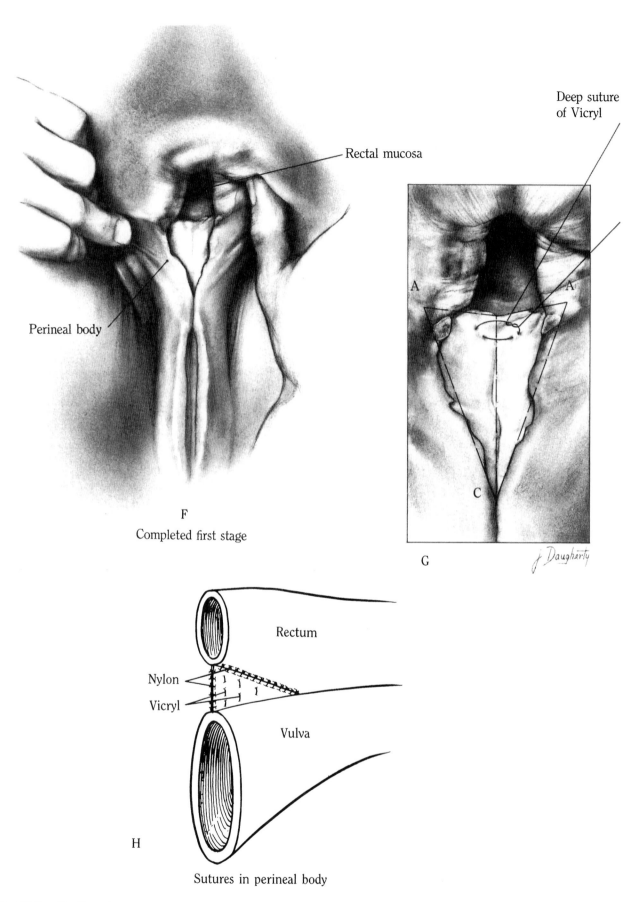

Rectal mucosa

Perineal body

F

Completed first stage

Deep suture
of Vicryl

A   A

C

J Daugherty

G

Rectum

Nylon

Vicryl

Vulva

H

Sutures in perineal body

Fig. 10-8. *Continued.*

are removed manually, and the perineal region is scrubbed with mild soap and water. The rectum and vagina are then cleansed with povidone-iodine solution (Betadine), and excess fluids are absorbed with moistened cotton.

During the first phase of the surgery, two temporary retaining sutures are placed on each side of the laceration, one at the level of the anal sphincter and one near the dorsal commissure of the vulva. These sutures are tied to the skin 8 to 10 cm lateral to the normal position of the anus and vulva. If assistants are available during surgery, they can use a pair of malleable retractors to enhance visualization of the surgical site (Figure 10-8B).

Instrumentation

General surgery pack
Malleable retractors
Long-handled needle holders, thumb forceps, and scalpel handles

Surgical Technique

Stage One

An incision is made along the scar tissue at the junction of the rectal and vaginal mucosa, commencing at the cranial end of the shelf and moving caudad toward the operator. The completed incision should extend from the shelf formed by the intact rectum and vagina, along the scar-tissue margin, to the level of the dorsal commissure of the vulva (Figure 10-8B).

The vaginal mucous membrane and submucosa are reflected ventrad from the line of the incision to form a flap of tissue approximately 2.5 cm wide. At the shelf, the rectum and vaginal mucosa are separated craniad for a distance of 2 to 3 cm. Hemorrhage from the incision is usually minimal and is not a problem.

At this point, the surgeon should determine whether further dissection is necessary by estimating the ease with which the vaginal mucosa can be brought into apposition. The mucosa should form the vaginal roof with minimal tension on the suture material.

Closure of the shelf is commenced by apposing the vaginal roof, using no. 0 polyglyconate, and tying on the midline of the vaginal roof just cranial to the defect. The knot becomes the cranial end of a continuous horizontal mattress suture pattern, inverting the vaginal mucosa and forming the first layer of the repaired roof of the vagina (Figure 10-8C and D).

The suture pattern should penetrate the edges of the vaginal mucous membrane and should be continued caudad for one-third to half the laceration. The suture is tied and is tucked into the vagina until it is needed later in the repair (Figure 10-8C).

A second row of sutures of no. 0 or 1-polyglyconate (Maxon) is placed between the rectum and the vaginal wall. The suture is essentially a purse-string pattern,

passing through the rectal submucosa, perivaginal tissue, and vaginal submucosa on both sides of the common vault. Each suture is tied immediately after it is placed (Figure 10-8E).

When the interrupted sutures are placed as far caudally as the newly sutured vaginal roof, the continuous horizontal mattress pattern of polyglyconate is resumed, and the vaginal mucosa is sutured in a caudal direction to the dorsal commissure of the vulva (Figure 10-8C). The interrupted sutures are continued caudad to the dorsal commissure of the vulva; one should keep the overall direction of this row horizontal. This method avoids narrowing of the rectal lumen. Sutures should not be placed in the rectal mucous membrane (Figure 10-8F).

Following the first stage of the operation, the mare should receive antibiotics for about 5 days. Approximately 2 weeks of healing should be allowed before proceeding with the second stage of the operation. Any exposed polyglactin 910 sutures should be removed a few days before the second operation. Conversely, the second stage can be performed immediately. A single stage repair is preferred by the author.

Stage Two

Surgical preparation and anesthesia for the second stage of the procedure are similar to those for the first stage. The retrovestibular shelf is examined for healing, and if a small, granulating fistula remains, the second stage should be delayed until it is healed. When a large fistula remains, the shelf is converted to a third-degree perineal laceration, and the first stage is repeated. Local infiltration of lidocaine can be used, rather than epidural anesthesia.

To obtain fresh surfaces for reconstruction and healing of the perineal body, the newly formed epithelialized tissue must be removed. An incision that commences at the cranial margin of the perineal body is made; it extends peripherally along the scar tissue margin and ends at the dorsal commissure of the vulva, forming two sides of a triangle. An incision is made on the opposite side, and a superficial layer of epithelium is removed, creating two raw, triangular surfaces. The skin of the perineum is undermined and is reflected laterad to permit subsequent closure of the skin without undue tension (Figure 10-8G). This step is not necessary if the reconstruction is performed in a single stage.

Closure of the deep layers of the perineal body should commence cranially with simple interrupted sutures of no. 0 or 1-polyglyconate (Maxon). This closure is completed with simple interrupted sutures of 2-0 polyglyconate placed within the epithelial edges of the rectum. The sutures are placed alternately until reconstruction of the perineal body is completed. No attempt is made to locate and to suture the ends of the anal sphincter muscle because they are usually surrounded by scar tissue. The dorsal portion of the vulvar lips is removed just as in Caslick's operation for pneumovagina. The skin of the perineum and lips of the vulva are closed with interrupted sutures of 2-0 nylon or polyglyconate (Figure 10-8H).

Postoperative Management

The mare is put back on a low bulk feed, such as Buckeye Maturity Senior, immediately after the operation. A stool softener, such as mineral oil, should be administered for at least a week. Antibiotics are administered for 5 days, and any nonabsorbable sutures in the perineum and lips of the vulva are removed 14 days after surgery.

Following healing, the mare should be examined for endometritis and treated accordingly. A uterine biopsy may be indicated. Natural service should be postponed for 6 months to allow the region to attain some strength. Some mares require artificial insemination because of a marked reduction in the size of the vulvar opening.

Complications and Prognosis

The complications of this surgery include dehiscence, abscessation and cellulitis, constipation, and fistula formation. Excessive straining after surgery can result from cystitis or fecal impaction of the rectum.[6] This should be treated with epidural analgesia or tranquilization. Urine pooling may occur due to excessive closure of the vulvar cleft or poor perineal conformation and may require one of the urethral extension operations described elsewhere in this chapter.

In most cases, the prognosis for future pregnancies following successful repair of a third-degree perineal laceration is excellent. A fertility rate of approximately 75% can be expected.[4] Recurrence of third-degree perineal lacerations at subsequent parturitions ranges from no injury to another third-degree perineal laceration. It is advisable to have an attendant present during future foalings to minimize the severity of damage in case dystocia occurs.[1]

References

1. Aanes, W.A.: Personal communication, 1981.
2. Aanes, W.A.: Surgical repair of third-degree perineal laceration and rectovaginal fistula in the mare. J. Am. Vet. Med. Assoc., *144*:485, 1964.
3. Aanes, W.A.: Progress in rectovaginal surgery. *In* Proceedings of the 19th Annual Convention of the American Association of Equine Practitioners in 1973: 1974, p. 225.
4. Colbern, G.T., Aanes, W.A., and Stashak, T.S.: Surgical management of perineal lacerations and rectovestibular fistulae in the mare: a retrospective study of 47 cases. J. Am. Vet. Med. Assoc., *186*:265, 1985.
5. Haynes, P.F., and McClure, J.R.: Eversion of the urinary bladder: a sequel to third degree perineal laceration in the mare. Vet. Surg., *9*:66, 1980.
6. Schumacher, J.: Perineal injuries of the horse. *In* Proceedings of the 6th Annual Convention of American College of Veterinary Surgeons in 1996, p. 205.

Chapter 11

SURGERY OF THE EQUINE UPPER RESPIRATORY TRACT

Objectives

1. Describe common upper respiratory surgical techniques, including tracheostomy, laryngotomy, two techniques for ventriculectomy and ventriculocordectomy, partial resection of the soft palate, and two surgical techniques for entry into the guttural pouches to facilitate drainage.
2. Discuss the indications and alternative treatments for each procedure.

Tracheostomy

Relevant Anatomy

The incision site for this procedure follows the ventral median of the proximal one-third of the neck, approximately 3 cm distad to the cricoid cartilage, or at the point where the sternocephalicus and omohyoideus muscle bellies diverge and converge, respectively. To visualize the trachea, the muscle bellies of the sternothyroideus and sternohyoideus, which lie on the ventral aspect of the trachea, will be separated. From this point, the tracheal rings will be visible. Dorsolateral to the proximal half of the trachea are the common carotid artery, the vagosympathetic trunk, and the recurrent laryngeal nerve, which are all enclosed in the carotid sheath.[4]

Indications

Tracheostomy may be performed on an emergency or an elective basis. Emergency situations include obstructions of the upper airway, such as those caused by rattlesnake bite, regional lymph node abscessation due to *Streptococcus equi* infection, nasopharyngeal neoplasia, excessive guttural pouch distention with inspissated pus, or postsurgical edema. Elective tracheostomy may be performed

following nasal surgery, such as nasal septum resection or laryngeal surgery, or whenever postoperative respiratory obstruction is anticipated. It is also indicated for retrograde pharyngoscopy and endotracheal intubation to permit arytenoidectomy or surgery in the oral cavity,[1] as well as to provide oxygen insufflation into the trachea during any hypoxic crisis.[3] In elective situations, the tracheotomy may be temporary or permanent as well.

Anesthesia and Surgical Preparation

Elective tracheostomy is usually performed with the horse sedated in a standing position, preferably in the stocks so that the head may be supported with the neck extended. A 3-in × 6-in rectangle of hair is clipped over the middle third of the neck and the area is scrubbed surgically. The surgical site is anesthetized by infusing local anesthetic in either a 10-cm line or an inverted "U" pattern beginning from about the 5th tracheal ring and extending dorsally over the 2nd tracheal ring[2] (Figure 11-1A).

Instrumentation

General surgery pack
Tracheostomy tube

Surgical Technique

The surgical site is variable, but it is generally at the junction of the middle and upper third of the neck (approximately the 2nd to 5th tracheal rings). With the operator standing on the right side of the horse (the reverse for a left-handed operator), a 10-cm incision is made through the skin and subcutaneous tissue; this is facilitated by tensing the skin at the proximal end of the incision with the left hand and making the skin incision with the right hand (Figure 11-1B). Following incision of the skin and subcutaneous tissues, the bellies of the sternothyrohyoideus muscles are visible. These muscle bellies are bluntly divided in the midline with scissors or the tip of a

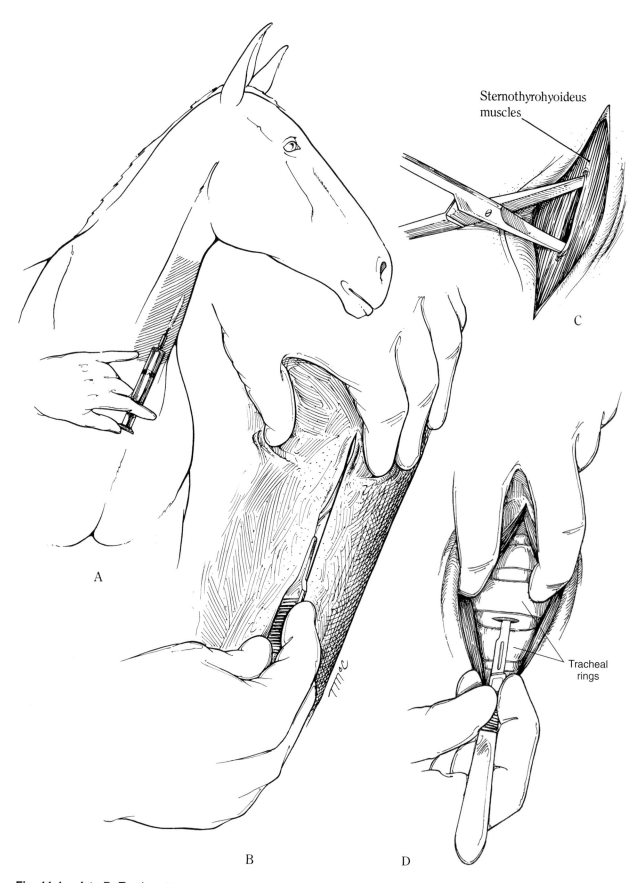

Sternothyrohyoideus
muscles

C

Tracheal
rings

A

B   D

Fig. 11-1. A to D, Tracheostomy.

hard-backed scalpel (Figure 11-1C). Then the tracheal rings are identified. The scalpel is inserted midway between two of the tracheal rings with a sharp thrust. This incision is made in a horizontal direction about 1 cm in either direction from the midline (no more than one-third the circumference of the trachea) (Figure 11-1D); when the incision is completed, the tracheostomy tube can be inserted. This method is used when a tracheostomy tube will be left in place for a short period of time. Generally, the incision is not closed and will heal well by secondary intention after the tracheostomy tube is removed.

Postoperative Management

The tracheostomy site should be cleaned daily with a sterile physiologic solution, such as saline solution. The area can be dressed with a suitable, nonirritating, triple antibiotic ointment at the same time. When the tracheostomy tube is in place, it should be removed and cleaned once or twice daily, depending on the amount of accumulated secretions. The site will usually heal uneventfully by secondary intention.

Complications and Prognosis

In an emergency situation, such as when the animal is in danger of suffocation, the surgeon may need to forego a complete aseptic preparation, which may predispose the animal to infection. Occasionally, subcutaneous emphysema develops where air is trapped between the wound edges and dissects along fascial planes. This condition is usually self-limiting, and its chances of occurrence are minimized by handling tissues gently and not dissecting around either side of the trachea. Tracheal stenosis is a potential complication of this surgery, and its likelihood depends on the length of time the tracheostomy tube is left in place and the width of the incision between the tracheal rings.

References

1. Gabel, A.A.: A method of surgical repair of the fractured mandible in the horse. J. Am. Vet. Med. Assoc., 155:1831, 1969.
2. McClure, S.R., Taylor, T.S., Honnas, C.M., Schumacher, J., Chaffin, M.K., and Hoffman, A.G.: Permanent tracheostomy in standing horses: technique and results. Vet. Surg., 24:231–234, 1995.
3. Moore, J.N., et al.: Tracheostomy in the horse. Arch. Am. Coll. Vet. Surg., 7:35, 1977.
4. Stick, J.A.: Trachea, In Equine Surgery, 3rd Ed. Edited by J.A. Auer and J.A. Stick. St. Louis, Saunders, pp. 608–615, 2006.

Laryngotomy, Laryngeal Ventriculectomy, and Ventriculocordectomy

Relevant Anatomy

The larynx is comprised of the unpaired cricoid, thyroid, and epiglottic cartilages and the paired arytenoid cartilages. The arytenoid cartilages articulate with the lateral surfaces of the cricoid cartilage, thus facilitating the dorsolateral and axial rotation of the arytenoids during adduction and abduction. This allows the glottis to completely close during swallowing and open maximally during exercise. If this movement is impaired, upper airway function during exercise may be compromised, resulting in respiratory noise (roaring), poor performance, and exercise intolerance. The arytenoid cartilages are particularly susceptible to inflammation and injury, which may result in exercise-induced respiratory noise, known as *roaring*, or paralysis in a condition known as *laryngeal hemiplegia*.

Indications

Laryngeal ventriculectomy is indicated for the treatment of laryngeal hemiplegia. It may be performed alone in some cases, or, in conjunction with laryngoplasty, which is described in *Equine Surgery: Advanced Techniques*.[9] Other surgical treatments for laryngeal hemiplegia include ventriculocordectomy, partial or full arytenoidectomy, and laryngeal reinnervation.[12] The degree of surgical treatment and the most appropriate technique necessary to produce the desired results in the patient are largely dependent on the use of the horse, the horse's level of performance, and the grade of laryngeal movements.[12] For the purpose of this text, ventriculectomy and ventriculocordectomy will be described.

Ventriculectomy, or sacculectomy, consists of the removal of the mucous membrane lining the laryngeal ventricle. This technique is accomplished by performing a laryngotomy through the cricoid membrane. Ventriculocordectomy is essentially a sacculectomy with the additional removal of a small wedge of tissue from the leading edge of the vocal fold.[13] Ventriculocordectomy is indicated for horses affected by vocal fold collapse and some show and draft horses with laryngeal hemiplegia. The technique of laryngotomy described here is also used for partial resection of the soft palate,[1] arytenoidectomy,[14] and the surgical treatment of epiglottic entrapment,[2] pharyngeal cysts,[2] or lymphoid hyperplasia.[2]

Ventriculectomy and ventriculocordectomy are not indicated alone for treatment of laryngeal hemiplegia in sport horses or racehorses, because they will not produce abduction of the arytenoid cartilages and alleviate airway obstruction in these horses.[12] These procedures are, however, appropriate in animals in which the arytenoid cartilage is not adducted beyond the normal resting position, so the larynx appears symmetric at rest. For some show horses, these treatments will provide satisfactory reduction of respiratory noise by reducing soft tissue collapse during exercise.[12] Laryngoplasty is used when endoscopic examination shows that the arytenoid cartilage is displaced medially from the resting position. In these cases, ventriculectomy alone will not provide sufficient abduction of the vocal cord. Laryngoplasty involves the additional insertion of a laryngeal prosthesis to abduct the arytenoid cartilage and vocal cord and is often indicated in severe cases of laryngeal hemiplegia.[8]

Laser-assisted ventriculectomy and ventriculocordectomy, either alone or in conjunction with laryngoplasty, are indicated for treatment of specific cases of laryngeal hemiplegia, as previously described. Although laser-assisted surgical techniques are considered advanced, they will be discussed here because they are important alternatives to many of the traditionally performed upper respiratory surgical techniques. This technique is usually performed using a neodymium:yttrium garnet or diode laser transendoscopically through an oral approach or by performing a laryngotomy. The transendoscopic laser-guided technique does not require a laryngotomy, and therefore it reduces anesthesia and convalescence time. Laser vocal cordectomy has been described as a potential treatment for laryngeal hemiplegia, but it has not been shown to reduce respiratory noise as effectively as ventriculocordectomy.[3]

Anesthesia and Surgical Preparation

Laryngotomy and ventriculectomy may be performed with the horse under general anesthesia and in dorsal recumbency or with the standing animal sedated and injected with local analgesic at the surgical site. Prior to surgery (ideally, 4 hours prior), patients are given 2 g of phenylbutazone intravenously to minimize postoperative laryngeal edema. The surgical area at the caudal aspect of the mandible is clipped and prepared aseptically (Figure 11-2A).

To perform the endoscopically guided ventriculectomy, the horse is placed in standing stocks and sedated with 0.3 mg xylazine HCl. A jugular catheter is placed and a continuous infusion of 20 mg detomidine in 1 L polyionic fluids is used to maintain sedation. A flexible endoscope is passed nasally, and 20 ml of 2% carbocaine is used to bathe the surgery area.

Instrumentation

General surgery pack
Self-retaining retractor (Gelpi, Weitlaner, or Hobday's roaring retractor)
Laryngeal bur
Tracheostomy tube
Laser with fiber (980 nm diode laser with 3 m/600 m fiber preferred)
Protective eyewear

Surgical Technique

Ventriculectomy and Ventriculocordectomy

A skin incision centered at the caudal aspect of the mandible, approximately 10 cm long, is made from the surface of the cricoid cartilage to beyond the junction of the thyroid cartilages (Figure 11-2A). In some instances, the triangular depression between the thyroid cartilages and cricoid cartilage can be felt before the skin incision is made. When this is not possible, the central area of the skin incision is located by placing a horizontal line across the area where the rami of the mandible merge with the neck. The skin incision exposes the midline between the sternothyrohyoideus muscles, which are separated with scissors to expose the cricothyroid membrane. After initial separation with scissors, the muscles may be retracted digitally for the length of the skin incision. The cricothyroid membrane is cleared of adipose tissue, and at this stage, it may be necessary to ligate a small vein that commonly is present in the surgical site. The cricothyroid membrane is then incised, commencing with a stab incision, to penetrate the laryngeal mucosa (Figure 11-2B). The incision is then extended longitudinally from the cricoid cartilage caudad to the junction of the thyroid cartilages cranially. The wings of the thyroid cartilages are retracted with a self-retaining retractor (Gelpi, Weitlaner, or Hobday's roaring retractor).

If a small-diameter, cuffed endotracheal tube is used, ventriculectomy may be performed with the endotracheal tube in place; otherwise, removal of the tube will be necessary for identification of the laryngeal saccule and ventriculectomy. The laryngeal ventricle is identified by sliding the index finger craniad off the edge of the vocal cord and turning the finger laterad and downward toward the base of the ear to enter the ventricle. The laryngeal bur is passed into the ventricle as deeply as possible and twisted to grasp the mucosa (Figure 11-2C). A sagittal section of the larynx showing the location of the laryngeal ventricle is illustrated in Figure 11-2D. When the operator believes that the mucosa is engaged in the bur, the bur is carefully withdrawn from the ventricle by everting the ventricular mucosa (Figure 11-2E). At this stage, it is advisable to place a pair of forceps on the everted mucosa to avoid tearing or slippage as the mucosa is fully retracted. The forceps are attached to the mucosa, the bur is untwisted and removed, and the ventricular saccule is completely everted using traction. With retraction maintained by Ochsner forceps or a similar instrument placed across the saccule, the everted mucous membrane is resected with scissors as close to the base as possible without damaging associated cartilage (Figure 11-2F). It is common to perform the ventriculectomy bilaterally, but the clinical problem is usually associated with the left side. Following excision of the ventricle, any tags of remaining mucous membrane are removed. To perform a ventriculocordectomy, an additional 2-cm long and

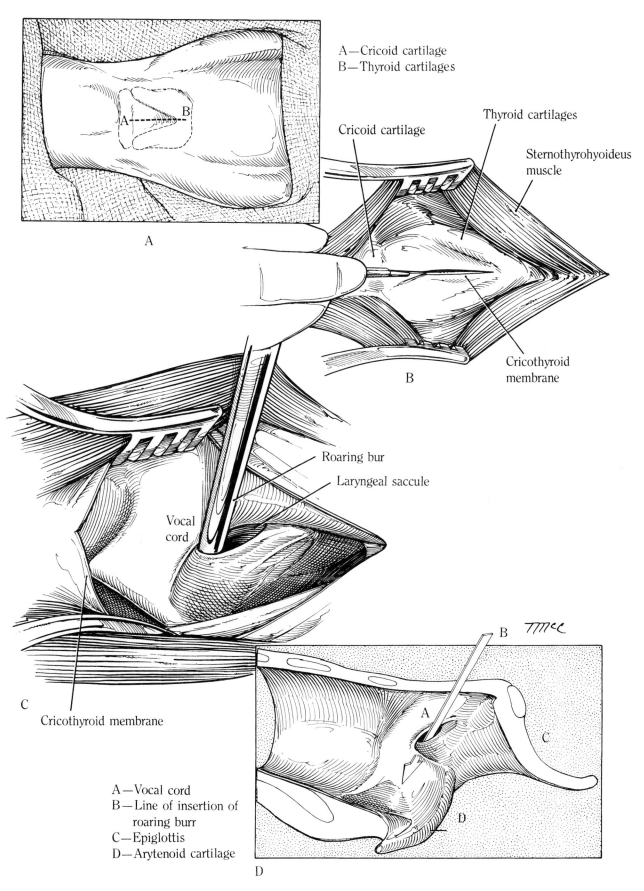

A—Cricoid cartilage
B—Thyroid cartilages

A

Cricoid cartilage

Thyroid cartilages

Sternothyrohyoideus muscle

Cricothyroid membrane

B

Roaring bur

Laryngeal saccule

Vocal cord

C

Cricothyroid membrane

B

A

C

D

A—Vocal cord
B—Line of insertion of roaring burr
C—Epiglottis
D—Arytenoid cartilage

D

Fig. 11-2. A to H, Laryngotomy, laryngeal ventriculectomy, laser ventriculocordectomy.

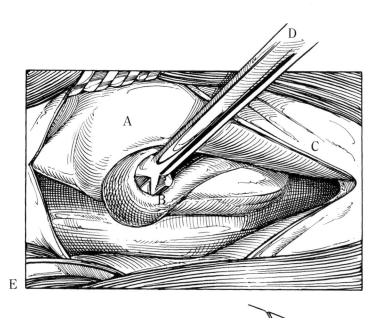

A—Vocal cord
B—Eversion of laryngeal
    saccule
C—Cricothyroid membrane
D—Roaring bur

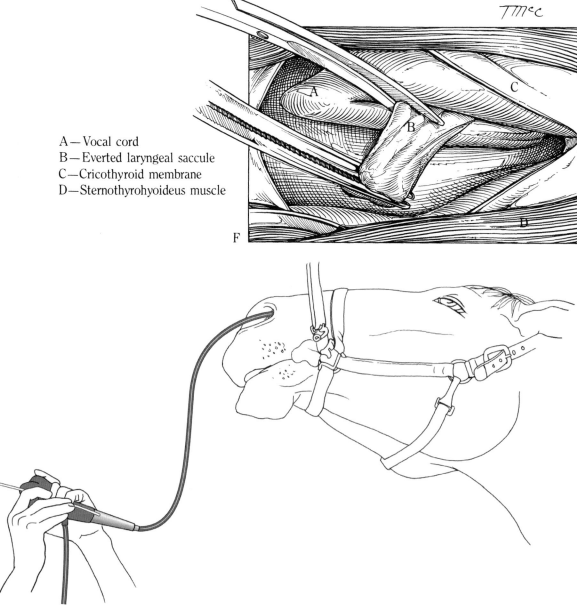

A—Vocal cord
B—Everted laryngeal saccule
C—Cricothyroid membrane
D—Sternothyrohyoideus muscle

Fig. 11-2. *Continued.*

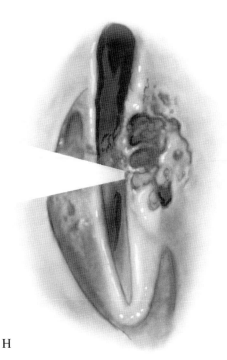

H

Fig. 11-2. *Continued.*

2-mm wide crescent-shaped wedge is excised from the leading edge of the adjacent vocal fold after performing ventriculectomy.[13] The abaxial edge of the vocal fold and the axial border of the ventricle may be opposed and sutured using 2-0 PDS. This serves to limit hemorrhage and lessen cicatrix formation and redundant tissue folds.[13] Many surgeons do not close the mucosa.

The cricothyroid membrane is closed using 3-0 polyglytone 6211 (Caprosyn). The rest of the laryngotomy incision is not sutured, but is left open, because the respiratory tract mucosa cannot be aseptically prepared, and contamination of the incision can occur with subsequent infection and abscessation as potential problems. The laryngotomy wounds heal satisfactorily by secondary intention; therefore, suturing this wound is not considered justifiable. Conversely, a tracheostomy tube can remain in the laryngotomy site while the horse recovers from anesthesia.

Laser Ventriculectomy/Ventriculocordectomy

The laser fiber is placed through the biopsy channel of the flexible endoscope and the endoscope placed into the nasal passage of the horse (Figure 11-2G). The laser is set at 15 watts, and the laser fiber extended through the end of the scope. The laser should never be fired if the fiber tip is not easily seen on the monitor. Because the fiber lasers create significant collateral damage, only the surface mucosa need be ablated (Figure 11-2H). In many instances, both ventricles are ablated along with the vocal cords to minimize noise after surgery. Care should be taken to avoid lasering the most ventral commissure of the vocal folds to reduce the chance of cicatrix formation. There is no laryngotomy incision to care for using this approach.

Postoperative Management

Antibiotics are not administered routinely. The laryngotomy wound is cleaned twice daily. The animal is confined for the 2 to 3 weeks it takes for the wound to heal. After this period, the horse is hand-walked. The horse may be put back to work 8 weeks following surgery.

The tracheostomy tube is usually left in the laryngotomy opening until the patient recovers from anesthesia. If there is undue trauma during surgery—more likely with some of the more involved procedures performed by a laryngotomy approach—it may be advisable to leave the tracheostomy tube in place in case laryngeal edema develops. We do not perform a separate tracheostomy without a specific, critical indication.

Complications and Prognosis

Ventriculectomy or ventriculocordectomy performed alone has less risk of complications than these procedures performed in conjunction with laryngoplasty, described in *Advanced Techniques of Equine Surgery*.[9] Overall, the success rate and prognosis for this procedure has improved over the last 30 years, but it is still generally subjective and varies with the individual's definition of a satisfactory result. A 1970 study reported improvement in 80% of horses that received ventriculectomies, but fewer than 10% had results in which the obstruction was relieved and rendered the horse's breathing "audibly indistinguishable, to the critical ear, from an unaffected horse at all paces."[7] Another study, which defined success of the operation by the horse's ability to perform work in a manner satisfactory to the owner, reported a success rate of 60 to 70%.[10] More recent studies report a higher success rate; in draft horses, ventriculectomy alone significantly improved athletic performance to a level deemed satisfactory by owners in 87% of these horses.[1] Postoperative complications are rare and generally minor.[4] The most common reported complication of laryngoplasty is coughing, which may be performance limiting in some horses.[5]

Complications associated with laser ventriculectomy and ventriculocordectomy are generally few, and in general, horses will ingest food and water without apparent discomfort in 6 hours postoperatively.[6,11] Thermal damage to surrounding tissue, inadequate removal of ventricular mucosa due to poor visualization, excessive tissue sloughing, mucocele formation, laser burns to the contralateral vocal cord, and arytenoid cartilage necrosis have been documented following laser ventriculocordectomy, however.[6,11] Complete healing of the surgical site was affirmed by endoscopic evaluation at 47 days postoperatively.[6]

References

1. Bohanon, T.C., Beard, W.L., and Robertson, J.T.: Laryngeal hemiplegia in draft horses. A review of 27 cases. Vet. Surg., 19:456–459, 1990.
2. Boles, C.: Treatment of upper airway abnormalities. Vet. Clin. North Am. (Large Anim. Pract.), 1:127, 1979.
3. Brown, J.A., Derksen, F.J., Stick, J.A., et al.: Laser vocal cordectomy fails to effectively reduce respiratory noise in horses with laryngeal hemiplegia. Vet. Surg., 34:247–252, 2005.
4. Brown, J.A., Derksen, F.J., Stick, J.A., et al.: Ventriculocordectomy reduces respiratory noise in horses with laryngeal hemiplegia. Eq. Vet. J., 35:570–574, 2003.
5. Davenport, C.L.M., Tulleners, E.P., and Parente, E.J.: The effect of recurrent laryngeal neurectomy in conjunction with laryngoplasty and unilateral ventriculocordectomy in Thoroughbred racehorses. Vet. Surg., 30:417–421, 2001.
6. Hawkins, J.F., and Andrews-Jones, L.: Neodymium:yttrium aluminum garnet laser ventriculocordectomy in standing horses. Am. J. Vet. Res., 62:531–537, 2001.
7. Marks, D., et al.: Observations on laryngeal hemiplegia in the horse and treatment by abductor muscle prosthesis. Eq. Vet. J., 2:159, 1970.
8. Marks, D., et al.: Use of a prosthetic device for surgical correction of laryngeal hemiplegia in horses. J. Am. Vet. Med. Assoc., 157:157, 1970.
9. McIlwraith, C.W., and Robertson, J.T.: McIlwraith & Turner's Equine Surgery: Advanced Techniques. Baltimore, Williams & Wilkins, 1998.
10. Raker, C.W.: Laryngotomy and laryngeal sacculectomy. 3rd Annual Surgical Forum: Chicago, 1975.
11. Shires, G.M.H., Adair, H.S., and Patton, S.: Preliminary study of laryngeal sacculectomy in horses, using a neodymium: yttrium aluminum garnet laser technique. Am. J. Vet. Res., 51:1247–1249, 1990.
12. Stick, J.A.: Larynx. In Equine Surgery, 3rd Ed. Edited by J.A. Auer and J.A. Stick. St. Louis, Saunders, 2006, pp. 608–616.
13. Stick, J.A.: Ventriculocordectomy. Ninth Annual ACVS Veterinary Symposium. Sept. 30–Oct. 3, 1999.
14. White, N.A., and Blackwell, R.B.: Partial arytenoidectomy in the horse. Vet. Surg., 9:5, 1980.

Partial Resection of the Soft Palate

Relevant Anatomy

The soft palate forms the floor of the nasopharynx and extends from the caudal border of the hard palate to the base of the larynx. The soft palate itself is comprised of oral and nasopharyngeal mucous membranes, the palatine gland and associated ductile openings, the palatine aponeurosis, and the palatinus and palatopharyngeus muscles.[4] At its most caudal-free margin, the soft palate continues dorsally to form two lateral pillars that join to form the palatopharyngeal arch, named for the palatinus muscle of which the pillars are composed.[4] The position of the soft palate is largely controlled by the surrounding intrinsic musculature; the tensor veli palatini, levator veli palatini, palitinus, and palatopharyngeus muscles. All are innervated by the pharyngeal branch of the vagus nerve except for the tensor veli palatinus muscle, which is supplied by the mandibular branch of the trigeminal nerve.[6]

Indications

Partial resection of the soft palate is indicated in certain cases of dorsal displacement of the soft palate (DDSP) or for the resection of granulomas and cysts from the caudal-free edge of the palate.[4] The etiology of DDSP is not completely understood, and it is probable that there are many inciting factors involved. DDSP may arise from a neuropathy of the pharyngeal branch of the vagus nerve[7] or secondary to conditions that involve the vagus nerves, such as guttural pouch mycosis or retropharyngeal lymphadenopathy, and in association with a hypoplastic epiglottis. The most common form of soft palate displacement is intermittent, however, and is usually associated with exercise.[1] It is a clinical impression that the condition may also accompany generalized inflammation of the pharynx. In these cases, the soft palate displacement may resolve itself on resolution of the inflammatory problem. Both so-called paresis and elongation have been postulated as causes, but not proved. Some horses with intermittent dorsal displacement of the soft palate above the epiglottis respond to tongue-tying, which prevents complete retraction of the tongue.[5] Cook has postulated that the basis of the condition is a temporary subluxation of the larynx, which becomes displaced in relation to the soft palate.[3]

Partial resection of the soft palate is not a panacea for dorsal displacement of the soft palate, but it has been described as a method of treatment in horses that do not respond to conservative therapy.[2] Surgical patients should be selected carefully. Other primary causes of the problem should be eliminated, and caution must be used because tranquilizers increase the tendency for soft palate displacement. A flexible endoscope in the caudal portion of the pharynx may interfere with the normal act of deglutition and may lead to an erroneous diagnosis. When the condition is the result of a hypoplastic epiglottis or guttural pouch mycosis with nerve involvement, soft palate surgery is not indicated.

Anesthesia and Surgical Preparation

The horse is prepared for laryngotomy as previously described. In this case, the surgery is always performed with the horse under general anesthesia and in dorsal recumbency.

Instrumentation

General surgery pack
Self-retaining retractor such as a Gelpi, Weitlaner, or
    Hobday's roaring retractor

Surgical Technique

Laryngotomy is performed as previously described. In some instances, the body of the thyroid cartilage may be sectioned to extend the laryngotomy incision and to provide additional exposure. If the thyroid cartilage is sectioned, one should be careful not to incise the epiglottis, which is in close association with the thyroid cartilage. Splitting the thyroid cartilage is not performed routinely in this procedure.

When laryngotomy is completed, the endotracheal tube must be withdrawn into the mouth to enable one to visualize the soft palate. The concave, U-shaped free border of the soft palate will be observed rostrally (Figure 11-3A). Allis tissue forceps are placed on each side of the soft palate, approximately 1 cm from the midline, and the positioning is checked for symmetry (Figure 11-3B). An incision into the soft palate with Metzenbaum scissors is made on the right side beside the forceps; this incision is extended toward the midline in a semicircular fashion so that, at the midline, it is about 1 cm from the central free border of the soft palate (Figure 11-3C). This procedure is repeated on the left side of the soft palate, so a piece of tissue approximately 2 cm × 1 cm is removed from the central free area of the soft palate. Hemorrhage is negligible, and no attempt is made to suture the soft palate. Alternatively, the resection of tissue can be made in a V-fashion, rather than in crescentic fashion. The cricothyroid membrane is closed with 3-0 polyglytone 6211 (Caprosyn) in a simple continuous pattern while the rest of the laryngotomy incision is left to heal by second intention.

Soft palate resection should be conservative. It is better to subject the animal to a second surgical procedure for resection of additional soft palate than to resect excessive tissue initially, because excessive resection can result in a bilateral nasal discharge of mucus and food material and, possibly, aspiration pneumonia.

Postoperative Management

The horse is confined to a stall until the laryngotomy incision is completely healed and should rest for 4 weeks before being placed into work. Antiinflammatory medication may be administered for 3 days and systemic antibiotic therapy may be administered for up to a week. The incision site should be cleaned twice daily until it is healed.

Complications and Prognosis

Based on his theory of the pathogenesis of dorsal displacement of the soft palate, Cook has advocated sternothyrohyoideus myectomy.[3] A preliminary study of this treatment in 21 racehorses showed that 17 of them (71%) benefited from this operation. Approximately two-thirds of horses undergoing resection of the soft palate have

improved sufficiently for racing purposes.[3] This operation is simple to perform, has fewer potential complications, and requires less convalescence than other procedures. It is described in *Advanced Techniques of Equine Surgery*.[8]

References

1. Boles, C.: Abnormalities of the upper respiratory tract. Vet. Clin. North. Am.: Large Anim. Pract., 1:89, 1979.
2. Boles, C.L.: Treatment of airway abnormalities. Vet. Clin. North Am.: Large Anim. Pract., 1:727, 1979.
3. Cook, W.R.: The biomechanics of choking in the horse. In Proceedings of the 40th Annual Conference for Veterinarians. Fort Collins, Colorado State University, 1979, p. 129.
4. Ducharme, N.G.: Pharynx. In Equine Surgery, 3rd Ed. Edited by J.A. Auer and J.A. Stick. St. Louis, Saunders, pp. 544–566.
5. Franklin, S.H., Naylor, J.R., and Lane, J.G.: The effect of a tongue-tie in horses with dorsal displacement of the soft palate. Eq. Vet. J. Suppl., 34:430–433, 2002.
6. Holcombe, S.J., Derksen, F.J., Stick, J.A., et al.: Bilateral nerve blockade of the pharyngeal branch of the vagus nerve produces persistent soft palate dysfunction in horses. Am. J. Vet. Res., 59:504–508, 1998.
7. Holcombe, S.J., Derksen, F.J., Stick, J.A., and Robinson, N.E.: Pathophysiology of dorsal displacement of the soft palate in horses. Eq. Vet. J. Suppl., 30:45–48, 1999.
8. McIlwraith, C.W., and Robertson, J.T.: McIlwraith & Turner's Equine Surgery: Advanced Techniques, 2nd Edition. Baltimore, Williams & Wilkins, 1998.

Surgical Entry and Drainage of the Guttural Pouches

Relevant Anatomy

The guttural pouches exist as paired, air-filled, diverticula of the eustachian tubes, which connect the middle ear to the pharynx. Guttural pouches are unique to horses and originate from the midline, dorsocaudal to the pharynx. The stylohyoid bone divides each pouch into lateral and medial portions, and a funnel-shaped opening, the pharyngeal orifice, serves to communicate with the pharynx.[4] The mucous membrane lining of the pouch contains the facial, glossopharyngeal, vagus, spinal accessory, and hypoglossal nerves as well as the cranial sympathetic trunk, internal carotid artery, and branches of the external carotid artery.[4]

Indications

Each of the three surgical approaches to the guttural pouches has particular uses, advantages, and disadvantages. Viborg's triangle approach is used mainly for drainage of the guttural pouch in cases of empyema. It may also be used for the treatment of guttural pouch tympany.[1]

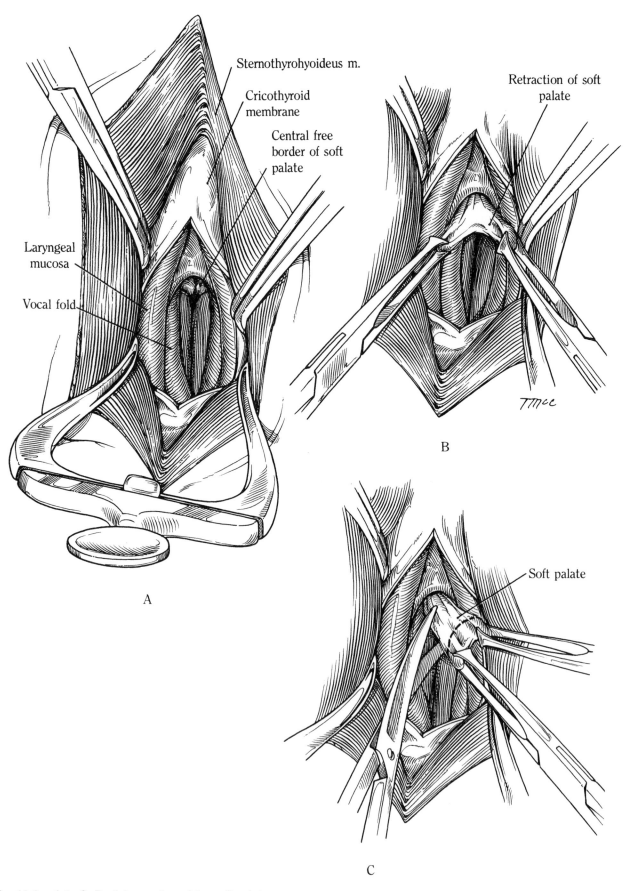

Sternothyrohyoideus m.

Cricothyroid
membrane

Central free
border of soft
palate

Laryngeal
mucosa

Vocal fold

Retraction of soft
palate

B

Soft palate

C

A

Fig. 11-3. A to C, Partial resection of the soft palate.

The hyovertebrotomy approach, also known as Chabert's approach, provides access through the dorsolateral aspect of the guttural pouch and is used for the removal of chondroids and inspissated pus. It is commonly combined with Viborg's triangle approach in the treatment of chronic guttural pouch empyema. A drain or seton may be placed through both incisions postoperatively. The hyovertebrotomy approach may also be used to ligate the internal carotid artery in the treatment of guttural pouch mycosis. Further details of the technique of internal carotid artery ligation are described elsewhere.[6]

The third approach is the ventral or Whitehouse approach (there is also a modified Whitehouse approach). This provides the best surgical exposure to the dorsal aspect of the guttural pouch for procedures such as ligation of the internal carotid artery within the pouch in the treatment of guttural pouch mycosis associated with epistaxis.[5] The Whitehouse approach may also be used to treat guttural pouch tympany.[2] Although the Whitehouse approach seems a logical choice for ventral drainage of the guttural pouch, temporary and permanent dysphagia has been experienced following the use of this procedure for the treatment of empyema. The dysphagia is presumably associated with compromise of the pharyngeal branches of the glossopharyngeal and vagus nerves that pass ventral to the guttural pouch. Because of the thickened nature of the guttural pouch in this inflammatory condition, these nerves may be difficult to identify, and the associated cellulitis may also compromise the nerves. Consequently, we are hesitant to recommend it as a drainage technique for guttural pouch empyema (details of the technique are available elsewhere[1,3]).

If the response to medical treatment of guttural pouch empyema is poor, surgical drainage of the guttural pouch will be indicated. Surgery is also indicated when the purulent material becomes inspissated or when chondroids have formed. In such cases, ventral drainage through Viborg's triangle is the approach of choice.

Anesthesia and Surgical Preparation

Viborg's triangle approach may be performed using local analgesia, but general anesthesia is preferred. General anesthesia is recommended for the hyovertebrotomy approach. The surgical sites, illustrated in Figure 11-4A, are clipped and prepared in a routine manner.

Instrumentation

General surgery pack
Blunt Weitlaner retractors
Drain or seton
Sponge forceps

Surgical Technique

Viborg's Triangle

Viborg's triangle is the area defined by the tendon of the sternomandibular muscle, the lingofacial (external maxillary) vein, and the caudal border of the vertical ramus of the mandible. A 4- to 6-cm skin incision is made just dorsal to and parallel with the linguofacial vein from the border of the mandible caudad. The subcutaneous tissue is separated, and the base of the parotid gland is reflected dorsad if necessary (Figure 11-4B). Care should be taken to avoid trauma to the parotid gland and duct, the lingofacial vein, and the branches of the vagus nerve along the floor of the guttural pouch. This procedure exposes the guttural pouch. Localization of the guttural pouch is facilitated by its distention when it is in a pathologic state. The guttural pouch membrane is grasped with forceps and is incised with scissors (Figure 11-4C). The wound is left open for drainage, or a drain is inserted. The surgical wound heals by granulation (secondary intention).

Hyovertebrotomy Approach

This approach, which gives access to the dorsolateral aspect of the guttural pouch, is more difficult and should probably be used only to access the arteries for ligation. Care should be taken because of the vessels and nerves within the surgical site. An 8- to 10-cm incision is made parallel and just cranial to the wing of the atlas (Figure 11-4A). The skin incision exposes the parotid salivary gland and the overlying parotidoauricularis muscle. The ventral part of the parotidoauricularis muscle is incised, and a dissection plane for the parotid gland is established by incising the fascia on its caudal border (Figure 11-4D). The parotid gland is reflected craniad. The caudal auricular nerve crosses obliquely in the dorsal aspect of the surgical field and is reflected caudad if necessary. Reflection of the parotid gland reveals the occipitohyoideus and digastricus muscles craniodorsally and the rectus capitis cranialis muscle caudodorsally (Figure 11-4E). The mandibular salivary gland may be identified ventrally. Blunt dissection through areolar tissue exposes the dorsolateral wall of the guttural pouch. The direction of dissection is caudal and then medial to the occipitohyoideus-digastricus muscle group.

The exact site of entry into the guttural pouch may vary, depending on the anatomic placement of the nerve branches overlying the surface. The position of the nerves seems variable and may also be influenced by pathologic distortion of the guttural pouch. Entry is usually made between the glossopharyngeal nerve rostrally and the vagus nerve caudally (Figure 11-4E). The internal carotid artery runs beneath the vagus nerve in this region and should be avoided. The guttural pouch is incised with scissors.

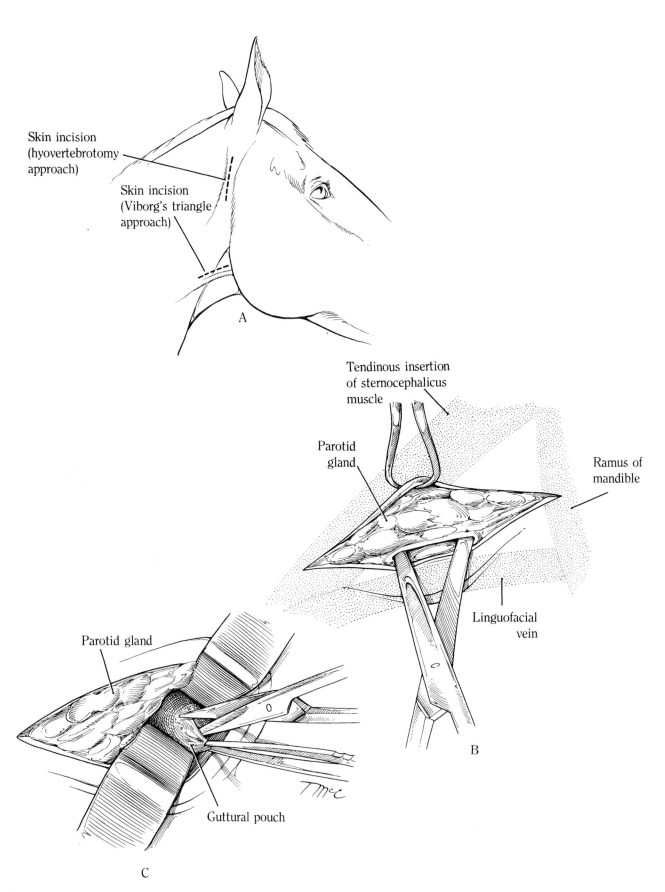

Skin incision
(hyovertebrotomy
approach)

Skin incision
(Viborg's triangle
approach)

A

Tendinous insertion
of sternocephalicus
muscle

Parotid
gland

Ramus of
mandible

Linguofacial
vein

B

Parotid gland

Guttural pouch

C

Fig. 11-4. A to E, Surgical entry and drainage of the guttural pouches.

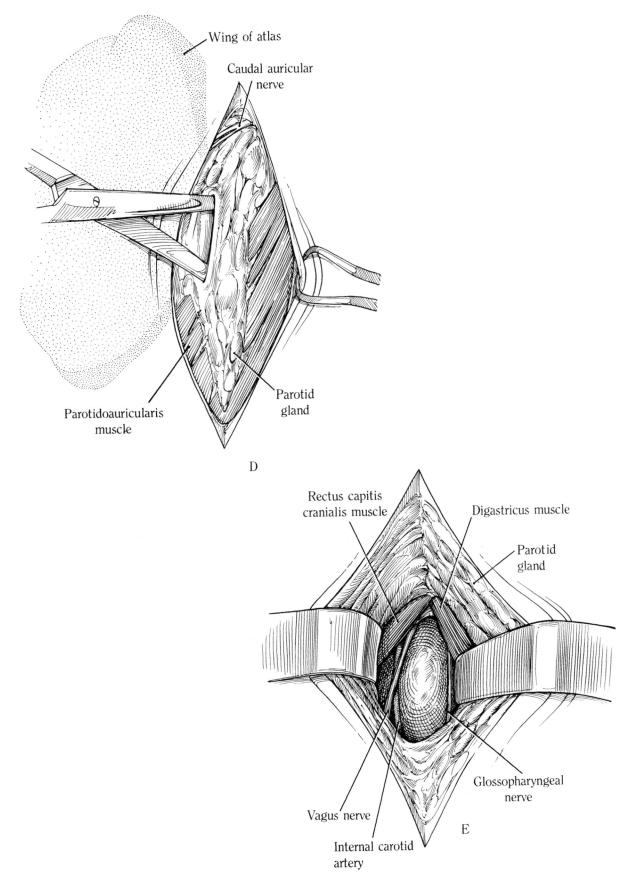

Wing of atlas

Caudal auricular
nerve

Parotidoauricularis
muscle

Parotid
gland

D

Rectus capitis
cranialis muscle

Digastricus muscle

Parotid
gland

Vagus nerve

Glossopharyngeal
nerve

Internal carotid
artery

E

Fig. 11-4. *Continued.*

197

The hyovertebrotomy incision may be closed primarily if contamination is not excessive and if a drain or seton is not going to be placed in the guttural pouch. The guttural pouch membrane is closed with simple interrupted sutures of synthetic absorbable suture material. One must be careful to avoid the adjacent nerves. The fascia associated with the parotid gland is also apposed with synthetic absorbable sutures. The skin is closed with nonabsorbable sutures.

Postoperative Management

Daily flushing of the pouch may be performed postoperatively. In some instances, removal of additional particulate debris may be necessary, and this can be performed by a combination of flushing and digital manipulation. When pus and debris are evacuated completely from the pouch, flushing is discontinued, any drains are removed, and the incisions are left to heal by secondary intention.

Complications and Prognosis

Some cases of guttural pouch empyema can be treated with the insertion of indwelling catheters to provide local therapy and to assist in drainage. Irritating solutions, however, including certain iodine compounds, should not be infused into the guttural pouches because of severe inflammatory changes. Even povidone-iodine diluted to a 10% solution (1% available iodine) causes considerable reaction.[7] We believe that the mechanical drainage of the contents of the pouch is more important than the antibacterial activity of the solutions placed in them. We advocate early surgical drainage, rather than extended periods of flushing using indwelling catheters.

References

1. Boles, C.: Treatment of upper-airway abnormalities. Vet. Clin. North Am.: Large Anim. Pract., *1*:143, 1979.
2. Cook, W.R.: Clinical observations on the anatomy and physiology of the equine respiratory tract. Vet. Rec., *79*:440, 1966.
3. Freeman, D.E.: Diagnosis and treatment of diseases of the guttural pouch. Part II. Compend. Contin. Educ. Pract. Vet., *2*:525, 1980.
4. Honnas, C.M., and Pascoe, J.R.: Guttural pouch disease. *In* Equine Internal Medicine, 2nd Ed. Edited by B.P. Smith. St. Louis, Mosby, Inc., 1996, pp. 610–615.
5. McIlwraith, C.W.: Surgical treatment of epistaxis associated with guttural pouch mycosis. VM/SAC, *73*:67, 1978.
6. McIlwraith, C.W., and Robertson, J.T.: McIlwraith & Turner's Equine Surgery: Advanced Techniques, 2nd Ed. Baltimore, Williams & Wilkins, 1998.
7. Wilson, J.: Effects of indwelling catheters and povidone-iodine flushes on the guttural pouches of the horse. Equine Vet. J., *17*:242, 1985.

Chapter 12

EQUINE DENTAL AND GASTROINTESTINAL SURGERY

Objectives

1. Discuss a technique for removal of the 1st molar in the equine upper arcade and the 3rd premolar in the lower arcade.
2. Provide a basic discussion of exploratory laparotomy in the horse, including indications, technique, and anatomy.
3. Discuss the advantages and disadvantages of two surgical approaches, ventral midline and flank laparotomy, for abdominal exploration in the horse.
4. Describe a surgical treatment of umbilical hernias in the foal.

Repulsion of Cheek Teeth

Relevant Anatomy

The equine dental formula for permanent teeth is I(3/3) – C(1/1) – PM(3/3 or 4/4) – M(3/3). There are a total of 36 to 44 teeth depending upon the presence of wolf teeth (PM1) and canines. Most of the tooth is composed of a cream-colored calcified tissue, called *dentin,* which is secreted by odontoblasts and functions to protect the pulp from infection.[4] The next external layer is the *cementum,* followed by the outermost and hardest layer of the tooth, the *enamel.* The elasticity of the underlying dentin and cementum prevents the brittle enamel from shattering and chipping by absorbing shock.[4]

The pulp of the tooth contains the pulpar nerves, capillaries, lymphatics, odontoblasts, and fibroblasts that support sensory capabilities and regenerative capabilities.[4] The crown of the tooth refers to the portion of the tooth extending from the root and is further divided into the visible crown and reserve crown, which lies below the gum line.

Blood supply to the teeth originates from the greater palatine artery, which courses around the periphery of the hard palate (2 to 3 mm medial to the lingual gingival margin of the maxillary teeth) and adjoins its counterpart rostrally.[4] This artery must be carefully avoiding during tooth extraction.

Nervous supply to the teeth is provided by the infraorbital and inferior alveolar nerves. The infraorbital nerve emerges from the infraorbital foramen approximately 5 cm dorsal to the rostral aspect of the facial crest. The infraorbital canal is in close proximity to the roots of the upper 8th, 9th, 10th, and 11th cheek teeth and must be carefully avoided when repelling cheek teeth.[4] The inferior alveolar nerve enters the mandibular canal and branches to innervate the teeth in the mandibular teeth, exiting out the rostral mental foramina.

Also in the vicinity of the surgical site are the parotid duct, facial artery, and facial vein, which follow the ventral edge of the mandible and run up the lateral aspect of the face near lower cheek teeth 10 and 11.

Indications

Cheek tooth repulsion is a method of tooth removal that is indicated when tooth preservation in not possible and extraction through the mouth with forceps is not feasible. Tooth removal is indicated in cases of infundibular necrosis, fractures extending into the reserve crown, or abscesses of teeth, periodontal disease, chronic ossifying alveolar periostitis, and tumors of the teeth. Infection of the teeth of either the upper or lower arcade may be secondary to fractures of the bones of the skull (mandible and maxilla) that involve the roots of the teeth also.

Repulsion of both upper and lower cheek teeth involves either trephining a hole or creating a maxillary sinus flap to gain access to the base of the tooth and driving the tooth from its socket into the mouth using a dental punch and mallet. It is the preferred technique for removal of maxillary cheek teeth 3–6 and all cheek teeth in the lower arcade.[5] Buccotomy extraction and vertical alveolar osteotomy techniques may also be used for cheek tooth extraction but are described in detail elsewhere.[5]

Buccotomy extraction involves a lateral approach and longitudinal sectioning of the tooth so that it may be removed piecemeal. Vertical alveolar osteotomy is similar to buccotomy but with a modification of the approach so that the incision is parallel to the parotid duct and linguofacial vein. This method is recommended for removal of mandibular cheek teeth 4 and 5.

All methods of tooth extraction in horses have a high documented rate of complications. Although not described here, surgical endonotic therapy is an alternative to tooth extraction that is relatively new to equine dentistry. By preserving the tooth, apicoectomy avoids problems associated with abnormal tooth wear and step formation along the occlusal table.

When the maxillary cheek teeth are involved (usually the 4th premolar or the 1st molar), signs of purulent nasal discharge are present because of secondary maxillary sinusitis. When the disease involves the mandibular teeth, swelling of, or chronic drainage from, the ventral border of the mandible is usually present. The teeth to be removed are ascertained by oral and radiographic examinations. In this chapter, repulsion of the 1st molar in the upper arcade and the 3rd premolar in the lower arcade are discussed.

Anesthesia and Surgical Preparation

Repulsion of teeth in the horse should be performed with the horse under general anesthesia. The horse is positioned with the affected tooth (teeth) uppermost. A mouth speculum is placed on the horse and is opened sufficiently to allow admission of the surgeon's hand. The hair is clipped over the surgical site, and routine surgical preparation is performed.

Instrumentation

General surgery pack
Mouth speculum
Molar forceps
Mallet or hammer
3/4-in and 1/2-in trephines
Molar cutters
Straight and curved dental punches
Bone curettes (sizes 1, 3, and 5)
Umbilical tape
Gauze roll, dental wax, or dental acrylic
Mild antiseptic solution, such as chlorhexidine
Bone saw (for the maxillary sinus flap)

Surgical Technique

In the case of trephination for the upper teeth, a curved incision should be made through the skin, with the apex pointing dorsad. The exact location of the incision depends on which tooth is to be repelled. Radiographs can be taken with radioopaque markers to help identify the proper location. The skin flap is reflected back, and the periosteum is incised and reflected from the bone to expose sufficient area to accept the trephine. A 3/4-in trephine should be used for the upper teeth. For the repulsion of lower teeth, a straight incision is made directly over the proposed site of trephination, and the edges of the skin are undermined to allow the trephine to be positioned on the lower border of the mandible. The periosteum is incised and reflected from the mandible. A 1/2-in trephine should be used for the lower teeth.

The trephine hole is begun by extending the center bit of the trephine 3 mm beyond the end of the trephine and fixing it to the bone. The trephine is turned back and forth in a rotary motion until it has cut a distinct groove in the bone. The center bit on the trephine is retracted, and cutting is continued until a disc of bone is detached (Figure 12-1A).

Locating the Trephine Opening for Upper Cheek Teeth

A line from the medial canthus of the eye to the infraorbital canal that continues forward past the roots of the 1st cheek tooth is the line of maximum height at which any trephining may be done for superior cheek teeth. This line marks the course of the osseous nasolacrimal canal. The trephine openings for all superior cheek teeth should be placed just below this line. In the case of old horses in which the teeth have grown out, it is permissible to drop down nearer to the facial crest. For the 1st and 2nd upper cheek teeth, which are straight, a line is drawn through the center of each tooth, and a trephine opening is made along each line. For the 3rd, 4th, and 5th upper cheek teeth, which have a caudal curvature, the trephination is made below the nasolacrimal canal, along a line directed over the posterior margin of the table surface of each tooth.

For repulsion of the 6th cheek tooth, a trephine hole must be made through the frontal sinus 4 cm lateral to the midline on a transverse line between the cranial margins of the orbits. It is necessary to go through the frontal sinus and the frontomaxillary opening into the maxillary sinus. The dental punch is passed lateral to the infraorbital canal to the root of the tooth. It is necessary to use a curved punch because the tooth has a tendency to lie under the infraorbital canal. The punch is seated on the base of the tooth, and the tooth is repelled. If the vein that lies above the infraorbital canal is severed, the area will have to be packed. This operation is difficult in young horses because of the marked caudal curvature of the tooth. Fortunately, this tooth does not require removal as frequently as other upper cheek teeth. Figure 12-1A and B shows trephination and repulsion of the 4th upper cheek tooth (1st molar).

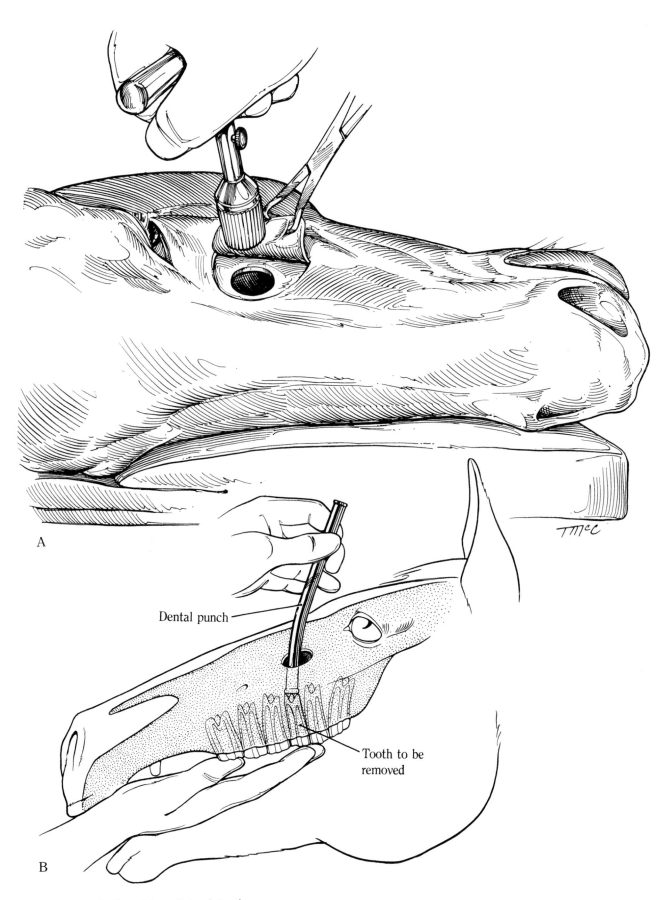

Dental punch

Tooth to be removed

A

B

Fig. 12-1. A to D, Repulsion of cheek teeth.

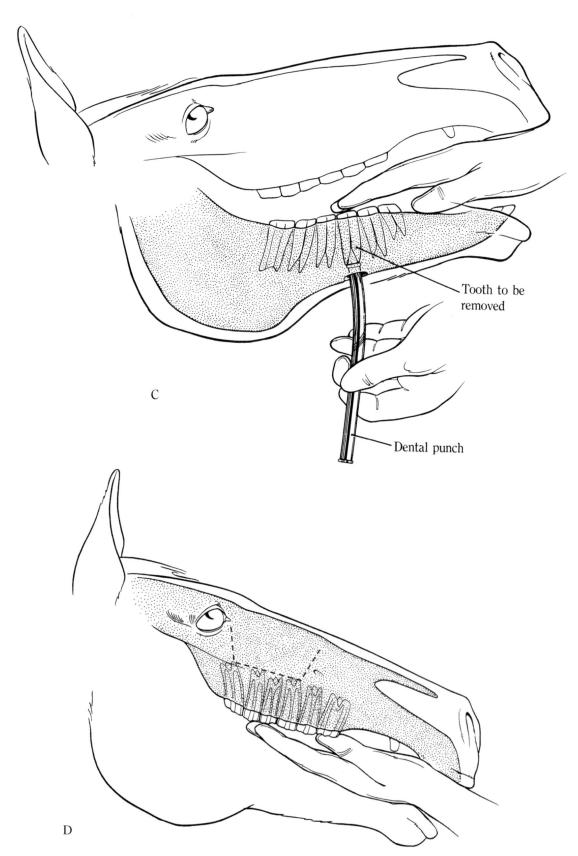

Tooth to be
removed

Dental punch

C

D

Fig. 12-1. *Continued.*

Locating the Trephine Opening for Lower Cheek Teeth

The trephine holes for repulsion of the lower cheek teeth are made on the ventrolateral border of the mandible. The inner and outer alveolar plates rest directly on the tooth, so it is necessary to align the punch with the long axis of the tooth to avoid punching toward the medial alveolar plate and fracturing it. For repelling the 1st cheek tooth, the trephine is centered directly below the table surface; for the 2nd to 5th cheek teeth, the opening is made below the caudal borders of the teeth because of their caudal curvature (Figure 12-1C); for horses older than 12 years, the opening can be made directly under the center of the table surface. Exposure of the trephine site for the 4th and 5th lower cheek teeth is complicated by the parotid duct and linguofacial artery and vein, which should be identified and retracted caudad. When a dental fistula is present on the lower border of the mandible, the trephine is positioned directly over the center of it because the fistula usually occurs opposite the affected alveolus.

The location of the 6th lower cheek tooth necessitates trephination over the lateral surface of the mandible. A line is drawn from the center of the table surface of the tooth to the point of greatest curvature of the ramus of the mandible. An incision is made on this line through the skin and masseter muscle over a bulging prominence where the two plates of bone that form the mandible are separated to accommodate the tooth. The muscle is separated from the bone by spreading it with wound retractors. The trephine opening is made and is elongated dorsad with a chisel to give better direction for the punch and to lessen the chances of fracturing the medial bony plate of the mandible. The skin-and-muscle incision is terminated at least 4 cm from the border of the mandible to avoid severing the branches of the facial nerve that spread out over the surface of the masseter muscle from above, ventrad, and rostrad. Further details of this technique are available in the advanced techniques textbook.[3]

Maxillary Flap Sinusotomy for Tooth Repulsion

In some cases, a larger opening is desired. The location of the flap is outlined in Figure 12-1D. The caudal border is just rostad to a line drawn from the medial canthus of the eye to the facial crest. The ventral border is just dorsal to the facial crest, and the rostral border just caudal to a line drawn from the rostad facial crest to the infraorbital foramen. The skin is incised down to the periosteum. The flap is cut on the caudal, ventral, and rostral sites with either an osteotome and mallet or an oscillating bone saw. The flap is lifted using the dorsal margin and periosteum as a hinge. The sinus is explored and lavaged.

After repulsion of the teeth, the flap is replaced and the periosteum sutured with 2-0 polyglyconate (Maxon) in a simple continuous pattern. The subcutaneous layer is closed similarly and the skin stapled. In some instances, the rostral ventral portion of the flap is left open for drainage.

Repulsion Following Trephination

The surgeon's hand is introduced into the patient's mouth, the diseased tooth is located, and the tooth's path in the sinus or jaw is determined. The punch is directed onto the root of the tooth, and an assistant begins to tap the punch with a mallet. The first few blows with the mallet should be sufficient to seat the punch into the root of the tooth. The trephine hole may have to be enlarged to allow the punch access to the diseased teeth.

Once the punch is seated, the assistant delivers steady blows to the punch. The mallet blows produce a characteristic ringing sound when the punch is seated properly, and the surgeon feels the vibrations of these blows transmitted through the tooth to his hand. If the punch slips off the tooth into alveolar tissue, it will need to be repositioned. After some time, the surgeon will feel the gradual loosening of the tooth with the hand that is in the patient's mouth. Subsequent blows with the mallet should be less forceful as the tooth is driven from the alveolus.

Following tooth repulsion, any fragments should be removed from the alveolus with forceps. The alveolus may require curettage if diseased bone surrounds the tooth. To prevent the socket from becoming packed with food, it should be filled with a suitable material until the socket is almost filled with granulation tissue. Dental wax, dental acrylic, gutta-percha, or gauze rolls may be used, depending on individual preference. The author prefers the use of Justi® hoof acrylic to fill the hole. If gauze rolls are used, a roll that will fit snugly into the hole is made and is tied around the center with umbilical tape, leaving two long ends. The ends are passed through the socket and trephine hole, the gauze is wedged firmly into the cavity, and the umbilical tape is brought to the exterior. The umbilical tape is then secured to the skin by tying it to another gauze roll. The ends should be kept long so that the gauze roll in the alveolus can be replaced without having to thread the new piece of umbilical tape back through the trephine hole.

Infected cheek teeth that are removed will usually require postoperative lavage of the associated sinuses with saline. Antibiotics can be left in the sinus after the lavage. For caudal cheek teeth, an additional 10 mm trephine hole is made into the ipsilateral frontal sinus after the maxillary bone flap is closed to facilitate postoperative irrigation.[2] For rostral cheek teeth, the maxillary septum can be fenestrated to allow accumulated serum and blood in the conchal sinus to drain to the rostral maxillary sinus and out the nares.

Postoperative Management

The horse should be placed on broad spectrum antibiotics preoperatively and for approximately 1 week following surgery. During the first few days, if a gauze pack is used, the pack is changed daily, and the sinus is flushed with a mild antiseptic solution if suppuration is present. The material used to pack the socket remains until the cavity is almost filled with granulation tissue. After a week, the material used to pack the socket can be changed every 2 or 3 days (if gauze is used). If the Justi® hoof acrylic is used, it will generally be pushed out of the socket in time and does not need to be removed.

Complications and Prognosis

Tooth repulsion is the traditional method for cheek tooth removal. However, all tooth extraction methods are associated with a high rate of complications as well as the inherent risks of general anesthesia in horses. Complication rates of maxillary cheek tooth repulsion have been near 50% in some studies with these horses requiring a second surgery.[1] Possible untoward sequelae of this procedure include punching out the wrong tooth, puncturing the hard palate by incorrect positioning of the punch over the tooth, rupturing the palatine artery, and breaking the alveolar plates of an adjacent tooth with the punch, which may lead to alveolar periostitis. Dixon et al. reported that 64% of horses treated with mandibular cheek tooth repulsion responded to a single surgical treatment.[2] Repulsion of maxillary cheek teeth was successful in 62% of horses (no continuation or recurrence of symptoms).

References

1. Dixon, P.M., and Dacre, I.: A review of equine dental disorders. Vet. J., 169:165–187, 2005.
2. Dixon, P.M., Tremaine, W.H., Pickles, K., Kuhns, L., Hawe, C., McCann, J., McGorum, B.C., Railton, D.I., and Brammer, S.: Equine dental disease. Part 4: a long term study of 400 cases: apical infections of cheek teeth. Eq. Vet. J., 32:182–194, 2000.
3. McIlwraith, C.W., and Robertson, J.T.: McIlwraith & Turner's Equine Surgery: Advanced Techniques, 2nd Ed. Baltimore, Williams & Wilkins, 1998.
4. Pence, P.: Equine Dentistry. Baltimore, Lippincott Williams & Wilkins, 2002.
5. Tremaine, W.H., and Lane, J.G.: Exodontia. In Equine Dentistry, 2nd Ed. Edited by Baker & Easely. Edinburgh, Saunders, 2005, pp. 267–279.

Ventral Midline Laparotomy and Abdominal Exploration

Relevant Anatomy

A discussion of relevant anatomy for this procedure is included in the description of surgical technique.

Indications

The ventral midline approach provides the greatest single incision exposure of the peritoneal cavity of the horse; it is also the quickest approach. It is particularly indicated for surgical management of acute equine abdominal disorders, although some surgeons use the paramedian technique.[6] This approach may also be used for bilateral ovariectomy or for removal of an ovarian tumor. Fears regarding the risk of dehiscence are not justified, and it is a practical approach that avoids both muscles and blood vessels. Although the scope of this text does not extend to detailed surgical management of patients with acute abdominal disorders, a basic discussion of exploratory laparotomy in the horse is appropriate.

Anesthesia and Surgical Preparation

This surgical procedure is performed with the patient in dorsal recumbency under general anesthesia. The ventral abdomen is clipped from the area of the pubis to the area of the xiphoid process extending at least 30 cm from the midline (this may be performed prior to the induction of anesthesia). The area of incision is shaved, and routine aseptic preparation is performed. Draping includes the use of hock drapes over the limbs to prevent contamination if the laparotomy sheet is displaced. An impervious drape is also used, so the bowel can be placed over it, to minimize soaking of the cloth drapes underneath.

Instrumentation

General surgery pack
Additional sterile lap sponges and gauze
Long-sleeved sterile gloves

Surgical Technique

The incision begins over the umbilicus and extends craniad; its length depends on the procedure, but it is generally 30 to 40 cm long (Figure 12-2A). Such an incision is used in patients with acute abdominal disorders, but cystotomies and ovariectomies require a more caudal incision. The skin incision extends through a layer of subcutaneous tissue, which is thin in most animals. When hemorrhage has been controlled, the linea alba is incised (it is preferable to maintain the incision within the linea alba) (Figure 12-2B). Slight divergence from the midline will result in entry into the rectus abdominis muscle, particularly in the cranial portion of the incision, but this event is generally of no consequence. Incision of the linea alba reveals the retroperitoneal adipose tissue deeply (Figure 12-2B). The retroperitoneal adipose tissue is cleared with a sponge to reveal the peritoneum, with the round ligament of the liver demarcating the midline (Figure 12-2C). The peritoneum is picked up and is incised with Metzenbaum scissors, and the incision may

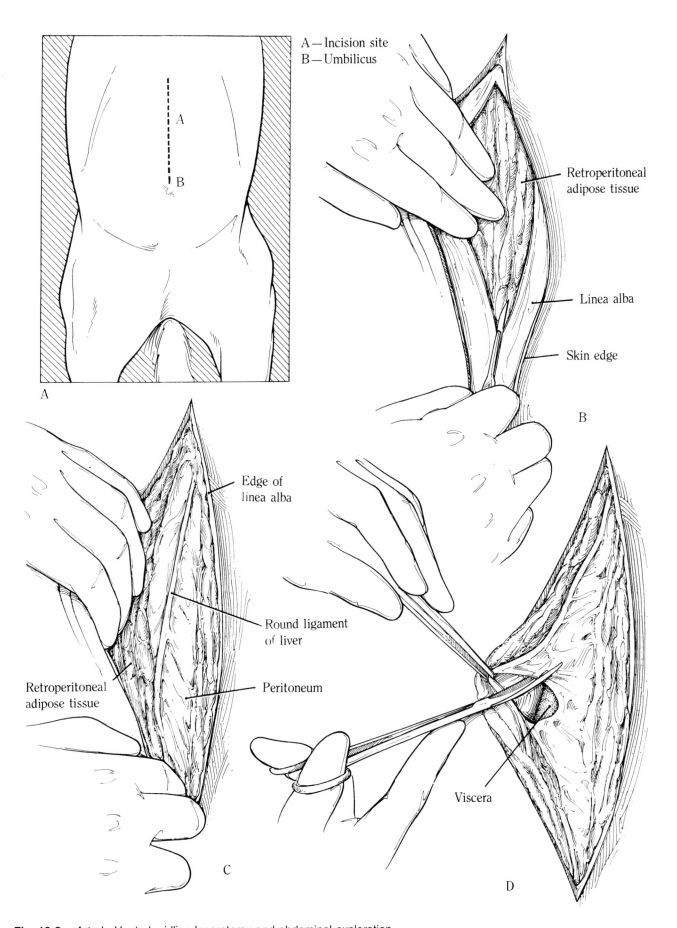

A—Incision site
B—Umbilicus

Retroperitoneal
adipose tissue

Linea alba

Skin edge

B

Edge of
linea alba

Round ligament
of liver

Retroperitoneal
adipose tissue

Peritoneum

C

Viscera

D

Fig. 12-2. A to L, Ventral midline laparotomy and abdominal exploration.

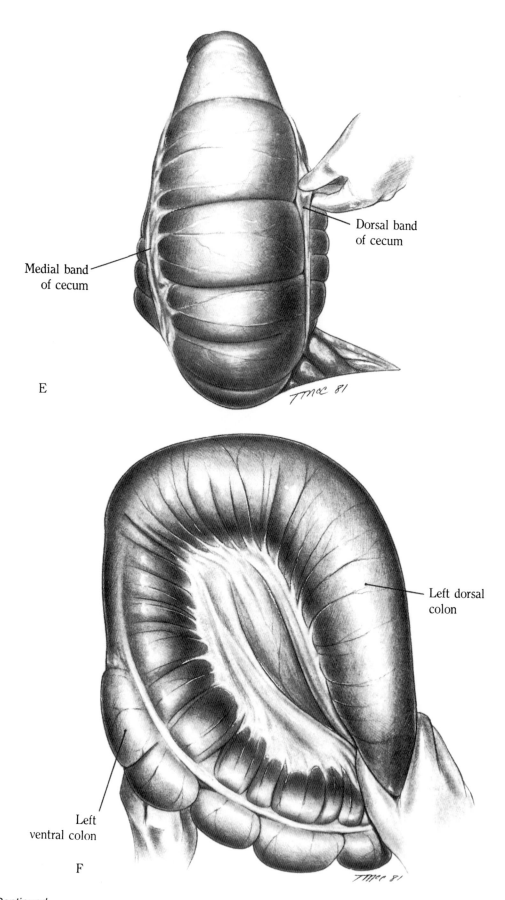

Medial band
of cecum

Dorsal band
of cecum

E

Left
ventral colon

Left dorsal
colon

F

Fig. 12-2. *Continued.*

206

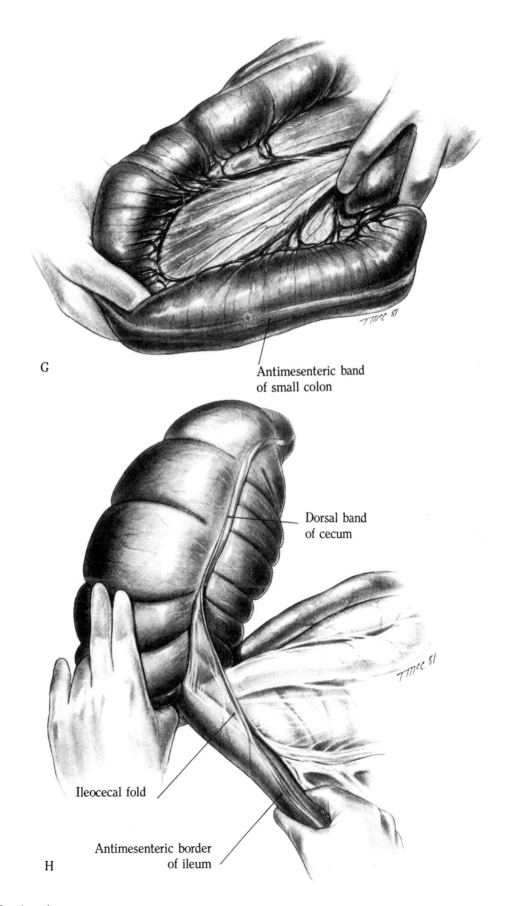

G

Antimesenteric band
of small colon

Dorsal band
of cecum

Ileocecal fold

Antimesenteric border
of ileum

H

Fig. 12-2. *Continued.*

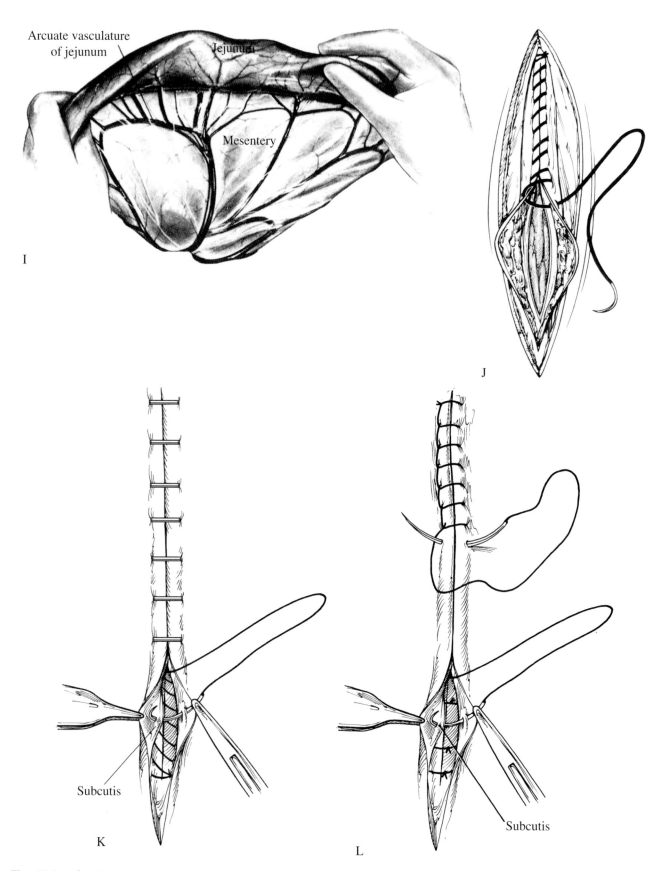

Arcuate vasculature
of jejunum

Jejunum

Mesentery

I

J

Subcutis

K

Subcutis

L

Fig. 12-2. *Continued.*

either be extended with the scissors (Figure 12-2D) or torn by hand. Retractors are not used routinely in exploratory laparotomy. Any exteriorized bowel is kept moist while systematic exploration of the abdomen is performed.

Upon opening the abdomen, the problem may be immediately obvious or may be determined quickly on cursory examination. In many instances, however, a systematic examination should be performed prior to closure of the abdomen. The systematic identification of normal, undisplaced viscera only is presented here.

If the cecum is not displaced (it lies ventrally, on the right side of the midline, with the apex directed craniad), it should be identified quickly after entering the peritoneal cavity (Figure 12-2E). The cecum is a reference point for systematic exploration of both the small and large intestine. The lateral band of the cecum is continuous with the cecocolic fold, which leads into the right ventral portion of the large colon. From this point, the large colon can be explored. The right ventral colon runs craniad and leads into the left ventral colon at the sternal flexure. The left ventral and left dorsal portions of the colon are the mobile parts and bend sharply at the pelvic flexure, which is located near the pelvic inlet (Figure 12-2F). The left dorsal colon passes forward from the pelvic flexure to the diaphragmatic flexure and becomes the right dorsal colon. This runs caudad in a dorsal position and, on reaching the medial surface of the base of the cecum, turns to the left, becomes narrower, and leads into the transverse colon. It joins the small colon ventral to the left kidney.

The small colon is characterized by two longitudinal bands, one within the mesentery and the other on the opposite (antimesenteric) side. It has two rows of sacculations and is attached to the sublumbar region by the colic mesentery (Figure 12-2G). The proximal small colon is also attached to the distal duodenum by the narrow duodenocolic fold of peritoneum. This fold is an identification point for the junction of the terminal duodenum and the proximal jejunum.

The small intestine is examined routinely by first locating the ileum. To do this, one retracts the cecum caudad to expose the dorsal band. This thin, avascular band runs into the ileocecal fold, which continues into the antimesenteric border of the ileum (Figure 12-2H). Using these landmarks, the surgeon can palpate the ileocecal junction deep in the abdomen; the junction cannot be exteriorized. The thin membranous fold called the antimesenteric border is 180° opposite the ileal mesentery and allows one positively to identify the ileum. Once the ileum is located, the small intestine may be examined systematically. Moving proximad, the entire length of the jejunum is explored until the duodenocolic fold, which is the junction between jejunum and duodenum, is reached. The jejunum has a mobile mesentery and is characterized by a lack of bands or sacculations (Figure 12-2I). The root of the mesentery may be palpated at this stage. The

duodenum also may be explored manually, not visually, because the duodenum's lack of mobility makes visualization difficult. The duodenum leads to the pylorus.

At this stage, the epiploic foramen should be palpated. It is most easily examined by standing on the patient's left side and using the left hand. If one holds the duodenum loosely between fingers and thumb with the dorsal surface of the fingers against the caudate lobe of the liver and moves laterad, the fingertips will locate the small opening of the epiploic foramen. This opening is larger in older horses.

The stomach and the spleen, which are in the left lateral quadrant, should be palpated. In a stallion, the internal inguinal rings that are ventrolateral to the femoral canals are palpated; in the mare, the uterus and ovaries are examined.

Further descriptions of how to deal with the various displacements and abnormalities of the equine gastrointestinal tract are presented in the advanced techniques textbook.[4]

The ventral midline incision is closed in three layers. A separate closure of the peritoneum is not necessary. The linea alba is closed with a simple interrupted or a simple continuous pattern. Simple interrupted sutures should be placed 1 cm apart (Figure 12-2J). If a simple continuous pattern is used, the suture should commence and should be tied beyond the extremities of the incision in the linea alba.[5] Five or six throws should be used in each knot. If the incision is less than 20 cm (8 in. approx), one length of doubled commercially available suture material is usually sufficient. If the incision is longer, two separate strands should be started beyond the commissure of the linea alba incision and directed to the center of the incision. Bites in the linea alba should be placed 0.75 to 1.00 cm apart (Figure 12-2K).

The choice of suture material depends on personal preference, but we have been most satisfied with synthetic absorbable materials such as polyglyconate (Maxon) or polyglactin 910 (Vicryl). The multifilament, nonabsorbable sutures have superior strength, but suture sinuses may be formed, depending on technique and degree of contamination. The subcutaneous tissue is closed with a simple continuous layer of 2-0 synthetic absorbable material (Figure 12-2L). The main purpose of this layer is to close dead space and cover the ends of the suture material, especially when an interrupted pattern is used. A continuous closure has fewer knots to cover with the subcutaneous layer and less chance that the ends of the sutures will protrude into the skin incision. Generally, the skin is closed with skin staples (Figure 12-2L). In most abdominal surgical procedures, speed is important; staples offer satisfactory closure as well as speed. Peritoneal drainage is not used routinely following abdominal surgery. The routine use of Penrose drains, in particular, is to be discouraged because of the risk of retrograde infection. If contamination is suspected or if bowel anastomosis has been performed, the abdomen should be irrigated and a fenestrated orthopedic drain should be inserted, mainly to drain the irrigation fluid. Generally, the drain is removed within 24 hours.

Postoperative Management

Nonsteroidal antiinflammatory drugs are administered at the end of surgery to decrease the immediate incisional (parietal) pain. Antibiotics and replacement fluids are used, the type and dosage depending on the particular surgical procedure. Additional drugs and supportive therapy may be necessary in patients with acute abdominal disorders. If a drain has been inserted, its patency must be checked regularly by applying negative suction to its end using a syringe. Bandaging is not used routinely, but a stent bandage may be indicated. Skin sutures or staples are removed in 12 to 14 days.

Complications and Prognosis

In the literature, incisional-related complication rates following ventral midline celiotomy range from 29% to 40%.[2,7] Incisional drainage is the most common, but other complications include periincisional edema, abscessation, suture sinus, and dehiscence. Reported rates of herniation following ventral midline celiotomy are relatively low (15 to 16%).[1,7] Horses that develop incisional drainage are more likely to develop incisional hernias than horses without incisional complications.[7] Other factors that are believed to contribute to the development of hernias include uncontrolled exercise, violent postoperative recovery, and early failure or weakening of suture material.

Generally, the prognosis for this procedure is good and the complications are relatively mild. Most survival rates in the literature are a reflection of the severity of the disease that necessitated surgery.

References

1. Gibson, K.T., Curtis, C.R., Turner, A.S., McIlwraith, C.W., Aanes, W.A., and Stashak, T.S.: Incisional hernias in the horse: incidence and predisposing factors. Vet. Surg., 18:360–366, 1989.
2. Kobluk, C.N., Ducharme, N.G., Lumsden, J.H., Pascoe, P.J., et al.: Factors affecting incisional complication rates associated with colic surgery in horses: 78 cases (1983–1985). J. Am. Vet. Med. Assoc., 195:639–642, 1989.
3. McIlwraith, C.W.: Complications of laparotomy incisions in the horse. In Proceedings of the 24th Annual Convention of the American Association of Equine Practitioners in 1978:1979, p. 209.
4. McIlwraith, C.W., and Robertson, J.T.: McIlwraith & Turner's Equine Surgery: Advanced Techniques, 2nd Ed. Baltimore, Williams & Wilkins, 1998.
5. Turner, A.S., et al.: Experience with continuous absorbable suture pattern in the closure of ventral midline abdominal incisions in horses. Eq. Vet. J. 20, 1988.
6. Vaughan, J.T.: Surgical management of abdominal crisis in the horse. J. Am. Vet. Med. Assoc., 161:1199, 1972.
7. Wilson, D.A., Baker, G.J., and Boero, M.J.: Complications of celiotomy incisions in horses. Vet. Surg., 24:506–514, 1995.

Standing Flank Laparotomy

Relevant Anatomy

A discussion of relevant anatomy for this procedure is included in the description of surgical technique.

Indications

The flank approach still is useful for some procedures. Although it is not recommended for patients with acute abdominal pain because it provides only limited exposure, it has been used in some instances. For example, the flank approach may be used for a standing exploratory laparotomy in a debilitated animal suspected of having neoplasia. In this instance, identification of a problem is all that is required, and complicated surgical manipulation is not performed. It is also a convenient approach for intestinal biopsies. For correction of other intestinal problems, except typhlectomy or cases of right dorsal colitis where access to the right dorsal colon is necessary, we favor the ventral midline approach. The standing flank approach can be used successfully for the correction of uterine torsion,[5] but it is not recommended for mares with a poor disposition because torsion on the ovarian pedicle is painful and may cause the horse to go down. The flank approach can also be used for removal of enteroliths, ovariectomy,[1] and cryptorchidectomy.[3,7]

The procedure is not recommended for patients with large ovarian tumors or tumors whose size cannot be determined on rectal examination.[2] For large ovarian tumors, a ventral midline approach is preferable.[6] The method is described in the advanced techniques textbook.[4] A right flank laparotomy has been performed to diagnose choleliths in horses,[8] and in smaller horses, choledolithotripsy is possible.[9]

Anesthesia and Surgical Preparation

Tranquilization of the patient is optional. The paralumbar fossa area is clipped, and the immediate area of the skin incision is shaved. The surgical area is prepared for aseptic surgery in a routine manner. Local analgesia is instituted by either a line block or an inverted L block; refer to Chapter 2, "Anesthesia and Fluid Therapy," for these techniques. The surgical area is then given a final preparation before surgery. With the standing procedure, aseptic preparation of a wide area and limited draping are preferred.

Instrumentation

General surgery pack
Long sterile gloves

Surgical Technique

A 20-cm skin incision is made midway between the tuber coxae and the last rib (Figure 12-3A). The dorsal limit of the incision is below the longissimus dorsi muscle and level with the tuber coxae. The incision is continued through the subcutaneous tissue, and any hemorrhage is controlled.

At this stage, there are two techniques for dividing the muscle layers. In the "grid" technique, all three layers may be divided along the direction of the muscle fibers. With the exception of the external abdominal oblique muscle, the fascial components of the flank muscles are weak, and splitting the muscles is preferred to transecting them. The grid technique, however, decreases the exposure. In most cases, a modified grid technique with a vertical incision through the fascia and muscle of the external abdominal oblique is used (the two alternate incisions in the external abdominal oblique muscle are illustrated in Figure 12-3B). The grid incision between the muscle fibers in a caudoventral direction is started with scissors and is completed with fingers (Figure 12-3C). In the modified grid approach, the fascia and muscle are incised with a scalpel (Figure 12-3D).

The remainder of the procedure is illustrated in a situation in which the external abdominal oblique muscle has been separated using the grid approach. In Figure 12-3E, the dotted line shows the line of cleavage in the internal abdominal oblique muscle where the fibers run cranioventrad. This layer is split to reveal the transverse abdominal muscle deeply (Figure 12-3F). A vertical split is made in the layer (the line of cleavage is indicated in Figure 12-3F). For this layer, the muscle should be tented with thumb forceps and nicked with scissors. The opening is enlarged to reveal retroperitoneal adipose tissue (Figure 12-3G), and the peritoneum is opened to expose the viscera (Figure 12-3H).

The surgeon should then don a sterile plastic sleeve to explore the peritoneal cavity. It is possible to exteriorize the small intestine, small colon, and pelvic flexure of the large colon. In addition, it is feasible to palpate the spleen, kidney(s), liver, stomach, cecum, large colon, cranial mesenteric artery, rectum, pelvic inlet, bladder, aorta, and reproductive tract.[10] The peritoneal surface is also examined.

The flank incision is closed in five layers. The peritoneum and transverse abdominal muscle are closed with simple interrupted sutures of no. 2-0 synthetic absorbable material. The internal abdominal oblique muscle is apposed with four or five simple interrupted or simple continuous sutures of no. 0 synthetic absorbable material (Figure 12-3I). A negative suction drain may be placed between the internal and external abdominal oblique muscles, and the last layer is closed with no. 0 or no. 1 synthetic absorbable material in a simple continuous pattern. Care is taken to ensure firm apposition of the fascia in the external abdominal oblique muscle. The suction drain, rather than a Penrose drain, is used to prevent seroma formation. However meticulous the closure is, a drain is generally necessary.

The subcutis is closed with a simple continuous pattern using synthetic absorbable sutures. The skin is closed with nonabsorbable sutures in a simple interrupted, simple continuous, or Ford interlocking pattern (Figure 12-3J).

Postoperative Management

Whether antibiotics are used and which type of antibiotics are used depend on the individual case. The negative suction syringe is taped over the patient's back and is emptied regularly. The drain is removed when the volume of aspirated contents decreases (2 to 3 days). The skin sutures are removed in 12 to 14 days.

Complications and Prognosis

Complications are similar to those described in the ventral paramedian approach. The major advantage to this approach for laparotomy is that it can be performed in standing. This may improve prognosis by decreasing contamination and avoiding the risks associated with general anesthesia.

References

1. Blue, M.G.: Enteroliths in horses: a retrospective study of 30 cases. Eq. Vet. J., 11:76, 1979.
2. Bosu, W.T.K., et al.: Ovarian disorders: clinical and morphological observations in 30 mares. Can. Vet. J., 23:6, 1982.
3. Burger, C.H.: The standing position for abdominal cryptorchidectomy in the horse. J. Am. Vet. Med. Assoc., 135:102, 1959.
4. McIlwraith, C.W., and Robertson, J.T.: McIlwraith & Turner's Equine Surgery: Advanced Techniques, 2nd Ed. Baltimore, Williams & Wilkins, 1998.
5. Pascoe, J.R., Meagher, D.M., and Wheat, J.D.: Surgical management of uterine torsion in the mare: a review of 26 cases. J. Am. Vet. Med. Assoc., 179:351, 1981.
6. Pugh, D.G., and Bowen, J.M.: Equine ovarian tumors. Symp. Contin. Educ., 7:710, 1985.
7. Scott, E.A., and Kunze, D.J.: Ovariectomy in the mare: presurgical, surgical and postsurgical complications. J. Eq. Med. Surg., 1:5, 1977.
8. Traub, J.L., et al.: Surgical removal of choleliths in a horse. J. Am. Vet. Med. Assoc., 182:714, 1983.
9. Traub, J.L.: Personal communication, 1987.

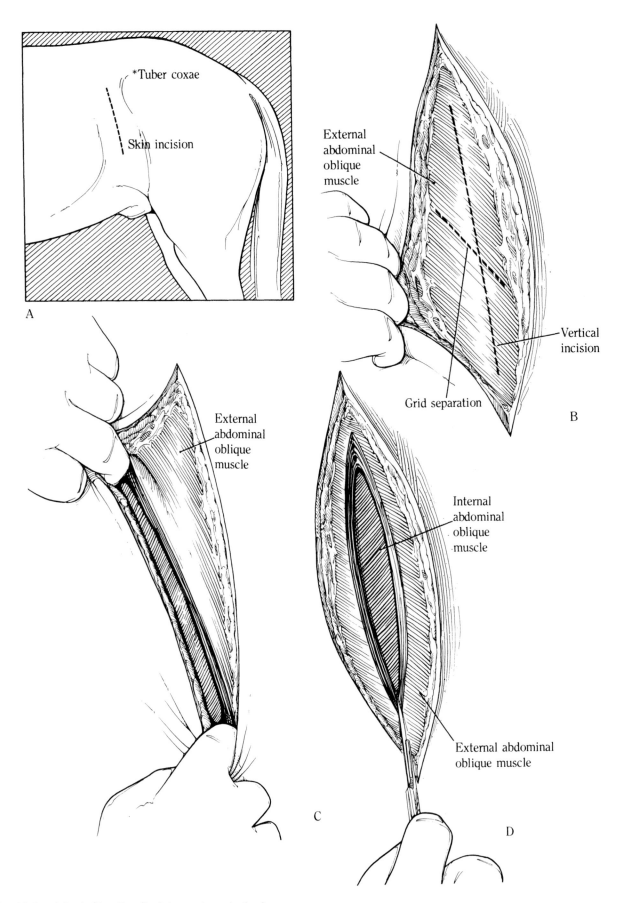

Fig. 12-3. A to J, Standing flank laparotomy in the horse.

Labels in figure:

A — *Tuber coxae, Skin incision

B — External abdominal oblique muscle, Vertical incision, Grid separation

C — External abdominal oblique muscle

D — Internal abdominal oblique muscle, External abdominal oblique muscle

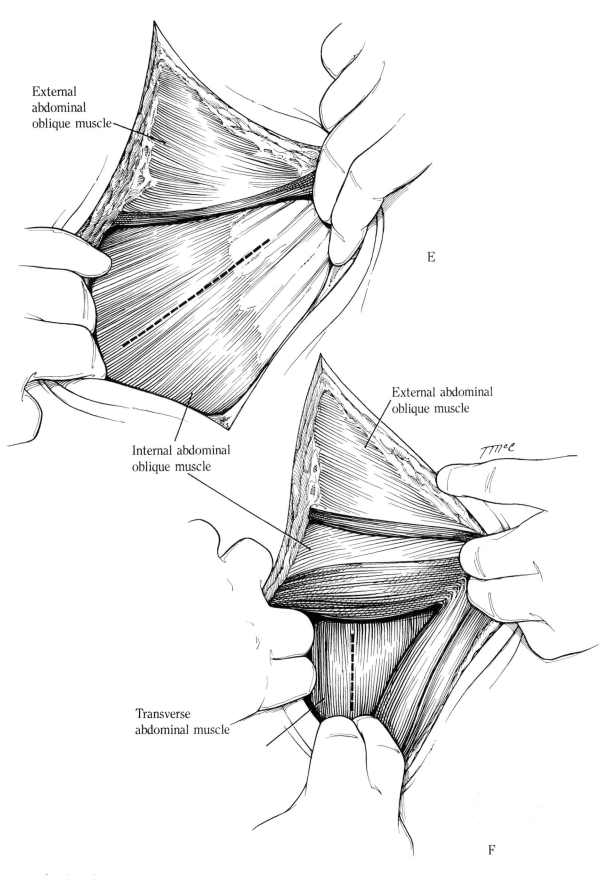

External
abdominal
oblique muscle

E

External abdominal
oblique muscle

Internal abdominal
oblique muscle

Transverse
abdominal muscle

F

Fig. 12-3. *Continued.*

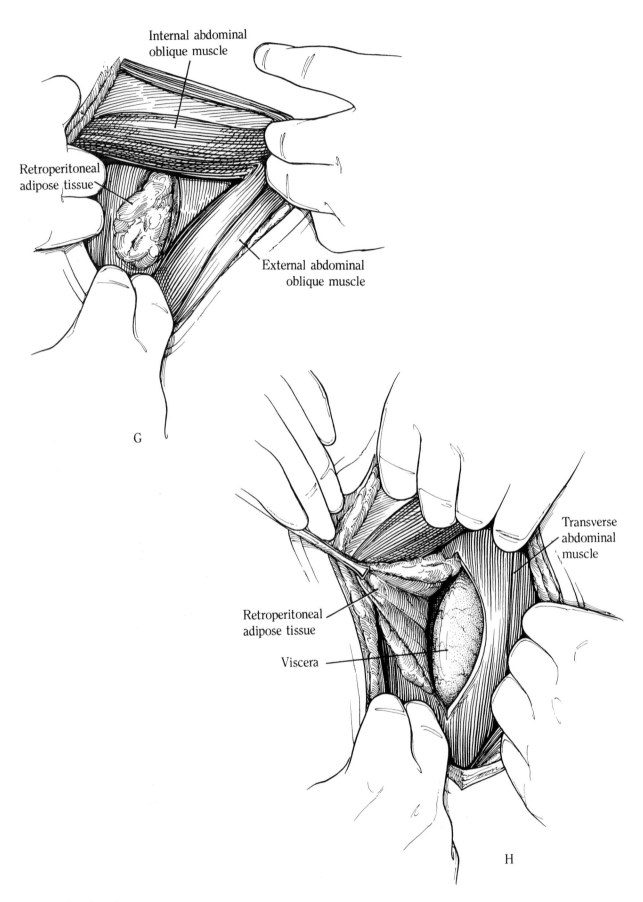

Fig. 12-3. *Continued.*

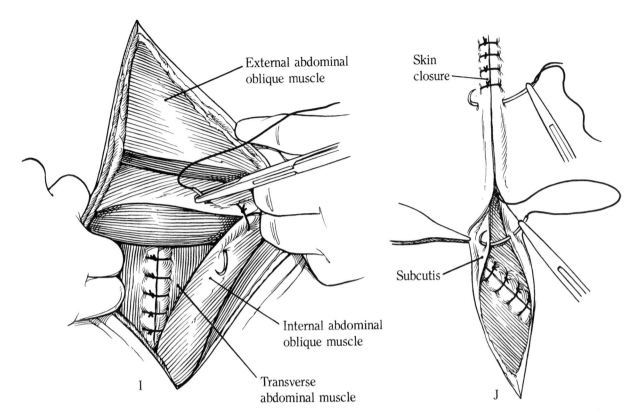

External abdominal
oblique muscle

Skin
closure

Internal abdominal
oblique muscle

Transverse
abdominal muscle

Subcutis

I

J

Fig. 12-3. *Continued.*

10. Vaughan, J.T.: Surgical management of abdominal crisis in the horse. J. Am. Vet. Med. Assoc., *161*:1199, 1972.

Umbilical Herniorrhaphy in the Foal

Relevant Anatomy

There is no further anatomy to discuss relevant to this section.

Indications

Umbilical hernias may be congenital or acquired and are seen in foals, calves, and pigs. Many small umbilical hernias may appear to resolve spontaneously, but large or strangulated umbilical hernias require surgical correction. Various methods are described in the literature for treatment of umbilical hernia: counterirritation, clamping, transfixation sutures, and even safety pins and commercially available rubber bands. The most popular of these techniques is the wooden or metal clamp technique (the clamps are illustrated in the discussion of instruments used in large animal practice in Chapter 3, "Surgical Instruments"). This method may result in infection, loss of clamps, or premature necrosis of the hernial sac. The last complication can lead to an open wound and, possibly, evisceration or formation of an enterocutaneous fistula. These methods are obviously unsuitable for the occasional strangulated hernia.

Ideally, surgery should be performed after one is sure that apparent external resolution is not going to occur and before the animal is too big (a typical hernia is represented in Figure 12-4A). Generally, the hernial sac is lined with peritoneum and contains some bowel (usually jejunum or ileum) or omentum. Another factor that the surgeon should always consider is possible heritability of hernias.

If the patient has large defects in the body wall or incisional hernias from previous abdominal surgery, it may be a candidate for the insertion of a prosthetic mesh. The application of this technique is described in the advanced techniques textbook.[1]

The incidence of incarceration of an umbilical hernia in foals is low, and signs include increased swelling of the hernia, which becomes firm and warm, and a plaque of edema surrounding the hernia sac. Colic is an inconsistent sign of hernial strangulation. Incarceration of only a portion of the intestinal wall (Richter's hernia) does not produce a complete obstruction of the lumen, but a Richter's hernia may progress to an enterocutaneous fistula.[2] When entire portions of the intestine are incarcerated, resection and anastomosis of the intestine may be required unless color and motility improve when the segment is freed.

The operation described here is also suitable for umbilical hernia repair in calves and pigs. Hernias in calves and pigs can be large and may be complicated by abscess formation. In such cases, pre- and postoperative antibiotics

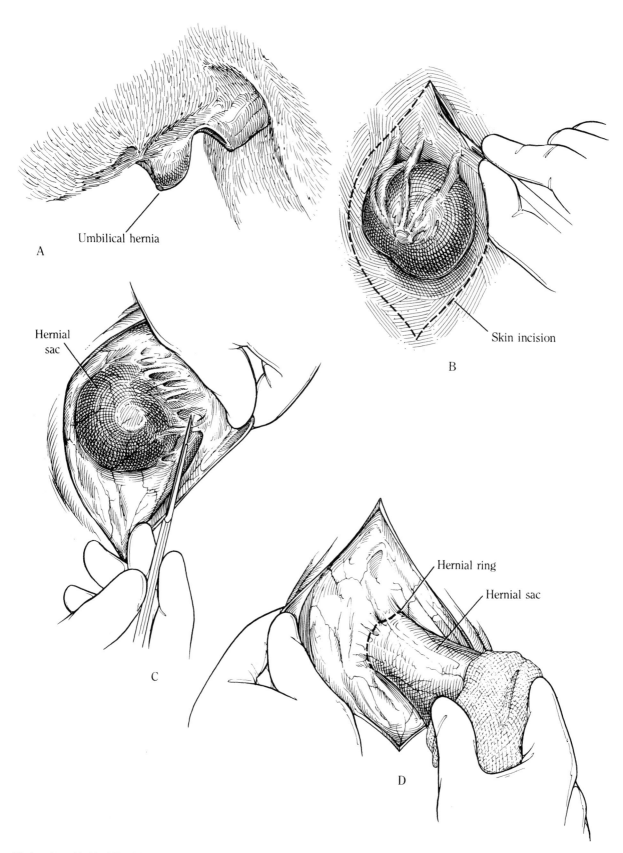

A

Umbilical hernia

B

Skin incision

Hernial
sac

C

Hernial ring

Hernial sac

D

Fig. 12-4. A to H, Umbilical herniorrhaphy.

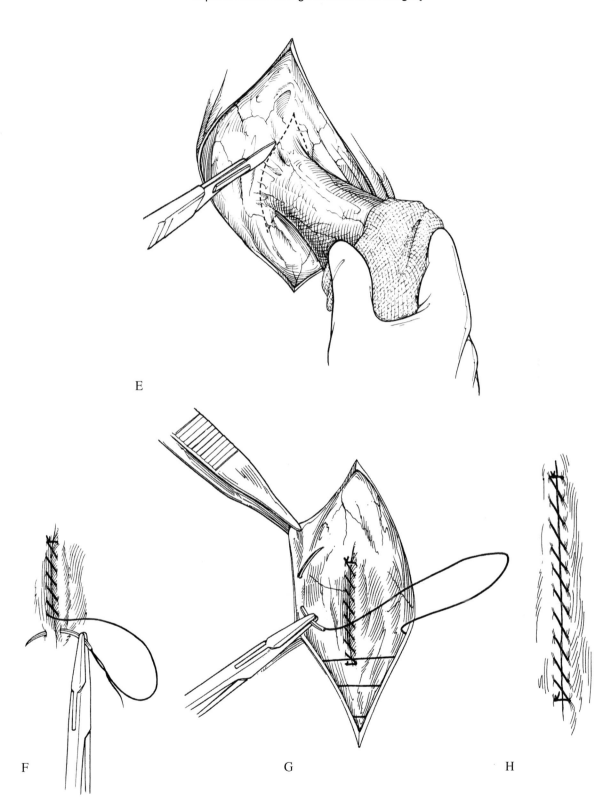

E

F   G   H

Fig. 12-4. *Continued.*

are indicated. It is also wise to resolve the abscess before attempting repair, especially if the abscess is large. If an abscess is present, the use of braided, synthetic nonabsorbable material should be avoided. For umbilical hernia repair in male pigs, the incision should avoid the preputial diverticulum and prepuce.

Anesthesia and Surgical Preparation

Inhalation anesthesia is preferable. Anesthesia in small foals can generally be induced with halothane administered by mask. Anesthesia in yearlings is induced intravenously and is maintained with an inhalation anesthetic.

The animal is placed in dorsal recumbency and is prepared for aseptic surgery in a routine manner.

Instrumentation

General surgery pack

Surgical Technique

A fusiform skin incision, pointed at both ends, is made around the hernial sac (Figure 12-4B). This shape avoids puckering or "dog ears" at the end of the wound at the time of skin closure. The shape of the incision should be such that sufficient skin remains at the wound edges to allow apposition without undue tension. Using either sharp dissection or blunt-tipped scissors, the surgeon dissects the subcutaneous tissue down to the hernial sac and ring (Figure 12-4C). Further sharp dissection around the base of the hernial sac delineates the hernial ring; this dissection should extend around the ring and outward for about 1 cm (Figure 12-4D). When the bowel has been incarcerated in the hernial sac, it is generally necessary to enter the sac carefully to replace the offending piece of bowel into the abdominal cavity. When opening the hernial sac, one must be careful not to cut through any adherent bowel because gross contamination of the surgical site will occur. If the surgeon cannot cut into the hernial sac without incising the bowel, the abdomen should be opened carefully along the linea alba, cranial to the hernial ring. This will allow the surgeon to identify the incarcerated portion of the bowel and to decrease the chance of inadvertent incision of the bowel.[1] There are two options available at this point for closure of the hernia. If the hernial sac has not been opened, a closed herniorrhaphy can be performed.

To perform a closed herniorrhaphy, often the hernial sac and ring have been freed of fascia, the sac is inverted into the abdomen, and the hernial ring is closed with a simple continuous pattern using a no. 1 or 2 synthetic absorbable suture material. Preferably, in the author's opinion, an open approach is used. In this technique, the hernial ring is sharply dissected and the entire hernial sac is removed (Figure 12-4E). The edges are then opposed using a simple continuous suture pattern with no. 1 or 2 synthetic absorbable suture material such as polyglyconate of polysorb (Figure 12-4F).

The subcutaneous tissue is closed using a simple continuous subcutaneous suture using no. 2-0 synthetic absorbable material (Figure 12-4G). Skin closure is performed with a nonabsorbable material of the surgeon's choice in ether a continuous interrupted or intradermal pattern (Figure 12-4H).

Postoperative Management

The decision to use antibiotics is left to the discretion of the surgeon. If the surgery is performed under aseptic conditions, antibiotics generally are not required. Preoperative antibiotics are also indicated if strangulation is suspected or if an enterocutaneous fistula has developed. Postoperative exercise seems to minimize swelling at the surgical site. Generally, a plaque of edema appears on the second or third postoperative day and persists for 2 to 3 weeks. Sutures are removed 10 to 14 days postoperatively. Some surgeons prefer trusses or belly bands to aid in the reduction of edema.

Complications and Prognosis

One study reported a complication rate of 19% in foals that received herniorrhaphy.[3] Of these foals, short-term complications included pneumonia in one foal and mild edema adjacent to the incision in two foals. No long-term complications occurred and all owners were satisfied with the cosmetic results. The prognosis for this procedure is good.

References

1. McIlwraith, C.W., and Robertson, J.T.: McIlwraith & Turner's Equine Surgery: Advanced Techniques, 2nd Ed. Baltimore, Williams & Wilkins, 1998.
2. Markel, M.D., Pascoe, J.R., and Sams, E.A.: Strangulated umbilical hernias in horses: 13 cases (1974–1985). J. Am. Vet. Med. Assoc., 190:692, 1987.
3. Riley, C.B., Cruz, A.M., Bailey, J.V., Barber, S.M., and Fretz, P.B.: Comparison of herniorrhaphy versus clamping of umbilical hernias in horses: a retrospective study of 93 cases (1982–1994). Can. Vet. J., 37:295–298, 1996.

Chapter 13

BOVINE GASTROINTESTINAL SURGERY

Objectives

1. Discuss the indications for flank laparotomy and abdominal exploration in reference to common bovine surgical conditions of the forestomach compartments and abomasum.
2. Describe the disadvantages and advantages of different laparotomy approaches in cattle.
3. Describe how to perform rumenotomy and ruminal fistulation in the standing cow.
4. Discuss the various surgical treatments of left- and right-sided abomasum displacements and volvulus, including right-flank omentopexy, with or without pyloropexy; ventral paramedian abomasopexy; and flank abomasopexy.

Principles of Laparotomy

Laparotomy is commonly performed either for exploratory purposes when a clinical diagnosis is still uncertain or for a specific purpose when a clinical diagnosis has already been made. Flank laparotomy performed on the standing animal under local anesthesia is the most common technique. Flank laparotomy through the left paralumbar fossa is commonly used for exploratory laparotomy if a problem is suspected on the left side, and the procedure is specifically indicated for left-sided abomasopexy, rumenotomy, and cesarean section. The right paralumbar approach is used for exploratory laparotomy if a problem is suspected on the right side, and it is specifically indicated for surgical conditions of the abomasum,

including right-sided omentopexy or abomasopexy, small intestine, cecum, and colon. The right paralumbar approach will provide the best access to the abdomen and the most complete exploratory in the adult ruminant. A right-flank approach may also be used for cesarean section when ruminal distention or right-sided positioning of the fetus causes the surgeon to consider the right side a superior approach to the left side. Although flank laparotomy is generally performed on the standing animal, general anesthesia may be indicated when surgery is to be performed through the right flank for a small intestinal or colonic problem, because the pain and shock associated with surgery may cause the animal to go down during the procedure.

Ventral paramedian laparotomy is an alternative that necessitates the animal being cast or sedated and placed in dorsal recumbency. The two main indications for this technique are for ventral abomasopexy and cesarean section, in which it offers advantages in the delivery of oversized or emphysematous fetuses and in complicated deliveries, including uterine tears. Another advantage of ventral paramedian laparotomy is less-visible postoperative scarring in feedlot heifers. The paramedian incision is parallel to the midline, between the midline and the subcutaneous abdominal vein. The incision for paramedian abomasopexy extends from the umbilicus craniad to the xiphoid process, as illustrated later in this chapter. The incision for paramedian cesarean section extends from the umbilicus caudad to the udder and is illustrated in Chapter 14, "Bovine Urogenital Surgery."

A third, less common laparotomy approach is the ventrolateral oblique incision, which may be performed on the right or left side and may also be indicated for cesarean section. As with the paramedian approach, fetal and uterine debris can be removed more efficiently, with less potential contamination of the peritoneum than with a flank approach. The ventrolateral oblique incision is considered advantageous to the paramedian incision in the high-producing dairy cow with large subcutaneous abdominal veins and the potential for severe hemorrhage.[3] This technique may be performed conveniently with the cow in lateral recumbency.

References

1. Ducharme, N.G.: Surgery of the bovine forestomach com-
    partments. Vet. Clin. N. Am. Food Anim. Prac., 6:371–396,
    1990.
2. Habel, R.E.: Ruminant digestive system. In The Anatomy of
    the Domestic Animals, Ed 5. Edited by S. Sisson and J.D.
    Grossman. Philadelphia, W.B. Saunders, 1975, p. 884.
3. Noorsdy, J.L.: Selection of an incision site for cesarean section
    in the cow. VM/SAC, 75:530, 1979.

Flank Laparotomy and Abdominal Exploration

Relevant Anatomy

In the ruminant, the most cranial forestomach, the reticulum, lies just caudal to the diaphragm and to the left of the midline, beneath the 6th through 8th rib.[1,2] The space left of the median, from approximately the 7th or 8th rib to the pelvis, is occupied by the rumen. On the right side of the ruminant lie the omasum and the elongated true stomach, the abomasum. The omasum lies near the ventral aspect of the 7th to the 11th ribs and the abomasum extends from the xiphoid region to the 9th or 10th rib, occupying primarily the right side except for the fundus, which deviates to the ventral aspect of the rumen atrium.[1,2]

Autonomic innervation of these structures is accomplished by a balance of both sympathetic and parasympathetic nervous inputs, supplied by the splanchnic nerves and the dorsal and ventral vagal trunks, respectively.

Indications

The following are indications for left-flank laparotomy: general exploratory laparotomy, particularly if a problem amenable to treatment from the left side is suspected; rumentomy; left-flank abomasopexy; and cesarean section when the viable fetus is only moderately oversized and the cow is capable of enduring the surgery in the standing position. The major advantage to the left-flank approach is that the bulk and position of the rumen generally precludes the risk of intestinal evisceration.

Right-flank laparotomy is indicated in the following instances: exploratory laparotomy when a problem amenable to treatment from the right side is suspected; right-flank abomasopexy and omentopexy; surgical correction of small intestinal, cecal, and colonic conditions; and cesarean section when, because of rumenal distention or fetal positioning, removal of the calf by a left-flank approach would be difficult or when hydrops amnii or allantois is present. Right-flank laparotomy is also chosen when the problem is unknown and a full exploratory is needed.

Anesthesia and Surgical Preparation

Typically, this surgical procedure is performed with the animal standing, and anesthesia is provided by a line block, an inverted L block, or a paravertebral block; refer to Chapter 2, "Anesthesia and Fluid Therapy," for these techniques. For surgery of the small or large intestinal tract, pain and shock associated with both the condition itself and the surgical manipulation may cause the animal to go down during surgery, with obvious compromise to aseptic technique. In such patients, general or high-epidural anesthesia may be used.

The surgical area is clipped and is prepared for aseptic surgery in a routine manner. Any bars on the stocks adjacent to the operative field are draped.

Instrumentation

General surgery pack

Surgical Technique

The site of the incision for left-flank laparotomy is illustrated in Figure 13-1A. A vertical incision is made in the middle of the paralumbar fossa extending from 3 to 5 cm ventral to the transverse processes of the lumbar vertebrae for a distance of 20 to 25 cm. For rumenotomy in a large cow, it may be advantageous to make the incision cranial to the midway point. For cesarean section, the incision may begin 10 cm ventral to the transverse processes and may extend 30 to 40 cm.

To incise the skin, reasonable pressure should be exerted on the scalpel to ensure complete penetration. This incision is continued ventrad so that the skin is opened in one smooth motion. Separation of the skin and subcutaneous tissue reveals fibers of the external abdominal oblique muscle and fascia (Figure 13-1B). This layer is incised vertically to reveal the internal abdominal oblique muscle (Figure 13-1C). A similar incision through the internal abdominal oblique muscle reveals the glistening aponeurosis of the transverse abdominal muscle (Figure 13-1D). Then the muscle is picked up with tissue forceps and is nicked with a scalpel in the dorsal part of the incision to avoid cutting the rumen. The incision through the transverse abdominal muscle and peritoneum may be extended with scissors or a scalpel for entrance into the peritoneal cavity (Figure 13-1E).

A thorough, systematic examination of the abdomen should always be carried out before specific surgical manipulation is performed on a viscus. Unless a left displacement of the abomasum is present, the rumen will be visible following completion of the left-flank laparotomy incision, and the color of its serosa may be noted (Figure 13-1F). The rumen is palpated to determine the nature of its contents. The left kidney is pendulous and also can be

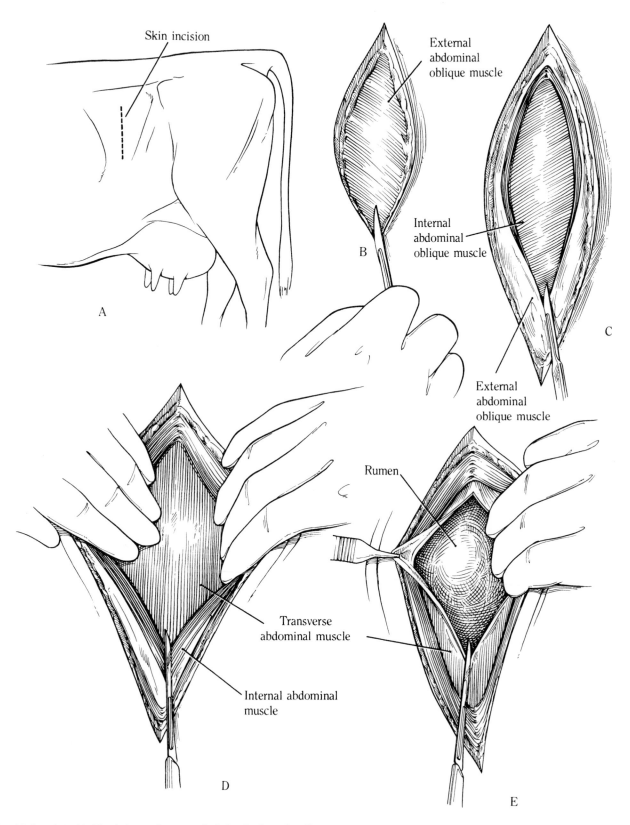

Fig. 13-1. A to H, Flank laparotomy and abdominal exploration.

Skin incision

A

External
abdominal
oblique muscle

Internal
abdominal
oblique muscle

B

External
abdominal
oblique muscle

C

Transverse
abdominal muscle

Internal abdominal
muscle

D

Rumen

E

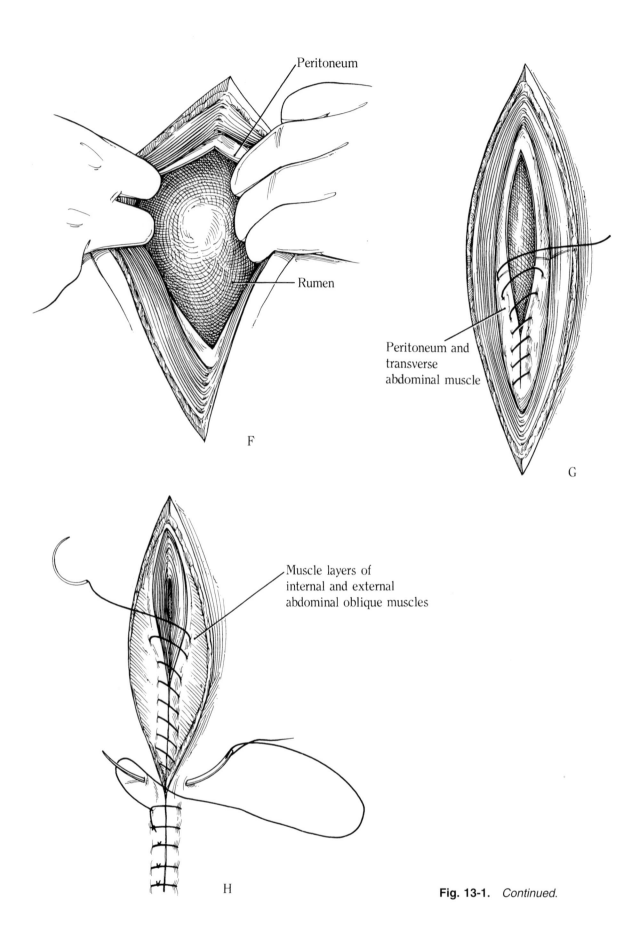

Peritoneum

Rumen

F

Peritoneum and
transverse
abdominal muscle

G

Muscle layers of
internal and external
abdominal oblique muscles

H

Fig. 13-1. *Continued.*

palpated straight in from the incision if the rumen is empty. If the rumen is full, the kidney is located by passing a hand around caudal to the dorsal sac of the rumen. Passing a hand forward on the left side of the rumen, the spleen, reticulum, and diaphragmatic area may be palpated, and the presence of adhesions or abscesses in this area may be ascertained. Moving behind the rumen over to the right side, the viscera within the omental bursa are palpated. Further forward on the right side, it is possible to palpate the caudate lobe of the liver and the gallbladder. The pelvic region, including the uterus (in a cow) and bladder, should also be palpated. It is questionable whether routine palpation of the ovaries and fimbriae of the uterine tubes is appropriate in the cow, especially if peritonitis is present in the abdomen. It is possible that local infection and adhesions could result in problems with reproduction. Following this exploration, any specific procedures indicated, such as rumenotomy or abomasopexy, are performed.

Abdominal exploration may be similarly performed through a right-flank incision. If the viscera are in normal position, the duodenum will be encountered running horizontally across the dorsal part of the incision with the mesoduodenum dorsal and the greater omentum ventral. The pylorus and abomasum can be palpated ventrally. The greater omentum may be reflected craniad to allow examination of the jejunum, ileum, cecum, and colon. The kidneys and pelvic region can also be palpated at this stage. The rumen can be palpated, but examination of the reticulum and diaphragm, as performed with left-flank laparotomy, is not possible. The omasum, liver (the right-flank approach allows complete palpation of this organ), gallbladder, and diaphragm can be palpated cranially on the right side. The anatomic peculiarities with abomasal displacements are discussed in the sections of this chapter on abomasopexy and omentopexy.

Routinely, a flank laparotomy incision is closed in three layers. The peritoneum and transverse abdominal muscles are closed together with a simple continuous suture pattern using no. 0 or 1 synthetic absorbable sutures (Figure 13-1*G*). Placing this suture layer in a ventral-to-dorsal direction is helpful to maintain the viscera within the incision, particularly on the right side. The internal and external abdominal oblique muscles may be closed with a second simple continuous layer using no. 1 synthetic absorbable sutures (Figure 13-1*H*). This suture line is anchored to the deeper transversus muscle at various intervals to obliterate dead space. It is also desirable to take even bites on either side with the muscle closures, so the muscles will come together without a defect and without wrinkling. If the external and internal abdominal oblique muscle layers are substantial in a large cow, closure should be performed in separate layers. Generally, skin closure is performed with a continuous Ford interlocking pattern using heavy polymerized caprolactam (Vetafil) (Figure 13-1*H*). At the surgeon's option, two to three simple interrupted sutures may be placed in the ventral aspect of the incision (Figure 13-1*H*); this measure allows easy drainage if infection develops in the incision. Such an event is possible in the compromised conditions under which this surgical procedure may have to be performed. If the skin incision has been obviously contaminated, as by the delivery of an emphysematous fetus, an interrupted suture pattern may be more appropriate.

Postoperative Management

Antibiotics are administered, if indicated, depending on the procedure. Supportive management is also instituted in accordance with the animal's condition. Sutures may be removed 2 to 3 weeks after surgery; at 10 to 14 days, the incision is still vulnerable to trauma, and in cattle housed together, a "popped" incision may occur if sutures are removed at this time.

Complications and Prognosis

Complications such as peritonitis and adhesions may arise following abdominal exploration. Cattle in particular may be more prone to incisional dehiscence and wound infection when housed together. The incidence of incisional infection can be greatly reduced when antibiotics are given preoperatively.

Rumenotomy

Relevant Anatomy

The rumen and reticulum accommodate most of the microbial fermentation during digestion. They are divided from each other by the same mechanism that partitions the rumen itself, by the internal pillae formed by internal projections of the rumenal wall.[4] Externally, the pillae appear as grooves. The ruminoreticular fold demarcates the rumen from the reticulum. The rumen itself is divided into dorsal and ventral sacs by the ruminal pillars, and cranial and caudal blind sacs by the coronary pillars. A cranial pillar further divides the dorsal sac into a ruminal atrium, which is most closely associated with the reticulum.[4] The reticular-omasal and esophageal orifices are located in the reticular groove, which runs down the right internal surface of the reticulum from the cardia to the fundus.

The mucosal lining of the reticulum is characterized by honeycomb shaped ridges that house a collection of short papillae.[4] This honeycombed appearance subsides at the ruminoreticular fold as it merges into the papillated mucosa of the rumen. These projections are associated with a subepithelial capillary plexus that facilitates the absorption of the volatile fatty acid by-products of microbial fermentation.[4]

Indications

Rumenotomy is indicated for the removal of metallic foreign bodies whose presence might cause traumatic reticulitis or traumatic reticuloperitonitis, materials such as baling twine or plastic bags that are obstructing the reticulo-omasal orifice, and foreign bodies lodged in the distal esophagus or over the base of the heart.

Rumenotomy is also indicated for evacuation of rumen contents in selected cases of rumen overload or following ingestion of toxic plants, spoiled roughages, or chemicals.[2] Finely ground feedstuffs readily pass into the omasal-abomasal region, but coarser, more fibrous material remains in the rumen for longer periods. Other indications for rumenotomy include rumen impaction and impaction and atony of the omasum or abomasum.[1]

There are several techniques described for performing a rumenotomy, including suturing the rumen to the skin prior to rumenotomy (described here), the use of fixation devices such as Weingarth's ring, the use of stay sutures, or the use of towel clamps to fix the rumen to the skin.[2] Although more time consuming than the alternatives, suturing the rumen to the skin prior to rumentomy provides the most secure seal between rumen and skin, is not easily displaced (as are the fixation devices), and has been shown to result in fewer postoperative compications.[2]

Anesthesia and Surgical Preparation

The left-flank area is prepared for aseptic surgery in a routine manner, and local anesthesia is instituted by line block, inverted L block, or paravertebral block.

Instrumentation

General surgery pack
Kingman tube to drain fluid from the rumen
Rumenotomy board or fixation ring if the rumen is not sutured to the skin as described here

Surgical Technique

Rumenotomy is performed through a left paralumbar incision (a 20-cm incision generally is sufficient) with the animal standing. The technique for left-flank laparotomy has been described previously. In large cows, the flank incisions for rumenotomies sometimes are made just caudal and parallel to the last rib, to place the incision closer to the reticulum. It is essential, however, to leave sufficient tissue caudal to the last rib for suturing (the incision should be approximately 5 cm (2 in) caudal to the last rib).

Following opening and systematic exploration of the peritoneal cavity (no attempt is made to break down firm adhesions in the region of the reticulum), it is necessary to anchor the rumen to the incision to avoid contamina-

tion of the abdominal musculature and peritoneum during the rumenotomy procedure. A technique for suturing the rumen to the skin prior to rumenotomy is illustrated in Figure 13-2A to D. A continuous inverting suture pattern (similar to a Cushings pattern) is used to pull the rumen over the edge of the skin incision (Figure 13-2A and B). This suture should be of heavy-gauge material such as nylon of polypropolene (Surgipro, Prolene). Two large, inverting sutures are placed at the ventral aspect of the incision so that the rumen projects well over the skin edge; this avoids contamination in the ventral region (Figure 13-2C). Alternate techniques for isolating the rumen and preventing contamination include the use of stay sutures, a rubber rumenotomy shroud, a fixation ring (Weingart's),[6] or a rumenotomy board. These alternatives are quicker than suturing the rumen, but they are also more easily displaced; the consequent contamination may be disastrous.

The rumen is incised with a scalpel, taking care to leave enough room dorsally and ventrally for closure at the end of the procedure (Figure 13-2D), and the operator, wearing long rubber gloves, evacuates and explores the rumen (Figure 13-2E). A rumen shroud or a wound edge protector (3M™ Steri-Drape™) may be placed in the incision to prevent ingesta from accumulating at the incisional site and compromising wound healing.[3,5] The inside of the rumen and the reticulum are explored, and if a foreign body is present, it is removed. A large-bore stomach tube, such as a Kingman tube, may be used to siphon out liquid contents.

To reach the reticulum from the rumenotomy incision, the dorsal wall of the rumen (where a natural air pocket exists) should be followed, until it becomes the ventral wall, at which point one is in the reticulum. Following a direct line from the incision, one encounters ingesta as well as the cranial pillar of the rumen and ruminoreticular fold. To help locate foreign bodies, the reticulum can be gently picked up with the hand. The area where the foreign body is located usually has extended adhesions and cannot be picked up. This is an ideal area to look for foreign bodies. Moreover, while exploring the inside of the reticulum, one should also feel for abscesses. Abscesses are frequently found on the medial wall of the reticulum near the reticulo-omasal orifice. If abscesses are found, they should be evaluated. If the cow's economic value justifies the surgeon to proceed, abscesses that adhere to the reticulum should be lanced or drained. This is best accomplished by carrying a scalpel or scalpel blade, attached to a piece of string or umbilical tape in case it is dropped, into the reticulum and lancing the abscess into the reticulum through the adhesion. Following this exploration, the reticulum may be swept with a magnet to pick up additional metallic debris. A magnet is placed (or replaced) in the reticulum, and fresh rumen contents (if available) are placed in the rumen. Alkalinizing products may be inserted at this stage in cases of rumen overload, and mineral oil may also be instilled when

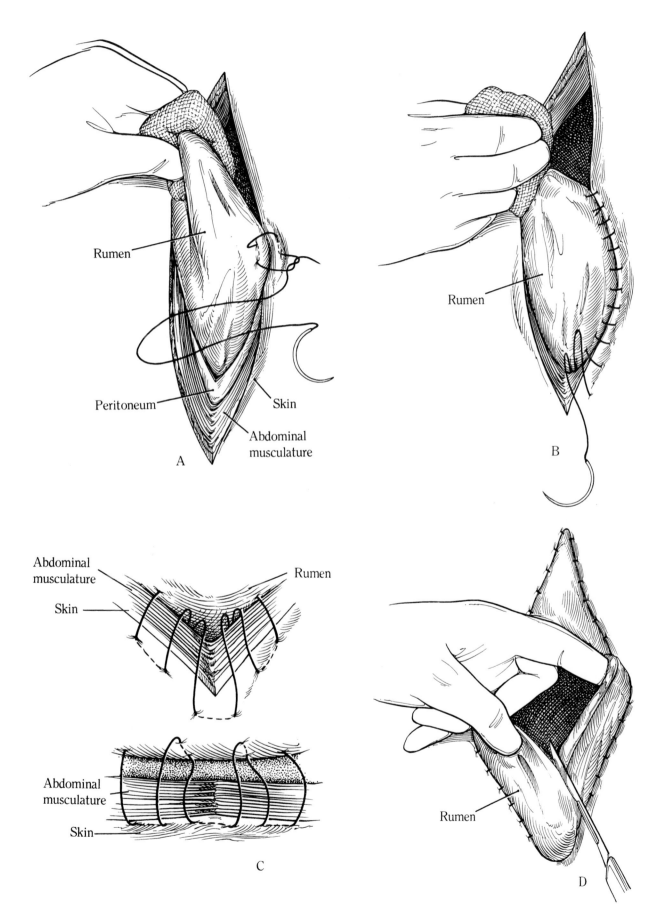

Rumen

Peritoneum   Skin

Abdominal
musculature

A

Rumen

B

Abdominal
musculature   Rumen

Skin

Abdominal
musculature

Skin

C

Rumen

D

Fig. 13-2. A to F, Rumenotomy.

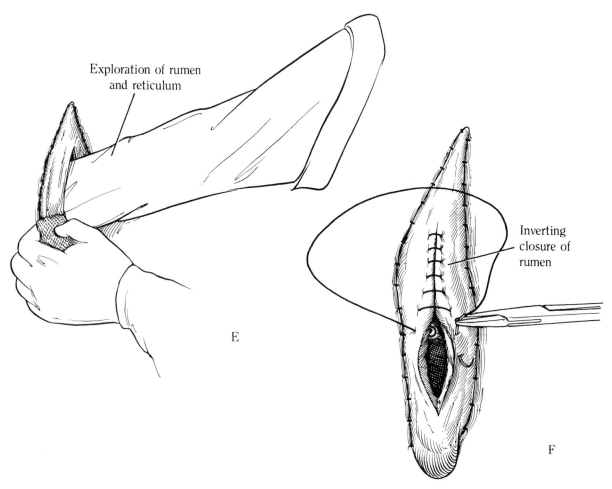

Fig. 13-2. *Continued.*

indicated. The surgeon's contaminated gloves are then discarded.

The rumen incision is closed with a simple continuous pattern using a no. 1 or 2 synthetic absorbable material (Figure 13-2F). A single layer can be adequate,[6] but a double row is generally used, with the second row an inverting pattern with similar suture material. The surgical site is then irrigated with polyionic fluid prior to removal of the rumen-fixation suture or apparatus. Closure of the laparotomy incision has been described previously.

Postoperative Management

Postoperative medication varies with the indication for the rumenotomy. Although rumen overload often requires intensive fluid therapy, traumatic reticulitis requires little intensive care. Antibiotics are indicated following the removal of foreign bodies from the reticulum. Oral fluids can be administered following rumenotomy, and mild osmotic laxatives, such as magnesium hydroxide, often promote gut motility.

Complications and Prognosis

Potentially fatal peritoneal contamination may occur if a fluid-tight seal is not created between the rumen and abdominal wall. This can be avoided by thoroughly palpating between suture bites for any gaps large enough to fit an index finger through.[5] These gaps should be eliminated by additional sutures. Incisional swelling and infection may also occur.[3]

Prognosis depends on the diagnosis of disease and the location and extent of perforations, if any, in the reticulum. Cases of traumatic reticuloperitonitis involving a perforation of the diaphragm have a very poor prognosis due to the risk of developing myocarditis, septic pericarditis, and thoracic abscesses.[3] Perforations on the right wall of the reticulum also carry a guarded prognosis due to their tendency to involve adhesions along the ventral branch of the vagus nerve, which may result in vagal sydrome.[3] Surgical treatment of perireticular abscesses secondary to traumatic reticuloperitonitis appears to be favorable in the literature.[3]

References

1. Baker, J.S.: Abomasal impaction and related obstructions of the forestomachs in cattle. J. Am. Vet. Med. Assoc., *175*:1250, 1979.
2. Dehghani, S.N.: Bovine rumenotomy: comparison of four surgical techniques. Can. Vet. J., *36*:693–697, 1995.
3. Ducharme, N.G.: Surgery of the bovine forestomach compartments. Vet. Clinics: Food An. Pract., *6*:371–396, 1990.
4. Dyce, K.M., Sack, W.O., and Wensing, C.J.G.: Textbook of Veterinary Anatomy, 2nd Ed. Philadelphia, W.B. Saunders, 1996, pp. 671–694.
5. Fubini, S.L., and Ducharme, N.G.: Bovine surgery, *In* Farm Animal Surgery. St. Louis, Elsevier, 2004, pp. 189–194.
6. Hofmeyr, C.F.B.: The digestive system. *In* Textbook of Large Animal Surgery. Edited by F.W. Oehme and J.E. Prier. Baltimore, Williams & Wilkins, 1974.

Rumenostomy (Rumenal Fistulation)

Relevant Anatomy

Anatomy relevant to this procedure is discussed in previous sections.

Indications

The techniques of rumenal fistulation have been developed for experimental purposes, as well as for the relief of chronic bloat. The experimental techniques use various types of cannulas to create a permanent opening, whereas the therapeutic technique provides temporary, symptomatic relief. Chronic bloating results from abnormal function of the parasympathetic nerve supply to the cardia of the stomach and dorsal sac of the rumen. This situation can result from reticuloperitonitis or fibrinous pneumonia-pleuritis involving the vagus nerve. Bloat may also develop secondary to enlarged lymph nodes or liver abscess; it is also observed occasionally in nursing cows and is thought to be associated with disturbed rumen metabolism. Another cause of bloat, especially in feedlot cattle, is altered rumen flora secondary to a rapid change from one feed to another. The technique of rumenostomy that we describe here is used as a therapeutic device in animals with chronic bloat.

Anesthesia and Surgical Preparation

This surgical procedure is performed with the animal standing. If rumenal tympany is present, it is relieved by a stomach tube; this measure will facilitate exteriorization of the rumen later. The left paralumbar fossa area is prepared surgically in a routine manner. A circular area immediately ventral to the transverse processes of the lumbar vertebrae and approximately 10 cm in diameter is infiltrated with local anesthetic.

Instrumentation

General surgery pack
Permanent fistula device

Surgical Technique

A circular piece of skin, approximately 4 cm in diameter, is removed to expose the underlying abdominal musculature (Figure 13-3A). The abdominal muscles and peritoneum are bluntly dissected to expose the rumen. It may be necessary to remove some of the external abdominal oblique muscle if it is thick and limits exposure of the rumen. The wall of the rumen is then grasped with forceps, and a portion of it is pulled through to the exterior. In this fashion, a "cone" of rumen is brought to the skin surface, where it is anchored to the skin with four horizontal mattress sutures of polymerized caprolactam or nylon (Figure 13-3B); these mattress sutures pass through rumen and skin. The central portion of the exposed rumen is removed (Figure 13-3B), and the incised edge of the rumen is sutured to the skin with simple interrupted sutures of nonabsorbable material (Figure 13-3C and D). The rumenal fistula that results from this procedure should be no larger than 2 to 3 cm in diameter. The muscle layers perform a valve-like function and help control seepage of rumenal ingesta while relieving gas accumulation in the rumen.

Postoperative Management

When surgery is performed properly, antibiotics need not be administered, and aftercare is not usually indicated. Many animals with chronic bloat fail to recover normal eructation, so the fistula should be permanent. If the fistula is made with the dimensions we have described, it should remain patent for a sufficient time. A smaller fistula will close earlier. With the valvelike function of the muscle layers, the fistula generally stays open as long as gas is expelled from it; however, it usually closes once the animal regains normal eructation.

Complications and Prognosis

Ruminal fistulation has not been shown to cause permanent effects on heart rate, respiratory rate, or EKG patterns. These effects have been temporary in the literature and may last an average of 20 days postoperatively. Temporary side effects include increases in ruminal pH, total volatile fatty acids, propionic acid, valeric acid, respiratory rate, and heart rate.[1] The prognosis for the procedure is good and complications are generally few and mild.

Reference

1. Rumsey, T.S., Putnam, P.A., Williams, E.E., and Samuelson, G.: Effect of ruminal and esophageal fistulation on ruminal parameters, saliva flow, EKG patterns and respiratory rate of beef steers. J. Anim. Sci., *35*:1248–1256, 1972.

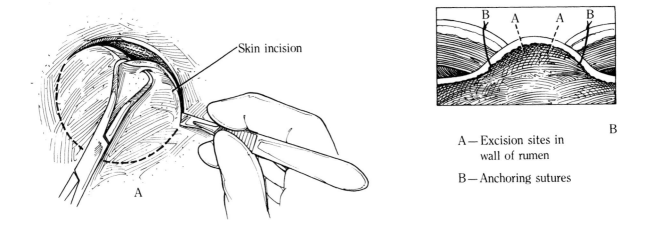

A—Excision sites in
   wall of rumen

B—Anchoring sutures

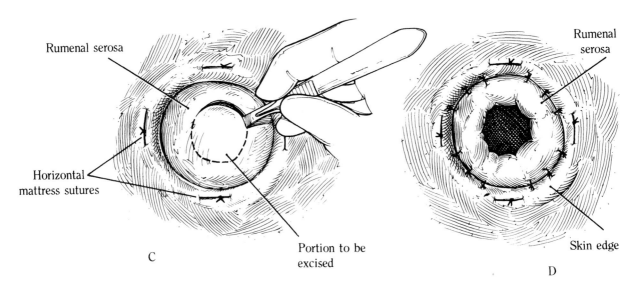

Fig. 13-3. A to D, Rumenostomy.

Surgical Corrections of Abomasal Displacements and Torsion

Relevant Anatomy

In general, the exact position of the abomasum in the living animal depends on the rate and size of contractions of the rumen and reticulum, the fullness of the other stomach compartments, the abomasum's activity, the presence of a pregnant uterus, and the age of the animal.[11] The body of the abomasum lies on the abdominal floor with the cranial aspect of the fundus anchored to the reticulum, atrium, and ventral sac by muscular attachments.[11] The pyloric part of the abomasum transverses the ventral abdomen toward the right body wall.

The lining of the abomasum is comprised of thick folds of glandular mucosa. The mucosa of the body and fundus contains peptic glands and the pyloric part secretes only mucous.[11] At the flexure of the abomasum, the folds diminish to low rugae, and a large, highly vascularized, thickening of the wall, called the *torus,* narrows the pyloric passage.

Indications

Dilation or displacement of the abomasum is considered to be one of the most common surgical conditions in bovine patients. Displacements may occur to the left or right side (LDA or RDA), although most occur to the left side and are more common during the first month after calving in Jersey, Guernsey, and Holstien-Friesan cows.[2,9,23] Abomasal displacement is believed to occur secondarily to abnormally high volatile fatty acid levels and excessive fermentation that lead to gas accumulation and distention. As a result of the gas, the abomasum may float up the abdominal wall on either the left or right side. Although less common, right torsion of the abomasum (RTA) may occur to varying degrees. If the torsion exceeds 180°, it is termed a *volvulus*. Abomasal volvulus is a serious condition that leads to complete obstruction of the outflow of ingesta to the duodenum. The etiology of RTA is not completely understood, but the condition is thought to occur secondary to some cases of right-sided displacement of the abomasum. Animals with RTA generally have more acute clinical signs. In addition, they may have marked electrolyte changes, particularly in the chloride and potassium levels.[24] The severity of RTA has been classified into four grades, on the basis of the volume of sequestered abomasal fluid, and this classification is useful and less subjective than the common clinical means.[24]

There are several surgical techniques described in the literature for correcting abomasal displacements.[1] Factors such as economy, cosmetics, surgical environment, number of assistants, and the reproductive stage and systemic condition of the patient affect the decision to choose one technique over another. Both LDA and RDA may be treated with right-flank omentopexy, with or without pyloropexy, and ventral paramedian abomasopexy.[18,20] In addition, right-flank omentopexy and ventral paramedian abomasopexy may be used to treat select cases of RTA. Right-flank omentopexy was developed when the only alternative was paramedian abomasopexy, which required the patient to be in dorsal recumbency. In some cows, this position was undesirable, so a surgical procedure that could be performed with the animal standing had obvious advantages. Recumbency should be avoided in animals with compromised systemic conditions, respiratory distress, or distended rumens, or those that are pregnant.[14,18, 20] The subsequent development of the flank abomasopexy techniques offered a third alternative.

Ventral paramedian abomasopexy has several advantages: The abomasum is brought into position more easily in most cases, and instantaneous repositioning commonly occurs; the abomasum is easily viewed for detailed examination and detection of ulcers; and strong, positive, long-lasting adhesions can be anticipated. The main disadvantage of this approach is that it is not performed in standing animals and requires more assistants.

Right-flank omentopexy involves suturing the superficial layer of the greater omentum in the region of the pylorus to the abdominal wall in the right flank. To perform pyloropexy, the technique is modified to include a portion of the pyloric antrum in the incisional closure.[6] Some surgeons believe this may increase the risk of penetrating the lumen during fixation, however, due to the strong adherence of the submucosa to the mucosa in this region.[14]

Right-flank omentopexy has a high success rate for the treatment of LDA.[17] A disadvantage to this approach is that the surgeon's access to a left-sided displaced abomasum is more limited than with the ventral paramedian

approach. The displacement can be exceedingly difficult to correct if movement of the abomasum is inhibited by focal adhesions or accumulations of fibrous tissue that may occur secondary to peritonitis.[8] Also, the maintenance of long-term fixation of the abomasum can be questioned, particularly with inexperienced surgeons. Adipose tissue is weak, and the trauma of a cow being knocked down could be sufficient to tear or stretch the omental attachment. Right displacement of the abomasum can also occur if the abomasum pivots around an intact omental adhesion.[17]

Left-flank and right-flank abomasopexies are used to correct LDA and RDA, respectively.[2,8] Right-flank abomasopexy may also be used to treat RTA.[5] These techniques have the advantage of offering direct fixation of the abomasum to the ventral body wall and are performed with the animal in the standing position. In addition, adhesions or ulceration of the displaced abomasum can be visualized and treated, and an exploratory rumenotomy can be performed if indicated. One disadvantage of these techniques is that the abomasal anchoring achieved with the flank approaches is not considered as secure as that achieved with the ventral paramedian technique. Furthermore, the site for abomasal fixation to the body wall can be difficult to reach in large cows or if the surgeon has short arms. Care is necessary to avoid puncturing viscera because the needle is carried to the floor of the abdomen; and in some cases, the abomasum may be lying in a cranioventral position and may be difficult to expose sufficiently for placement of the suture.[8] Auscultation during the clinical examination prior to surgery should identify the situation, and another approach may be considered.

Right-flank abomasopexy is generally preferred over a paramedian approach to treat cases of RTA in the severely affected cow. Fluid can be removed from the abomasum more easily through a flank incision, and there is less risk to a patient in a compromised condition if it is operated on in the standing position. However, in cases of severe RTA in which abomasal compromise is suspected, omentopexy should be considered because suture material may pull through the abomasal wall.[7] In animals that survive the surgery, however, this problem has not been observed.[4]

There are several alternative techniques for treatment of LDA that will not be described here. Blind stitch abomasopexy and toggle pin fixation (roll-and-toggle procedure) are two closed surgical techniques that are considered quick and inexpensive for the experienced surgeon.[2,6] However, these techniques require considerable precision and accuracy because the structures to be fixed are not directly visualized. A significant disadvantage to the closed techniques is the inability of the surgeon to assess other possible complications within the abdomen (e.g., adhesions, ulcers, fatty liver, etc.). An inexperienced surgeon will most likely find that the closed techniques are just as difficult to master as the open techniques. For this reason, many surgeons opt for an alternative approach through the paralumbar fossa. Right paramedian, left paramedian, and one-step laparoscopic approaches to abomasopexy have been described.[19,21] These procedures are described in detail elsewhere.[19,21]

Anesthesia and Surgical Preparation

Right-flank omentopexy, right-flank pyloropexy, and right- and left-flank abomasopexies are performed with the animal standing. The right or left paralumbar area is clipped and prepared surgically. Local anesthesia is instituted by performing a paravertebral block, inverted L block, or a line block. If a left-flank abomasopexy is to be performed, an area from the xiphoid process to the umbilicus and from the midline to the right subcutaneous abdominal vein is also prepared surgically. This second area is not anesthetized.

Ventral paramedian abomasopexy is performed in dorsal recumbency. The cow is sedated (xylazine HCl 15–30 mg i.v.) and is cast in dorsal recumbency. Acepromazine or butorphanol tartate are also appropriate sedatives. The cow's legs are tied, and its body is supported by a trough or weighted side frames. The patient should be tilted slightly to the right, to facilitate later closure of the incision. An area from the xiphoid process to the umbilicus is clipped and is surgically prepared in a routine manner. Local anesthesia is administered by local infiltration along the proposed incision or an inverted L block of the right paramedian area.

Instrumentation

General surgery pack
Sterile sleeves
14–16-gauge needle with sterile tubing attached
Large, straight, cutting needle or an S-curved cutting
   needle for abomasopexy
Sterile, medium-sized stomach tube

Surgical Technique

Right-Flank Omentopexy

The abdomen is entered through a 20-cm vertical incision in the right paralumbar fossa starting 4 to 5 cm ventral to the transverse processes of the lumbar vertebrae (Figure 13-4A). When the peritoneal cavity is entered in the case of an LDA, the duodenum will be vertical instead of in its normal horizontal position. Wearing sterile sleeves, the surgeon palpates the left side of the abdomen by deflecting the greater omentum craniad, and then passes his/her left arm caudal to the omentum and rumen to palpate the abomasum distended with gas on the left side of the rumen. This confirms the diagnosis of LDA. In addition, while palpating the displaced organ, one should feel for any evidence of adhesions.

The abomasum may be deflated using a 14–16-gauge needle with a length of sterile tubing attached. The needle is carried caudal to the rumen to the most dorsal part of the displaced abomasum and is inserted obliquely through the abomasal wall. Pressure is applied firmly with the forearm and the hand to release the gas or the tubing may be attached to a suction device. The needle is withdrawn and is carried back carefully, with the tubing folded to avoid contamination.

The abomasum is returned to its normal position by following the peritoneal surfaces ventrally with the hand between the rumen and the body wall. Once to the left of the rumen, the hand, with the fingers closed, is used to sweep the abomasum back to the right side of the abdomen. Gentle dorsocraniad pulling on the omentum, which has also been displaced to the left, is also helpful in this manipulation. If the rumen is full, it may be necessary to elevate the caudal ventral blind sac of the rumen with the inside of the elbow to allow the abomasum to be pulled along under the rumen. Once the abomasum is returned to its normal position, the duodenum resumes its normal horizontal position (Figure 13-4B) and is commonly observed to fill with gas. The greater omentum, which is observed through the abdominal incision, also feels loose (Figure 13-4B). Unnecessary handling of the duodenum during these manipulations may cause postoperative duodenitis.

If the surgery is performed for the treatment of an RDA or RTA, care should be taken not to incise the dilatated abomasum when entering the peritoneal cavity. The various right-sided malpositions of the abomasum when using a right-flank approach are detailed in the section on right-flank abomasopexy. The abomasum commonly requires evacuation before the displacement can be corrected. An RTA usually has large quantities of fluid. Correct positioning of the abomasum is recognized in the same fashion as in LDA. Once the abomasum has been returned to its correct position, the technique of omentopexy is the same whether it is an LDA, RDA, or RTA.

The omentum is grasped and pulled out through the incision. It is gently retracted dorsad and caudad until the pylorus can be visualized. This fold of omentum may be held by an assistant or attached to the upper part of the skin incision with towel forceps while the anchoring sutures are placed. Two mattress sutures of no. 1 or 2 synthetic absorbable suture material (one cranial to the incision and one caudal to it) are placed through the peritoneum and transverse abdominal muscle and through both layers of the fold of omentum (Figure 13-4C). The sutures are placed about 3 cm caudal to the pylorus. The peritoneum and transverse abdominal muscle are then sutured in a simple continuous pattern with no. 1 or 2 synthetic absorbable suture, and the omentum is incorporated into the suture line in the ventral two-thirds of the incision (Figure 13-4D). The internal and external abdominal oblique muscle layers and the skin are closed as in a routine flank laparotomy.

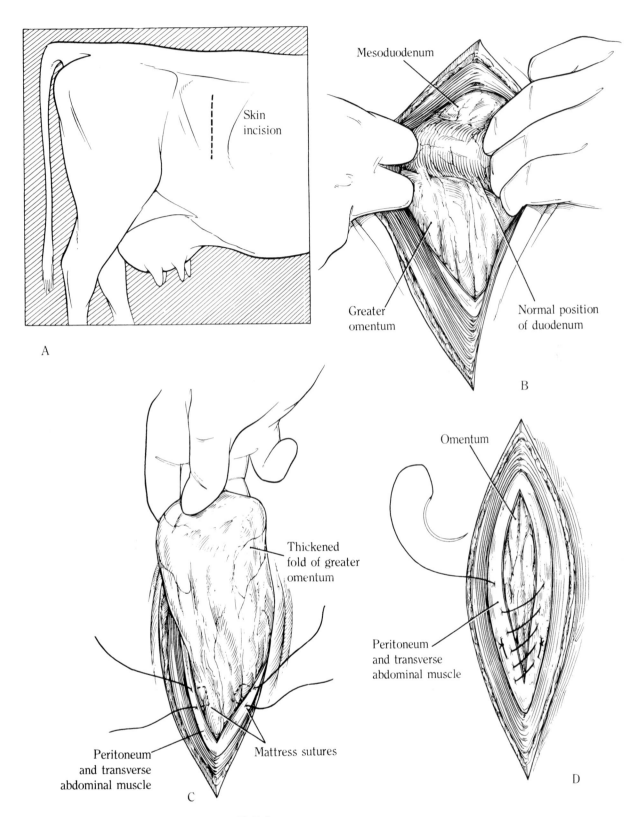

Fig. 13-4. A to D, Right-flank omentopexy. E, Pyloropexy.

231

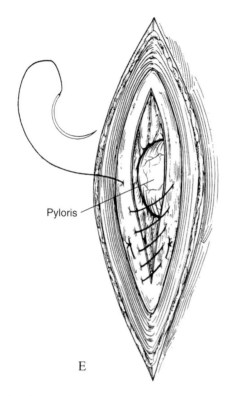

Pyloris

E

Fig. 13-4. *Continued.*

Pyloropexy

One to two sutures are placed in a cruciate pattern through all the muscle layers and the peritoneum cranioventral to the incision site and through the torus pyloricus muscle (Figure 13-4E).[13] The omentum caudal to the pylorus may be included in the suture line of the ventral two-thirds of the closure incision as described above. Theoretically, the pyloropexy is more secure than an omentopexy. However, care must be taken to not penetrate the lumen with the sutures.

Left-Flank Abomasopexy

A left-flank laparotomy is performed using a 20- to 25-cm incision in the paralumbar fossa, as previously described. Caution should be exercised when entering the abdomen because a distended abomasum may lie immediately within the incision area. Usually, the abomasum is visible through the incision. An 8- to 12-cm simple continuous or interlocking suture line of heavy polymerized caprolactam, nylon, or polypropylene is placed in the greater curvature of the abomasum 5 to 7 cm from the attachment of the greater omentum (Figure 13-5A). The suture bites pass through the submucosa, and a meter of suture material should extend from each end of the suture line. Hemostats are placed on these suture ends in such a fashion that the cranial and caudal ends are easily identified. The abomasum may then be deflated using a 12-

gauge needle and rubber tubing (Figure 13-5A) if this is considered necessary. The needle is placed into the dorsal portion of the abomasum and is inserted at an angle to obviate leakage when the needle is withdrawn. It is important that the abomasum not be deflated prior to the insertion of the suture; otherwise, the site for suture placement may be retracted from the incision.

The cranial end of the suture is attached to a large, straight, cutting needle or to an S-curved cutting needle; this needle is carried along the internal body wall to a position right of midline, but medial to the subcutaneous abdominal vein and 15 cm caudal to the xiphoid process. The forefinger protects the end of the needle, and the lateral fingers reflect the viscera away from the body wall and ahead of the needle. An assistant can apply upward pressure on the abdominal wall in the area where the needles are to be inserted through the body wall. An empty syringe case works well for this purpose.

The needle is inserted quickly through the ventral body wall (Figure 13-5B). The assistant grasps the needle, and the caudal suture is placed through the body wall 8 to 12 cm caudal to the cranial suture. The assistant then grasps the two suture ends and applies gentle traction; at the same time, the surgeon pushes the deflated abomasum into its normal position. When the sutured area of the abomasum is lying against the floor of the abdomen, the assistant ties the suture ends together (Figure 13-5C). The flank laparotomy incision is closed routinely. The suture is left in place for 4 weeks; the ends are then cut as close to the skin as possible. This time is considered necessary to allow the development of adhesions sufficient to prevent redisplacement.

Right-Flank Abomasopexy

The right-flank approach to the bovine abdomen has been described previously. A 20- to 25-cm incision is made. At this stage, the particular problem needs to be recognized, and certain guidelines can be stated. In a simple RDA, the greater omentum comes into view through the laparotomy wound in the right flank as in a normal animal. The greater omentum may be looser because the distance between the abomasum and the descending duodenum is less than normal. The fundus will typically have moved caudolaterad and will appear uncovered by omentum. Abomasal torsions (*volvulus* may be a better term) occur counterclockwise when viewed from the rear and counterclockwise when viewed from the right flank. The omentum is usually wrapped in the torsion site, and the abomasum therefore appears at the incision without omentum covering it.

The color of the abomasal serosa is ascertained before one attempts to deflate the abomasum or correct its position. If the serosa appears viable and the organ is tightly distended, a 12-gauge needle with rubber tubing attached is inserted to relieve the gaseous pressure and to facilitate further exploration and manipulation. It is easier to

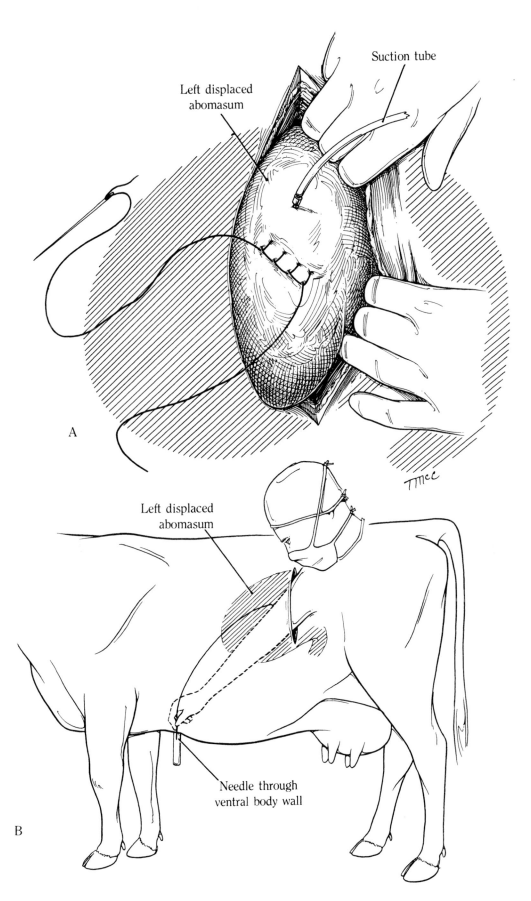

Suction tube

Left displaced
abomasum

A

Left displaced
abomasum

B

Needle through
ventral body wall

Fig. 13-5. A to C, Left-flank abomasopexy.

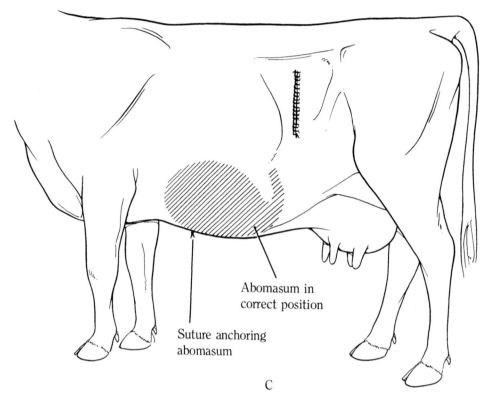

Fig. 13-5. *Continued.*

Abomasum in
correct position

Suture anchoring
abomasum

C

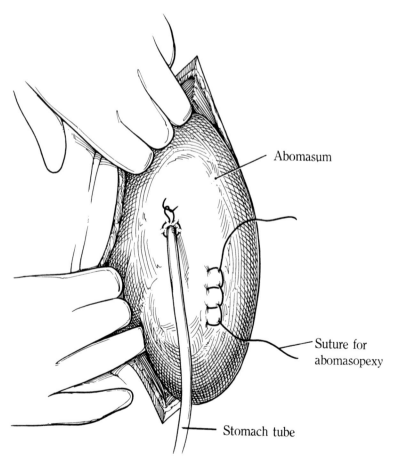

Abomasum

Suture for
abomasopexy

Stomach tube

Fig. 13-6. The fluid within the abomasum is
removed using a medium-sized stomach tube.

remove gas and fluid before detorsion because the aboma-sum is closer to the incision. Early or less-severe torsion may not even require fluid removal, but severe torsion may require fluid removal before the torsion can be reduced. Placement of the suture requires careful thought, to ensure correct positioning at the completion of the procedure. An interlocking suture is placed in the middle of the greater curvature of the abomasum near the attach-ment of the greater omentum in the manner previously described and illustrated for left-flank abomasopexy (Figure 13-5A to C). If absolutely necessary, a purse-string suture can be placed in the abomasal wall, a stab incision is made, and a sterile, medium-sized stomach tube inserted into the abomasum (Figure 13-6). The fluid within the abomasum is then removed. If the fluid is dif-ficult to drain, lavage may be performed. At the end of abomasal drainage, 2 to 3 L of mineral oil are instilled into the abomasum, the tube is withdrawn, and the purse-string suture is tied. The abomasopexy is completed as described for left-flank abomasopexy.

Ventral Paramedian Abomasopexy

A 20-cm incision is made between the midline and the right subcutaneous abdominal vein, starting approxi-mately 8 cm behind the xiphoid process and ending immediately cranial to the umbilicus (Figure 13-7A and B). The small branches of the subcutaneous abdominal vein that are cut when incising the skin and subcutaneous tissue need to be ligated because the lack of muscle tissue in this region inhibits natural hemostasis, and may result in hematoma and seroma formation. The incision is con-tinued through the external rectus sheath (aponeuroses of external and internal abdominal oblique muscles) (Figure 13-7C) and the rectus abdominis muscle to reveal the fibers of the internal rectus sheath (the transverse abdominal aponeurosis) running crosswise in the inci-sion line. The transverse abdominal aponeurosis and peritoneum are incised (Figure 13-7D). The transverse aponeurosis may be cut separately with a scalpel and the peritoneum may be entered using scissors, or both layers may be opened together with scissors.

In most cases of LDA, the abomasum will have returned to a relatively normal position during the casting proce-dure. If necessary, the abomasum should be returned to its normal position. Rarely, in the case of an RDA or RTA, it may be appropriate to empty gas with a 12-gauge needle and rubber tubing (Figure 13-7E). This is probably unnec-essary with an LDA. Once the correct position of the abomasum has been ascertained, the lateral aspect of the greater curvature of the abomasum (where it is free of omentum) is incorporated with the peritoneum and internal rectus sheath in a simple continuous suture pattern with no. 1 or 2 synthetic absorbable suture mate-rial (Figure 13-7F). Care must be taken to not penetrate the abdominal mucosa. The heavy, external rectus sheath

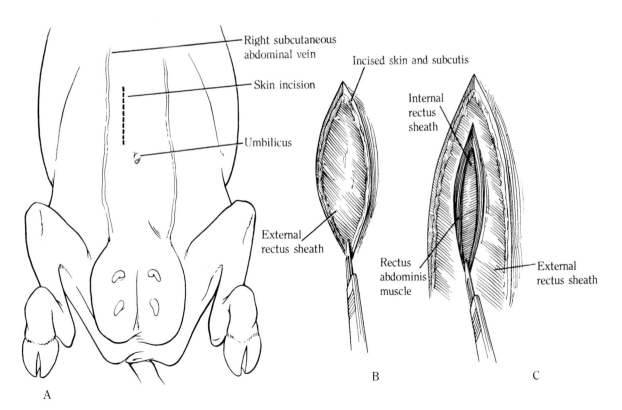

Fig. 13-7. A to G, Ventral paramedian abomasopexy.

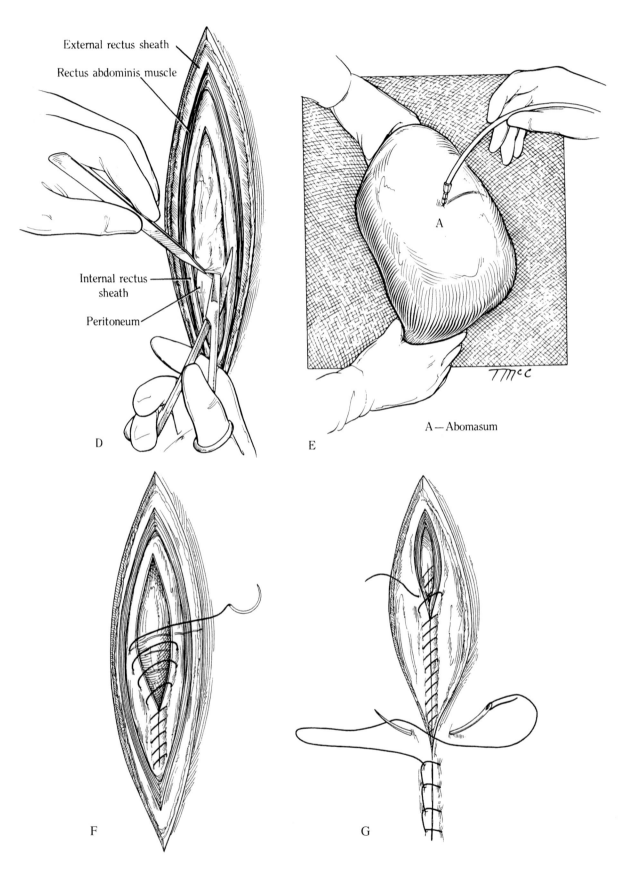

External rectus sheath

Rectus abdominis muscle

Internal rectus sheath

Peritoneum

A

A — Abomasum

D

E

F

G

Fig. 13-7. *Continued.*

is closed with a simple continuous pattern of no. 1 or 2 synthetic absorbable suture (Figure 13-5G), and the skin is closed with a Ford interlocking suture using heavy polymerized caprolactam (Figure 13-5G). The patient is rolled into left lateral recumbency, followed by sternal recumbency.

Postoperative Management

Postoperative management depends on the individual case. Some animals require little or no aftercare; other animals may have septic metritis, mastitis, or ketosis, and may also have been deprived of feed and water. Correction of metabolic disturbances subsequent to left abomasal displacements may necessitate the administration of electrolytes, calcium salts, and fluid therapy.

Animals operated on for RTA are in particularly critical condition and require a more gradual, cautious return to feed and water. These patients should be monitored regularly for clinical signs, milk production, and urine ketones. Antibiotics are administered postoperatively. Many of these animals need intense fluid therapy with particular emphasis on replacement of the chloride deficit (see Chapter 2). For this purpose, 0.9% sodium chloride solution is generally appropriate; supplementation with potassium chloride may also be indicated. With adequate fluid and electrolyte therapy in the presurgical and early postsurgical periods, the metabolic effects of RTA generally can be controlled. In severely affected cows, the abomasum's inability to regain normal function is often more important. The abomasum becomes filled and impacted if its function is not restored.[24] Typically, cases of abomasal torsion appear to improve in the first 24 to 48 hours and then deteriorate at 48 to 72 hours, with abomasal atony. Motility stimulants, such as neostigmine, have been recommended, but neostigmine must be used repeatedly to have any effect above the pylorus, and even then its benefit is minimal. If the animal's appetite has not returned in 2 days, a rumen inoculation may be appropriate. Oral supportive therapy, in which sodium chloride and potassium chloride are added to water, can be used in a patient capable of absorbing the fluid.

Complications and Prognosis

One of the most common complications of right-flank omentopexy and pyloropexy is recurrence.[2] Recurrence can be due to incorrect placement of sutures during fixation—for example, fixing the omentum too far dorsal or caudal to the pylorus—or due to stretching or disruption of the omentopexy.[2] Even in the hands of experienced operators, however, redisplacement may occur in the long term. Because of potential rotation of the abomasum around the omental attachment, the technique is certainly questionable for the treatment of RDA or RTA.

Abdominal fistulas may occur subsequent to abomasopexy if nonabsorbable sutures are used for fixation or closure of the external rectus sheath. Nonabsorbable sutures that penetrate the lumen of the abomasum may potentiate bacterial colonization of the abdominal wall resulting in fistulation. In the author's experience, catgut is satisfactory. Acute wound dehiscence with evisceration and redisplacements are considered rare complications of this procedure. Left-flank abomasopexy, in particular, is associated with an increased risk of puncturing viscera or accidentally catching omentum while carrying the needle to the floor of the abdomen. The surgeon must ensure accurate placement of fixation sutures; otherwise, redisplacement may occur or other abdominal structures may be inadvertently pinned between the abomasum and abdominal wall. Again, multifilament nonabsorbable sutures should be avoided due to the risk of abomasal fistulation. Other large animal surgeons have cited inadvertent damage to the milk vein and partial outflow obstruction due to improper positioning of the abomasum as common complications encountered in this procedure.[14]

The success rate of right-flank omentopexy for the treatment of LDA is high; ranging from 87% to 100% in dairy cows.[8,13,17,23] The complication rate that was reported in one of the studies was also low (3.3%), with the primary complication being peritonitis. The success rate of this procedure for cases of RDA is lower overall than that of LDA—74.5% reported by Rohn et al.; however, this is influenced by whether abomasal volvulus is present.[22] There are few statistical evaluations of omentopexy performed in conjunction with pyloropexy in the literature. One study reported a 67% success rate of right-flank pyloro-omentopexy for treatment of LDA in dairy cows, which was significantly lower than the 84% success rate for cows treated with the roll-and-toggle procedure.[6]

Some surgeons believe that their success in treating cows with RTA was due largely to not opening the abomasum prior to surgery.[15] Now this claim generally is considered invalid. Whether acidic fluid high in chloride is easily absorbed from the abomasum following detorsion is questionable. In addition, any fluid deficit sustained by draining the abomasum can be replaced by intravenous fluid therapy; this is considered more reliable than anticipating reabsorption of the fluid from the abomasum after detorsion. The rationale for removing fluids that potentially contain endotoxins is logical, but its validity is controversial. Whether deposition of mineral oil directly into the abomasum inhibits further toxin reabsorption is uncertain, and its value is equally controversial. One author believes that this measure has contributed to his success,[5] whereas another author does not think that this measure improved the prognosis for severely affected cows.[24]

Prognosis and survival rates for right-flank abomasopexy are not well documented. The prognosis for cases of abdominal volvulus is much less favorable than that of uncomplicated cases of RDA. Several studies have reported prognostic indicators that may be useful at the time of surgery for ascertaining outcome, such as whether fluid decompression is performed in addition to gas decompression, the presence of venous thrombosis, and blue or black discoloration of the abomasum.[10,15] Some surgeons believe that not performing fluid decompression is advantageous because the abomasum is allowed to resorb electrolytes, and the surgical time and risk of peritonitis is decreased.[10,18] Indeed, clinical studies show higher survival rates for cows that do not receive fluid decompression. However, this may be incorrectly correlated because cows with a greater duration of torsion will not only have accrued more fluid in the abomasum, but are also more likely to have greater tissue damage and necrosis, which could account for the much lower survival rate that is observed.

The prognosis for ventral paramedian abomasopexy is comparable to that of right-flank omentopexy. In a comparison study of right-flank omentopexy and right paramedian abomasopexy for treatment of LDA, survival rates were 81.5% and 87% at 6 months for abomasopexy and omentopexy, respectively.[13] However, this varies greatly with complicated cases or cases of RDA. In these instances, prognosis depends greatly on the extent of tissue damage and the amount and duration of volvulus.

References

1. Ames, S.: Repositioning displaced abomasum in the cow. J. Am. Vet. Med. Assoc., *153*:1470, 1968.
2. Aubry, P.: Routine surgical procedures in dairy cattle under field conditions: abomasal surgery, dehorning, and tail docking. Vet. Clin. Food. Anim., *21*:55–71, 2005.
3. Baker, J.S.: Displacement of the abomasum in dairy cows: part II. Pract. Vet., *Summer/Fall:*1, 1973.
4. Baker, J.S.: Personal communication, 1980.
5. Baker, J.S.: Right displacement of the abomasum in the bovine: a modified procedure for treatment. Bov. Pract., *11*:58, 1976.
6. Bartlett, P.C., Kopcha, M., Coe, P.H., Ames, N.K., Ruegg, P.L., and Erskine, R.G.: Economic comparison of the pyloroomentopexy versus the roll-and-toggle procedure for the treatment of left displacement of the abomasum in dairy cattle. J. Am. Vet. Med. Assoc., *Apr15;206(8)*:1156–1162, 1995.
7. Boucher, W.B., and Abt, D.: Right-sided dilatation of the bovine abomasum with torsion. J. Am. Vet. Med. Assoc., *153*:76, 1968.
8. Buckner, R.: Surgical correction of left displaced abomasum in cattle. Vet. Rec., *136*:265–267, 1995.
9. Constable, P.D., Miller, G.Y., Hoffis, G.F., Hull, B.L., and Rings, D.M.: Risk factors for abomasal volvulus and left abomasal displacement in cattle. Am. J. Vet. Res., *53*:1184–1192, 1992.
10. Constable, P.D., St. Jean, G., Hull, B.L., Rings, D.M., and Hoffsis, G.F.: Prognostic value of surgical and postoperative findings in cattle with abomasal volvulus. J. Am. Vet. Med. Assoc., *199*:892–898, 1991.
11. Dyce, K.M., Sack, W.O., and Wensing, C.J.G.: Textbook of Veterinary Anatomy, 2nd Ed. Philadelphia, W.B. Saunders, 1996, pp. 671–694.
12. Espersen, G.: Dilatation and displacement of the abomasum to the right flank, and dilatation and dislocation of the cecum. Vet. Rec., *76*:1423, 1964.
13. Fubini, S.L., Ducharme, N.G., Erb, H.N., and Sheils, R.L.: A comparison in 101 dairy cows of right paralumbar fossa omentopexy and right paramedian abomasopexy for treatment of left displacement of the abomasum. Can. Vet. J., *33*:318–324, 1992.
14. Fubini, S.L., and Ducharme, N.G.: Bovine surgery, *In* Farm Animal Surgery. St. Louis, Elsevier, 2004, pp. 208–217.
15. Fubini, S.L., Ducharme, N.G., Erb, H.N., and Sheils, R.L.: A comparison in 101 dairy cows of right paralumbar fossa omentopexy and right paramedian abomasopexy for treatment of left displacement of the abomasum. Can. Vet. J., *33*:318–324, 1992.
16. Fubini, S.L., Grohn, Y.T., and Smith, D.F.: Right displacement of the abomasum and abomasal volvulus in dairy cows: 458 cases (1980–1987). J. Am. Vet. Med. Assoc., *198*:460–464, 1991.
17. Gabel, A.A., and Heath, R.B.: Correction and right-sided omentopexy in treatment of left-sided displacement of the abomasum in dairy cattle. J. Am. Vet. Med. Assoc., *155*:632, 1969.
18. Gabel, A.A., and Heath, R.B.: Treatment of right-sided torsion of the abomasum in cattle. J. Am. Vet. Med. Assoc., *155*:642, 1969.
19. Lee, I., Yamagishi, N., Oboshi, K., and Yamada, H.: Left paramedian abomasopexy in cattle. J. Vet. Sci., *3*:59–60, 2002.
20. Lowe, J.E., and Loomis, W.K.: Abomasopexy for repair of left abomasal displacement in dairy cattle. J. Am. Vet. Med. Assoc., *147*:389, 1965.
21. Newman, K.D., Anderson, D.E., and Silveira, F.: One step laparoscopic abomasopexy for correction of left-sided displacement of the abomasum in dairy cows. J. Am. Vet. Med. Assoc., *227*:1142–1147, 2005.
22. Rohn, M., Tenhagen, B.A., and Hofman, W.: Survival of dairy cows after surgery to correct abomasal displacement: 1. Clinical and laboratory parameters and overall survival. J. Vet. Med. Assoc., *51*:294–299, 2004.
23. Seeger, T., Kumper, H., Failing, K., and Doll, K.: Comparison of laparoscopic-guided abomasopexy versus omentopexy via right flank laparotomy for the treatment of left abomasal displacement in dairy cows. Am. J. Vet. Res., *67*:472–478, 2006.
24. Smith, D.F.: Right-side torsion of the abomasum in dairy cows: classification of severity and evaluation of outcome. J. Am. Vet. Med. Assoc., *173*:108, 1978.
25. Van Winden, S.C.L., Brattinga, C.R., Muller, K.E., Noordhuizen, J.P.T.M., and Beynen, A.C.: Position of the abomasum in dairy cows during the first six weeks after calving. Vet. Rec., *151*:446–449, 2002.

Chapter 14

BOVINE UROGENITAL SURGERY

Objectives

1. Discuss the indications for various urogenital surgical techniques in the bovine.
2. Describe the disadvantages and advantages of different castration approaches in cattle.
3. Describe various penile, preputial, and inguinal surgical interventions including hematoma evacuation, and teaser bull preparation.
4. Describe the various surgical treatments involved with dystocia.

Calf Castration

Relevant Anatomy

The anatomy of the testes and associated structures is basically the same as in the horse (described in Chapter 10, "Equine Urogenital Surgery"). In the bull, the scrotum is located between the cranial parts of the thighs. On the cranial face of the scrotum are small, rudimentary teats that vary in number and spacing. In contrast to the horse, the testes are situated vertically rather than horizontally within the scrotum. The epididymis runs along the caudomedial border of the testes. At the distal pole of the testes, the ductus deferens begin at the tail of the epididymis and ascend the medial border of the testes. The spermatic cord may be palpated at the scrotal neck.

Indications

Castration of beef calves is a routine management procedure that is used to improve the quality of the carcass, prevent unintended births, and improve the safety and ease of herd management. There are three primary methods of castration: physical, chemical, and hormonal.[6] Chemical castration, which involves the injection of a toxic subject into the testes, is associated with a 25% failure rate and is not generally accepted as a useful technique.[1,5,6] Hormonal castration, which involves immunizing the bulls for gonadotrophin-releasing hormone, is not used frequently because of its limited practicality and consumer concerns.[3] All physical methods, including surgical castration, Burdizzo clamps, and latex bands, are associated with pain and discomfort to the animal as well as substantial potential complications. Generally, surgical castration is preferred because it is associated with rapid wound healing and a low failure rate, although the method of castration used by beef cattle operations varies with region and is fairly subjective.[4,6]

This procedure should be performed early in a calf's life. It is recommended that nursing calves are castrated at 1 to 4 weeks of age. Bucket-reared calves should probably be castrated 3 to 4 weeks later because of their slower start nutritionally and inferior condition. Sometimes it may be necessary to wait longer on an individual calf. Some calves will be held to weaning before castration if progeny testing for weight gain is performed.

Anesthesia and Surgical Preparation

In the beef industry, it has been traditional practice to perform surgical castration quickly without anesthesia or skin preparation based on the economics, convenience, and circumstances of the procedure. The humaneness of this practice has become a significant consumer concern and has garnered further research into improving intra- and postoperative analgesia for surgical castration. In some countries, it has led to revisions of welfare legislation that prohibit the surgical castration of male ruminants without local or general anesthesia, postoperative pain relief, and a veterinarian to perform the procedure.[8]

Evidence suggests that nonsteroidal antiinflammatory drugs, such as ketoprofen, may have a more beneficial effect in alleviating postoperative pain and inflammation in surgically castrated calves than local anesthetic alone due to their systemic analgesic properties. Although local anesthesia minimizes pain-related behavioral responses during surgical castration, it does not significantly reduce cortisol responses. A combination of local anesthetic and intravenous ketoprofen, however, significantly reduces both the behavioral responses and the rise in mean plasma cortisol concentrations during the first 8 hours post-operatively.[6] Ketoprofen has also been shown to reduce acute phase protein responses, and by inference, inflammation associated with the procedure.[2]

A tranquilizer or sedative may be administered, and local infiltration analgesia is performed. Following surgical preparation of the area, the skin is infiltrated on a line 1 cm from the median raphe with 10 ml of local analgesic solution; this infiltration is continued into the subcutaneous tissue. Local analgesia can be injected directly into the testis. It is also important to infiltrate the spermatic cord in the region of emasculation with a long 18- to 20-gauge needle. Ketoprofen may be administered intravenously to provide better analgesia.

Additional Instrumentation

General surgery pack
Emasculators

Surgical Technique

The scrotum is grasped, and a horizontal incision is made through skin and fascia at the widest part of the scrotum (junction of middle and distal thirds). The entire distal segment of the scrotum is transected (Figure 14-1A), and the common vaginal tunic is left intact. Traction is then placed on the testes, and the skin is pushed proximad so that the fascia is separated from the spermatic cords enclosed in the common tunics (Figure 14-1B). The operator's hands should not touch the proximal regions of the spermatic cords.

The spermatic cords are emasculated (site of emasculation is illustrated in Figure 14-1B). It is important that the emasculators are pushed proximad and that tension on the cord be relaxed when emasculation is performed (Figure 14-1C). Following removal of the emasculators, any redundant adipose tissue is removed (Figure 14-1D). The incision may be sprayed with a topical antibacterial powder, and at the discretion of the operator, this powder may also be put up inside the incision.

Postoperative Management

The wound is left open to heal by secondary intention. Concurrent immunization for black leg and malignant edema is recommended. Prior immunization would be preferable, but it is often not practical. Exercise of the calves is important following castration. Calves should be monitored for signs of hemorrhage for approximately 24 hours.

Complications and Prognosis

The prognosis for surgical castration is good and complications are usually mild and infrequent. Potential complications include hemorrhage, excessive swelling, tetanus, and infection. Infection may occur 5 to 15 days following the procedure and often arises much later than would be anticipated. Infections usually manifest as acute cellulitis and require prompt treatment with drainage and antibiotics.

References

1. Coventry, J., McEwan, D., and Bertram, J.D.: Sterilization of bulls with lactic acid. Aust. Vet. J., 66:156–157, 1989.
2. Earley, B., and Crowe, M.A.: Effects of ketoprofen alone or in combination with local anesthesia during the castration of bull calves on plasma cortisol, immunological, and inflammatory responses. J. Anim. Sci., 80:1044–1052, 2002.
3. Finnerty, M., Enright, W.J., Morrison, C.A., and Roche, J.F.: Immunization of bull calves with a GNRH analog human serum-albumin conjugate—effect of conjugate dose, type of adjuvant and booster interval on immune, endocrine, testicular and growth-responses. J. Repro. Fertil., 101:333–343, 1994.
4. Fisher, A.D., Knight, T.W., Cosgrove, G.P., Death, A.F., Anderson, C.B., Duganzich, D.M., and Matthews, L.R.: Effects of surgical or banding castration on stress responses and behavior of bulls. Aust. Vet. J., 79:279–284, 2001.
5. Hill, G.M., Neville, W.E., Richardson, K.L., Utley, P.R., and Stewart, R.L.: Castration method and progesterone-estradiol implant effects on growth rate of suckling calves. J. Dairy Sci., 68:3059–3061, 1985.
6. Stafford, K.J., and Mellor, D.J.: The welfare significance of the castration of cattle: a review. N. Zeal. Vet. J., 53:271–278, 2005.
7. Stafford, K.J., Mellor, D.J., Todd, S.E., Bruce, R.A., and Ward, R.N.: Effects of local anaesthesia or local anaesthesia plus a non-steroidal anti-inflammatory drug on the acute cortisol response of calves to five different methods of castration. Res. Vet. Sci., 73:61–70, 2002.
8. Thuer, S., Mellema, S., Doherr, M.G., Wechsler, B., Nuss, K., and Steiner, A.: Effect of local anesthesia on short- and long-term pain induced by two bloodless castration methods in calves. Vet. J., Mar;173:333–342, 2005.

Urethrostomy

Relevant Anatomy

The urethra in male ruminants is described in two parts, the pelvic urethra, which lies over the pelvic symphysis, and the penile urethra. The pelvic urethra may be fully palpated rectally. It is surrounded by the urethralis muscle, with the exception of the dorsal aspect where it is replaced by the aponeurotic plate. The urethral diverticulum is located at the level of the ischial arch. Just proximal to the diverticulum is a fold of urethral mucosa that acts as a

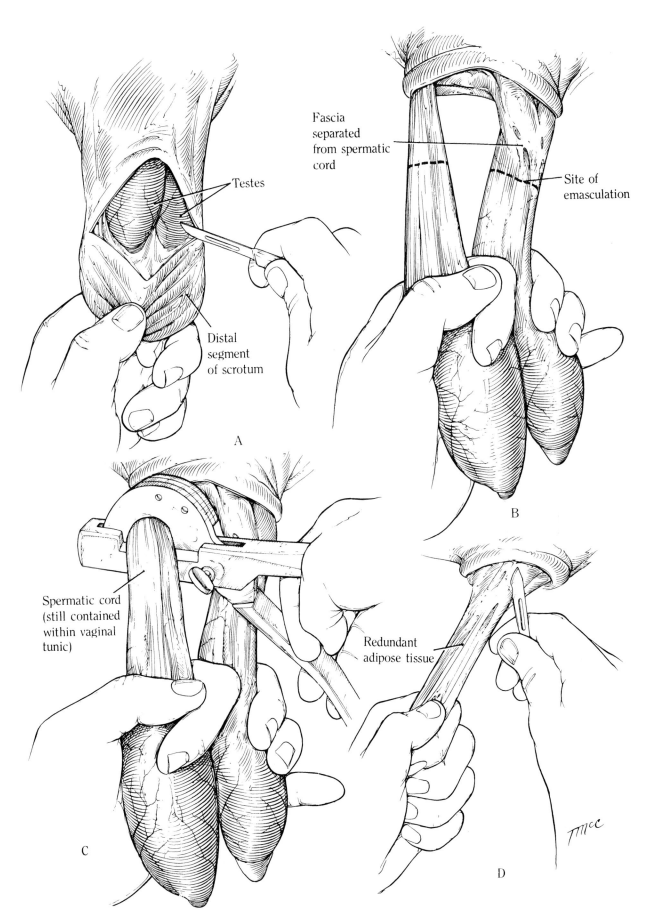

Testes

Distal
segment
of scrotum

A

Fascia
separated
from spermatic
cord

Site of
emasculation

B

Spermatic cord
(still contained
within vaginal
tunic)

C

Redundant
adipose tissue

D

Fig. 14-1. A to D, Calf castration.

valve to prevent retrograde flow of urine into the pelvic urethra.[2,3] The excretory ducts of the bulbourethral glands empty into the urethra at the diverticulum.

The lumen of the urethra in ruminants is relatively small and is further decreased in diameter by the dorsal ridge of the bladder and longitudinal mucosal folds. The lumen of the penile urethra becomes progressively smaller and is most pronounced at the distal sigmoid flexure of the penis. Hence, urethral calculi frequently become lodged at the distal sigmoid flexure of the penis, near the attachments of the retractor penis muscles, or at the urethral process.

Indications

Urethrostomy is most commonly performed in steers because of obstruction by urethral calculi, a condition known as urolithiasis. The occurrence of urethral obstruction in steers, as opposed to bulls, is influenced by the smaller diameter of their urethrae. The chemical composition of the urethral calculi may vary, depending on the steer's diet. Silicate calculi, which are rough and hard, occur in steers grazing stubble and pastures consisting largely of grasses.[1] Phosphate calculi, which are soft, smooth, and often multiple, are more common in steers in feedlots.[5]

Failure to relieve the obstructed urethra can result in rupture of the bladder and subsequent uroperitoneum, or rupture of the urethra, resulting in subcutaneous infiltration of urine in the perineal region. Attending cellulitis, septicemia, and death may follow. The following technique generally is regarded as a salvage procedure to remove urine. It is usually performed to buy time until the animal's condition can be stabilized sufficiently to permit slaughter.

Anesthesia and Surgical Preparation

This surgical procedure is performed using caudal epidural anesthesia with the animal in the standing position or cast in dorsal recumbency. Sometimes xylazine hydrochloride (Rompun) is used for sedation. The positioning of the animal for surgery is determined by the surgeon. The animal may be cast in dorsal recumbency with its legs tied cranially and the surgeon kneeling behind it (Figure 14-2A). This method may produce unwanted, additional pressure on an already distended urinary bladder. It is preferable to operate on large steers and bulls in the standing position. When the animal is positioned, the surgical site is clipped and is prepared for surgery in a routine manner.

Urethrostomy in steers and bulls may be performed at several sites. If it is performed just ventral to the anus at the level of the floor of the pelvis (perineal or high urethrostomy), severe scalding and matting of the escutcheon and medial aspects of the limbs result; generally, the animal is penalized at market with a lower value for slaughter. The other site for urethrostomy is in the region of the distal flexure of the sigmoid flexure of the penis (low urethrostomy). The advantage of the low incision, described here, is that the penis can be directed so the urine is forced caudad, away from the medial aspects of the limbs, to reduce damage from urine scald. In addition, an incision in this region is more likely to expose the calculi because they most commonly lodge in this region.

A low urethrostomy may also be performed cranial to the scrotum or scrotal remnant.

Instrumentation

General surgery pack
Urinary catheter

Surgical Technique

The penis is palpated immediately caudal to the remnants of the scrotum. The scrotal remnant is grasped and is stretched craniad, and the distal flexure of the sigmoid flexure is located. A 10-cm skin incision is made on the midline directly over the penis (Figure 14-2A and B), and blunt dissection is then performed to locate the penis. In Figure 14-2A to G, the patient is in dorsal recumbency. Generally, the penis is deeper than one would anticipate and is a firm fibrous structure about the thickness of the index finger. During the dissection, the surgeon encounters subcutaneous adipose tissue and several layers of elastic tissue surrounding the penis. With traction, a portion of the penis is exposed through the skin incision (Figure 14-2C). The retractor penis muscles should be identified because they serve as a useful guideline to the location of the ventral surface of the penis. Care should be taken not to twist the penis and thereby to lose the relationship of the retractor penis muscles and ventral surface of the penis. At this point, it may be possible to palpate the calculi in the urethra.

Several options exist at this point, depending on the severity of inflammation of the urethra and surrounding tissues. If inflammation of these structures is minimal and the calculi can be located, a small incision is made directly over the calculus (calculi) on the ventral aspect of the penis (Figure 14-2D). The calculus (calculi) is then removed. Prior to closure of the urethra, a catheter should be inserted up the urethra, both proximally and distally, to search for further stones and to ensure urethral patency. The urethra may be sutured if there is no urethral necrosis. A catheter may be placed in the urethra to minimize stricture formation during closure. Simple interrupted or simple continuous sutures of an absorbable suture material (polyglytone 6211, Caprosyn) are inserted. The sutures should go down to, but not through, the urethral mucosa. The penis is replaced in its normal position, and the dorsal third of the skin incision is closed (Figure 14-2E). The remainder of the incision may be left open to heal by secondary intention.

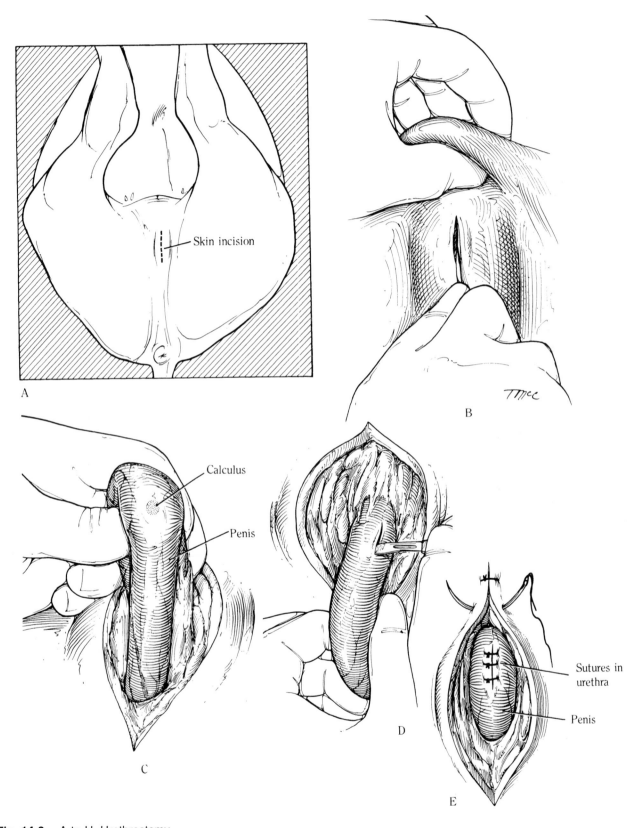

Fig. 14-2. A to H, Urethrostomy.

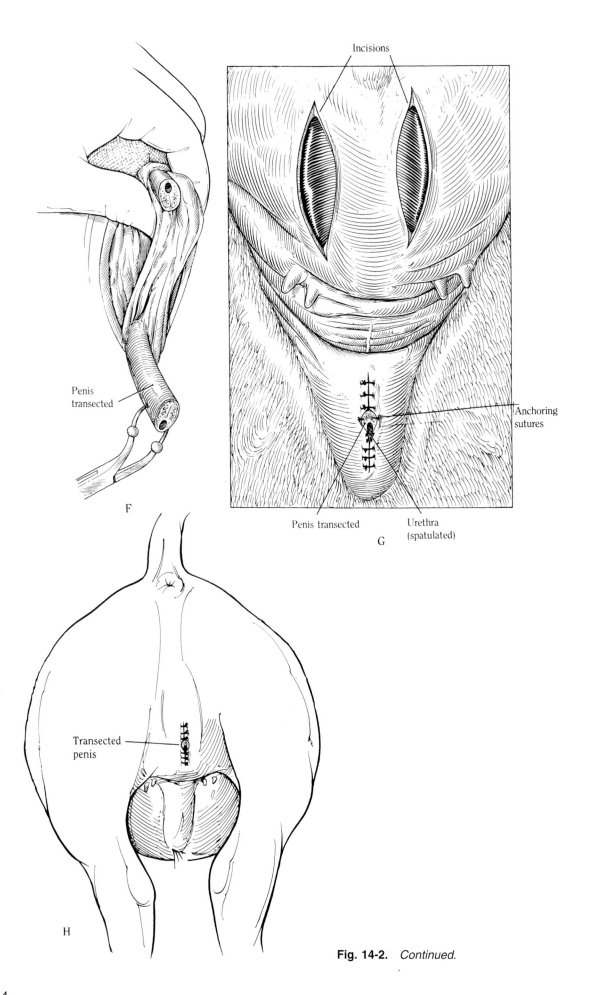

Penis
transected

F

Incisions

Anchoring
sutures

Penis transected

Urethra
(spatulated)

G

Transected
penis

H

Fig. 14-2. *Continued.*

If there is any necrosis of the urethra and if the urethra's ability to hold sutures is in question, the urethra and skin incisions may be left to heal by secondary intention.

If damage to the penis and surrounding tissues is extensive with rupture of the urethra, transection and extirpation of the penis are performed. The penis is dissected carefully from the dorsal arteries and veins of the penis and is transected to leave an 8- to 12-cm proximal stump (Figure 14-2F). The length of the penis varies with the size of the patient. From the surgeon's view, the arteries and veins appear ventral to the exposed stump of the penis. These vessels are ligated (some surgeons do not consider this necessary). It is a common error to isolate an insufficient amount of penile stump prior to anchoring it to the skin. The stump should be of sufficient length that when it is sutured to the skin there is no infolding of skin because of excessive tension. The stump of the exposed penis is directed caudoventrad and is anchored to the skin and two sutures. The sutures should pass through the skin, tunica albuginea, and corpus cavernosum penis. Care is taken to ensure that the urethral lumen is not compromised. The stump of the penis should not be bent because iatrogenic urethral obstruction might occur. The urethra at the end of the penile stump is split, and the edges are sutured to the lateral aspects of the penis (Figure 14-2G). This part of the technique is not performed routinely by all surgeons. Figure 14-2H shows a completed urethrostomy with the patient standing.

In animals with urethral obstruction and signs of subcutaneous edema and cellulitis, urethral rupture has usually occurred. The urine accumulation in the tissues causes a violent inflammatory response that may result in sloughing of the skin of the ventral abdomen. To facilitate drainage, the surgeon should make several bold, longitudinal incisions lateral to the prepuce with a scalpel, being careful to avoid the subcutaneous abdominal veins (Figure 14-2G). This procedure assists in resolution of the inflammatory process.

Postoperative Management

Unless the animal is destined for immediate slaughter, antibiotics should be administered. Other supportive measures, such as intravenous fluids, diuretics, and general therapy for shock, may also be indicated. The animal should be sent to slaughter as soon as it is judged that the carcass would be acceptable.

Complications and Prognosis

This procedure is intended to salvage the animal until slaughter, and long-term survival rates are poor. Out of 85 cattle that underwent urethrostomies, only 35% were slaughtered at normal body weight or were kept for their intended purposes.[4] The remaining 65% died or were euthanized during surgery or within 2 weeks postopera-

tively because of recurrence. Another study deemed urethrostomy successful in fewer than half of the cases.[3] The rest of the cattle suffered relapses, were sold after a low gain of body weight, or died of unknown causes. The postoperative mortality rates in cattle that undergo urethrostomy and surgical repair of a ruptured bladder are high; most cattle survive fewer than 2 weeks.[4]

References

1. Blood, D.C., Henderson, J.A., and Radostits, O.M.: Veterinary Medicine, 5th Ed. Philadelphia, Lea & Febiger, 1980.
2. Dyce, K.M., Sack, W.O., and Wensing, C.J.G.: Textbook of Veterinary Anatomy, 3rd Ed. Philadelphia, W.B. Saunders, 1996.
3. Gasthuys, F., Martens, A., and De Moor, A.: Surgical treatment of urethral dilatation in seven male cattle. Vet. Rec., 138:17–19, 1996.
4. Gasthuys, F., Steenhaut, M., De Moor, A., and Sercu, K.: Surgical treatment of urethral obstruction due to urolithiasis in male cattle: a review of 85 cases. Vet. Rec., 133:522–526, 1993.
5. Walker, D.F.: Penile surgery in the bovine: part I. Mod. Vet. Pract., 60:839, 1979.

Hematoma Evacuation of the Bovine Penis

Relevant Anatomy

The fibroelastic bovine penis is approximately 1 m long with a quarter of the total length involved in the sigmoid flexure. The body of the penis is comprised of three columns of erectile tissue, the dorsally paired crura and the urethra. The crura arise independently from one another at the ischial arch and converge in the body of the penis. The tunica albuginea encases the cavernous tissue of the crura to form the corpus cavernosum. The urethra and its surrounding vascularized tissue, the corpus spongiosum, run in a ventral groove formed by the union of the crura.

Penile hematomas usually result from a rupture of the tunica albuginea on the dorsal aspect of the distal bend of the sigmoid flexure, opposite the insertion of the retractor penis muscles.[4,5] Swelling due to a hematoma will usually occur near the distal sigmoid flexure, which in standing bulls is located near the base of the scrotum, or in the proximal half of the sheath.[4] The size of the defect in the tunica albuginea varies and is probably related to the amount of intracorporeal blood pressure at the time of rupture. The amount of extravasated blood is probably related to the length of time erection is maintained after injury.

Indications

Penile hematomas occur during breeding when the bull fails to achieve intromission into the female prior to the copulatory thrust, resulting in a bending of the erect penis.[4] Preputial prolapse frequently accompanies penile hematomas and has been reported as one of the most common presenting complaints from owners.[2,4] Medical treatment of penile hematomas consists of hot packs, warm hydrotherapy, penicillin therapy for 2 weeks, and ultrasound therapy to speed resorption of the hematoma.[4] Generally, the decision for surgery is made on the basis of the size of the hematoma and the length of time elapsed between the accident and treatment. It is believed that, with larger hematomas, more of the peripenile fascial layers are damaged or involved (this may be obvious at surgery); consequently, the incidence of adhesions or the risk of adhesion formation is greater. With a large hematoma, the attachment region of the retractor penis muscles is also involved; if palpation reveals involvement to this extent, surgical treatment will be necessary. Mechanical interference with penile extrusion may be a problem with a large hematoma.

The ideal time for surgery is probably an hour after injury. It is believed that bleeding quickly ceases after relaxation of the penis; therefore, waiting for so-called organization of the hematoma is not necessary. After 7 to 10 days, extensive granulation and increased fibrosis in the peripenile areas make surgery difficult. Although organization of the fibrous tissue may make the surgery easier after 25 days, as compared to 10 to 25 days, difficulty can still be anticipated. Clinical studies show that the success rate of surgery decreases greatly when the injury is more than 14 days old[2] and medical treatment may be more effective.

Anesthesia and Surgical Preparation

The surgery is performed with the animal sedated with xylazine (see Chapter 2, "Anesthesia and Fluid Therapy"), cast in lateral recumbency, and with local infiltration (line block) at the surgical site (Figure 14-3A), or under general anesthesia, if available.

Surgical Technique

A skin incision approximately 13 cm long is made in a cranioventral direction over the most prominent part of the swelling (Figure 14-3A and B), and this incision is continued through the subcutaneous tissues into the hematoma. Care should be taken not to incise the penis because it may be deflected by the hematoma and may be closer to the skin than anticipated. Care should also be taken to avoid any additional damage to the dorsal nerves of the penis. The clots of the hematoma are removed manually (Figure 14-3C). In an acute case, the rent in the tunica albuginea is easily identified. If fibrin deposition and granulation tissue formation have occurred, however, careful dissection through the fascial layers surrounding the penis might be necessary to locate the rent in the tunic (Figure 14-3D). At this stage, any peripenile adhesions

need to be broken down. The penis is grasped firmly, distal to the tunic defect, and all peripenile adhesions are broken down (Figure 14-3E). With manual rotation of the penis, the retractor penis muscles may be identified, and any adhesions in this area also removed. A nonsterile assistant then grasps the penis through the prepuce and extrudes it so that the surgeon can ascertain the free motion of the penis and can locate any further adhesions.

The edges of the rent in the tunica albuginea are debrided and are sutured with simple interrupted sutures of no.0 or 2-0 synthetic absorbable suture (Figure 14-3F). Although secondary-intention healing and fibrous union of the defect would be anticipated without suturing, it is probably preferable to suture the defect because vascular shunts may form between the corpora cavernosa penis and the dorsal vessels.[6] Although a rupture, if it recurs, will probably recur at the same site,[1,5] it is questionable whether suturing the defect will actually reduce the chances of recurrence. Some authors have proposed suturing of the tunica albuginea to be unnecessary.[3] The fascial layers of the penis are sutured with no. 2-0 synthetic absorbable sutures in a simple continuous pattern. The skin is closed with simple interrupted or vertical mattress sutures of nonabsorbable material (Figure 14-3G).

When preputial inflammation, swelling, or prolapse is present and problems with manual retraction of the penis are anticipated postoperatively, an umbilical tape suture is placed through the dorsal aspect of the penis (Figure 14-3H) and tied. Care should be taken to ensure that the tape is not passed through the urethra. This tape facilitates postoperative manipulation of the penis.

Postoperative Management

Penicillin is administered postoperatively to reduce the possibility of abscess formation after the injury. If extensive swelling of the prepuce is present, it should be reduced by hot packs and bandaging; diuretics may also be appropriate. If the swelling has caused a preputial prolapse, ointment should be applied to the exposed mucosa. The penis is extended daily for 10 days. If the umbilical tape is used for this purpose, care should be taken not to place undue tension on the tape or it may tear out of the penis.

Drainage of a seroma at the surgery site may be necessary, but seromas generally resorb spontaneously. The recommended period of sexual rest appropriate following surgery varies and ranges from 45 days.[1] Another study reported a 40% recurrence of penile hematomas in bulls that underwent a period of sexual rest shorter than 2 months.[2]

Complications and Prognosis

Hematomas may recur when the bulls are returned to service. In this case, the early hematomas are probably

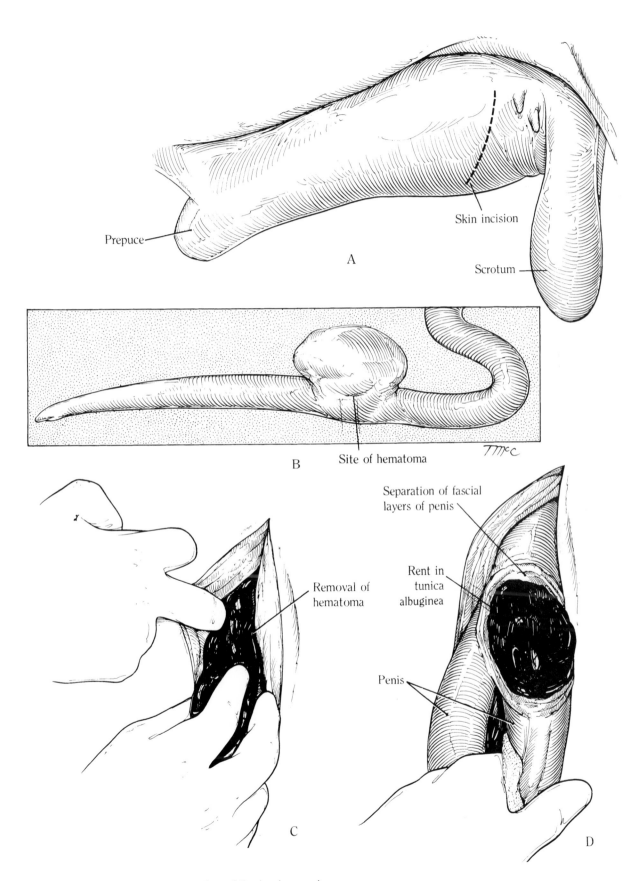

Prepuce

Skin incision

Scrotum

A

Site of hematoma

B

Removal of hematoma

Separation of fascial layers of penis

Rent in tunica albuginea

Penis

C

D

Fig. 14-3. A to H, Hematoma evacuation of the bovine penis.

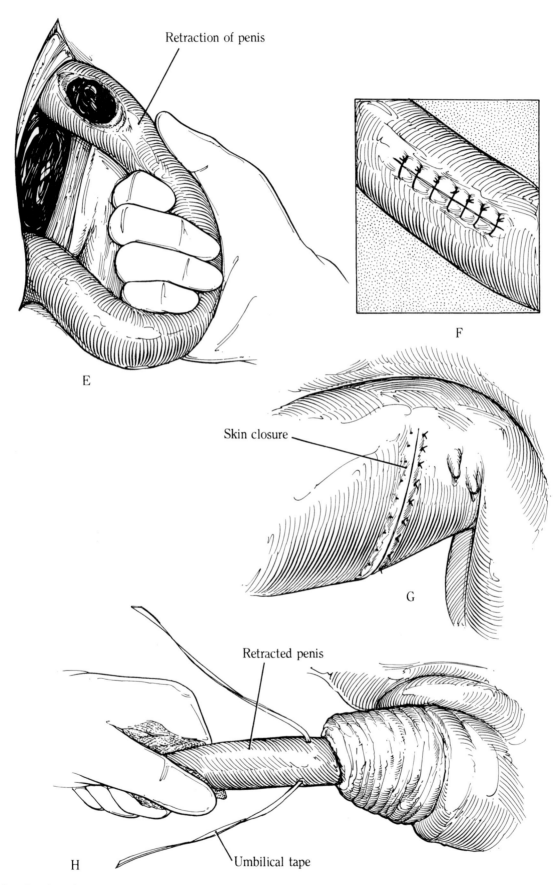

Fig. 14-3. *Continued.*

248

associated with tearing of adhesions in the area of the original rupture site; the ones that arise at a later time may be associated with reinjury unrelated to the original rupture. Injury of the dorsal nerves of the penis may cause failure to ejaculate or copulate, but recoveries up to 18 months later have been observed.[1] Thrombus formation in the corpora cavernosa and formation of vascular shunts have also been proposed as causes of nonerection postoperatively,[6] although these problems also occur following conservative treatment.

The literature supports a more favorable prognosis for surgical treatment of penile hematomas than medical treatment. One study reported that bulls that received surgical treatment were 2.8 times more likely to have a successful outcome than bulls treated medically.[2] Of the bulls with large hematomas (>20 cm wide), surgical treatment had an 80% success rate compared to the 33% success rate in medically treated bulls.[2] The method of treatment for small hematomas (<20 cm wide) did not affect their respective success rates. Surgical evacuation of the hematoma may reduce the formation of adhesions and the risk of infection by removing a potential medium for bacteria.[2]

References

1. Aanes, W.A.: Personal communication, 1980.
2. Musser, J.M.B., St. Jean, G., Vestweber, J.G., et al.: Penile hematoma in bulls: 60 cases (1979–1990). J. Am. Vet. Med. Assoc., 201:1416, 1992.
3. Pearson, H.: Surgery of the male genital tract in cattle: a review of 121 cases. Vet. Rec., 91:498, 1972.
4. St. Jean, G.: Male reproductive surgery. Vet. Clin. North Am.: Food Anim. Pract., 11:55–91, 1995.
5. Walker, D.F., and Vaughan, J.T.: Bovine and Equine Urogenital Surgery. Philadelphia, Lea & Febiger, 1980.
6. Young, S.L., Hudson, R.S., and Walker, D.F.: Impotence in bulls due to vascular shunts in the corpus cavernosum penis. J. Am. Vet. Med. Assoc., 171:643, 1977.

Preputial Amputation (Circumcision) in the Bull

Relevant Anatomy

Anatomy relevant to this procedure is discussed in previous sections of this chapter.

Indications

Preputial amputation (circumcision) is indicated in selected cases of preputial prolapse with fibrosis and ulceration of the prepuce. The breeds most often affected are the Bos indicus breeds (Brahman and Santa Gertrudis) and the polled Bos taurus breeds (notably Angus and Polled Hereford).[3] The two reasons advanced for the breed differences are a pendulous sheath and the absence of the retractor muscles of the prepuce in the polled breeds.[1,4] Protrusion of the parietal preputial lining followed by trauma or other irritation may produce inflammatory changes that ultimately prevent retraction of the prepuce.[1] Conservative treatment may be successful, but prolapse frequently recurs and eventually leads to chronic prolapse that requires surgical treatment. Prophylactic circumcision is also practiced in some areas.

Anesthesia and Surgical Preparation

Presurgical conservative treatment is usually necessary to reduce swelling and to improve the condition of the tissue. Prior to surgery, fibrosis and edema are reduced to a minimal level, decreasing the risk of postoperative infection and failure. Feed is withheld from the bull 24 hours prior to surgery. Surgery is performed with the bull in right-lateral recumbency, either under general anesthesia or with a combination of xylazine HCl sedation and local analgesia. The surgical area is prepared for aseptic surgery in a routine manner.

Instrumentation

General surgery pack

Surgical Technique

The prolapsed portion of the prepuce to be resected is extended with the left hand, the index finger of which is placed inside the prepuce (the line of amputation is indicated in Figure 14-4A). Note that the amputation line is oblique, rather than transverse, so the resulting orifice is oval, rather than circular. This precaution reduces the danger of phimosis developing during healing. A row of horizontal mattress sutures of no. 0 or 1 synthetic absorbable suture is placed around the prolapse immediately proximal to the proposed line of amputation (Figs. 14-4A and B). The sutures are placed in such a manner that they overlap one another around the entire circumference and are passed from the exposed preputial membrane completely through to the preputial cavity and back through both layers of the prepuce (Figure 14-4B). These sutures are tied to oppose the tissue, and the prepuce is amputated just distal to the suture line (Figure 14-4C). The preputial edges are then apposed with a simple continuous pattern suture line using a no. 0 synthetic absorbable suture material (Figure 14-4D).

It is convenient for the surgeon to perform this procedure on half of the prepuce at a time. The completed amputation (circumcision) is illustrated in Figure 14-4E.

Postoperative Management

The bull is placed on antibiotics, and the preputial cavity is infused daily with antibacterial agents until healing is complete.

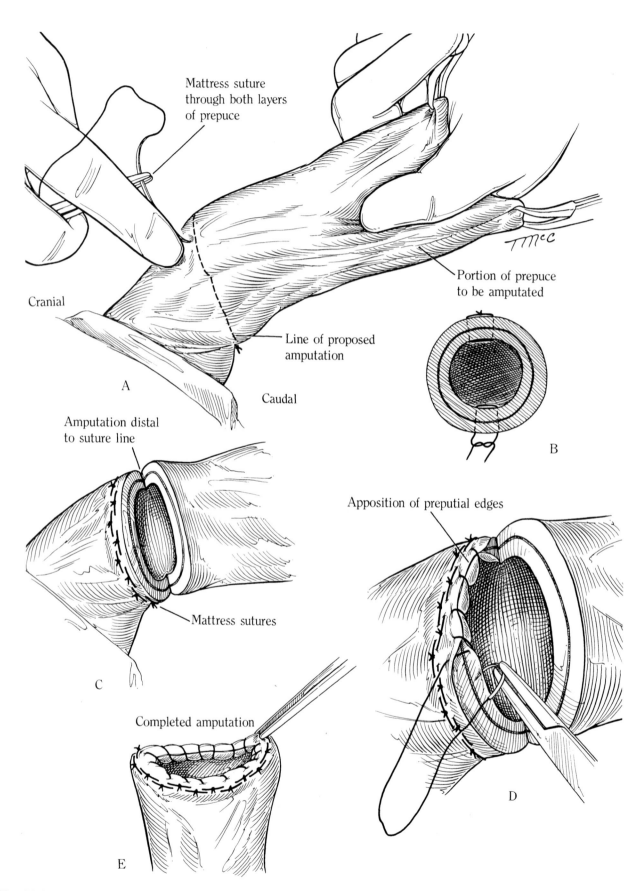

Fig. 14-4. A to E, Preputial amputation (circumcision) in the bull.

The following labels appear in the figure:

- Mattress suture through both layers of prepuce
- Portion of prepuce to be amputated
- Line of proposed amputation
- Cranial
- Caudal
- A
- B
- Amputation distal to suture line
- Mattress sutures
- C
- Apposition of preputial edges
- D
- Completed amputation
- E

Complications and Prognosis

A study of 33 beef bulls that received circumcisions as treatment for preputial prolapse reported a 76% return to breeding soundness for 1 or more years after surgery.[2] Of the 33 bulls, 11 bulls developed one or more postoperative complications, including incisional dehiscence, suture abscesses, and focal incisional hematomas.[2] In general, this technique of amputation is less successful in European (*Bos taurus*) breeds because the preputial membrane is too short. The loss of preputial membrane following surgery may prevent adequate extension of the penis to allow breeding. In less-severe cases, preputial prolapse may be treated by conservative resection of the preputial membrane (*reefing*) and suturing the healthy internal preputial membrane near the preputial orifice. A V-shaped incision pattern is used to reduce the danger of stenosis. Larsen and Bellenger point out that circumcision results in the loss of equal amounts of the external and internal linings of the prolapsed portion of the prepuce even though the internal lining is frequently not seriously involved in the inflammatory process.[3] These authors advocate conservative resection to preserve as much of the unaffected inner lining of the prolapsed prepuce as possible and thereby increase the bull's chances of returning to service.

A technique for amputation of the prolapsed prepuce that is claimed to have advantages for the practitioner with limited facilities involves the insertion of a plastic ring into the preputial cavity.[5] The ring is fixed with sutures and a tourniquet-like effect is produced; the prolapsed portion is sloughed in 1 to 2 weeks.

References

1. Arthur, G.H.: Wright's Veterinary Obstetrics, 4th Ed. Philadelphia, Lea & Febiger, 1975.
2. Baxter, G.M., Allen, D., and Wallace, C.E.: Breeding soundness of beef bulls after circumcision: 33 cases (1980–1986). J Am. Vet. Med. Assoc., *194*:948–952, 1989.
3. Larsen, L.H., and Bellenger, C.R.: Surgery of the prolapsed prepuce in the bull: its complications and dangers. Aust. Vet. J., *47*:349, 1971.
4. Long, S.E., and Hignett, P.G.: Preputial eversion in the bull: a comparative study of prepuces from bulls which evert and those which do not. Vet. Rec., *86*:161, 1970.
5. Walker, D.F., and Vaughan, J.T.: Bovine and Equine Urogenital Surgery. Philadelphia, Lea & Febiger, 1980.

Surgical Techniques for Teaser Bull Preparation

Relevant Anatomy

Anatomy relevant to this section is discussed in previous procedures.

Indications

The role of teaser bulls for the detection of heat in cattle is uncertain. It is possible to use steers that have had testosterone administered to them; in addition, the increased use of prostaglandins may obviate the need for teaser bulls in an artificial breeding program. In the meantime, various techniques have been developed to render the bull sterile or incapable of coitus. The techniques that render the bull incapable of coitus seem to be more acceptable. In this chapter, we describe two popular techniques, penile translocation and penile fixation. As a precaution, these techniques should be accompanied by a sterilization procedure, such as bilateral caudal epididymectomy, which is also described in this section.[5] One should consider making a new teaser bull every year about 30 days before the breeding season considering the economics of wintering a nonproductive teaser bull and the higher libido of the younger animal.

It has been reported that teaser bulls prepared by penile translocation can occasionally serve a cow. Considering this possibility, we also describe the method of penile fixation, which produces an adhesion of the penis to the lower abdominal wall that prevents protrusion of the penis.[2] A third technique is described elsewhere that involves the injection of acrylic into the corpus cavernosum, which creates an artificial thrombus.[4]

Anesthesia and Surgical Preparation

This surgical procedure is performed with the animal under general anesthesia or heavy sedation and local analgesia. The bull is placed in dorsolateral recumbency and is tilted with its left side uppermost. A large area of the midline and ventral left-flank area, including the preputial orifice, is clipped and is prepared for aseptic surgery in a routine manner.

Penile fixation is usually performed with the animal tranquilized and under local anesthesia. The surgery can be done on a commercially manufactured operating table, if one is available, or it can be done with the animal cast in lateral recumbency. If done on the floor with the animal in lateral recumbency, the patient's feet must be tied for the safety of the surgeon. The ventral abdominal wall from the end of the sheath to the base of the scrotum is clipped and is prepared for aseptic surgery. A line block of local anesthesia (about 30 ml) is placed along a line where the sheath joins the body wall and about midway between the end of the sheath and the base of the scrotum (Figure 14-6A). Epididymectomy is generally performed with the animal standing in a chute. The distal area of the scrotum is clipped and is prepared for surgery in a routine manner. Local infiltration of analgesia is administered over the tail of the epididymis.

Instrumentation

General surgery pack
Sponge forceps
Sterile rubber gloves
Sterile obstetric sleeve
Sterile stomach tube for insertion within the prepuce to
　　prevent urine contamination

Surgical Technique

Penile Translocation

The incision sites are illustrated in Figure 14-5A. A skin incision is made around the preputial orifice approximately 3 cm from the opening, and a ventral midline skin incision is extended caudad from this. The midline incision extends to the base of the penis (Figure 14-5A). This incision is continued through the subcutaneous tissue, and the penis, prepuce, and surrounding elastic tissue are dissected free from the abdominal wall in preparation for translocation (Figure 14-5B). A sterile stomach tube placed within the preputial orifice helps to delineate the prepuce during dissection and may also help to prevent urine contamination of the surgical area during surgery. During the dissection, it is important to maintain the integrity of the blood supply of the penis. Bleeding is controlled by ligation.

A circular skin incision is then made in the ventral left-flank area where the preputial orifice is to be moved (Figure 14-5B). Using a pair of sponge forceps, a tunnel is made from the circular incision through the subcutaneous tissues to the caudal end of the midline incision (Figure 14-5C). This tunnel must be large enough to permit the relocation of the penis and prepuce without restriction. A sterile rubber glove or plastic sleeve is placed over the preputial orifice (Figure 14-5D). This prevents contamination of the subcutis from the preputial orifice as it is drawn through the tunnel. If a tube had been positioned previously within the preputial orifice, it is removed at this stage. The penis and prepuce are drawn through the tunnel, and the skin of the preputial orifice is sutured to the circular skin incision (Figure 14-5E). Two layers of sutures are placed here: one in the subcutaneous tissue, and one in the skin. Before suturing is performed, it is also important to ascertain that no twisting has occurred during the translocation process. This possibility can be prevented by preplacing an identifying suture in the skin of the prepuce prior to its removal (Figure 14-5B). The ventral midline incision is then closed with nonabsorbable sutures. Although closely placed simple interrupted sutures are illustrated in Figure 14-5E, an argument can be made for bringing the edges together with widely spaced sutures and allowing drainage. It is believed that the latter technique eliminates the problem of postoperative edema.

Because of the excess skin and pendulous sheath in Indian breeds of cattle, it is possible to transpose the penis

and prepuce along with the encircling skin, rather than to dissect the penis and prepuce free from the skin.

Penile Fixation

A 10-cm longitudinal incision is made midway between the end of the prepuce and the base of the scrotum at the junction of the prepuce and the ventral body wall (about 2 cm lateral to the midline) (Figure 14-6A). This incision is made through the skin, subcutaneous tissue, and cutaneous trunci muscle. Blunt dissection through the loose connective tissue brings one to the dorsal surface of the penis. At this point, it is important to identify the urethra (urethral groove) within the penis. If the penis has not been rotated during the surgery, the urethral groove should be on the ventral surface of the penis. Because one must always be aware of the urethra during this procedure, it is often helpful to place a towel clamp around the urethra and its adjacent portion of the penis. This serves to identify the urethra and also as a traction device.

The penis is exteriorized through the incision, and the preputial reflection is identified. The dorsal surface of the penis is cleared of its elastic tunics commencing at the preputial reflection and extending caudad for about 10 cm. This exposes tough fibrous tunica albuginea. Once tunica albuginea has been exposed, the linea alba is cleared of all of its loose connective tissue. The tunica albuginea of the dorsal surface of the penis is now apposed to the linea alba. Before placing the sutures, one should be sure that the glans penis and prepuce are not protruding through the preputial orifice. No. 2 nylon sutures are placed through the dorsal third of the penis (Figure 14-6B) and then through the linea alba. This suture apposes the linea alba and tunica albuginea (Figure 14-6C). Figure 14-6D illustrates in cross section the placement of the sutures. Care should be taken not to enter the preputial reflection and not to involve the urethra, to avoid iatrogenic urethral obstruction. Usually, three interrupted sutures are adequately placed about 1 to 2 cm apart. It is helpful to preplace these sutures and then tie them simultaneously. The skin is closed with no. 1 or 2 monofilament synthetic suture.

This technique results in a permanent adhesion between the tunica albuginea and the linea alba. Ideally, the bull should have 2 to 3 weeks of sexual rest before use, to allow this adhesion to develop.

Epididymectomy

The testis is forced manually to the distal segment of the scrotum, and a 3-cm skin incision made over the tail of the epididymis. This incision is continued through the common vaginal tunic until the tail of the epididymis is extruded (Figure 14-7A). The tail of the epididymis is dissected free from its attachment to the testis using scissors (Figure 14-7B). The ductus deferens is identified and clamped with forceps, and a ligature of nonabsorbable suture material is placed proximal to the forceps (Figure

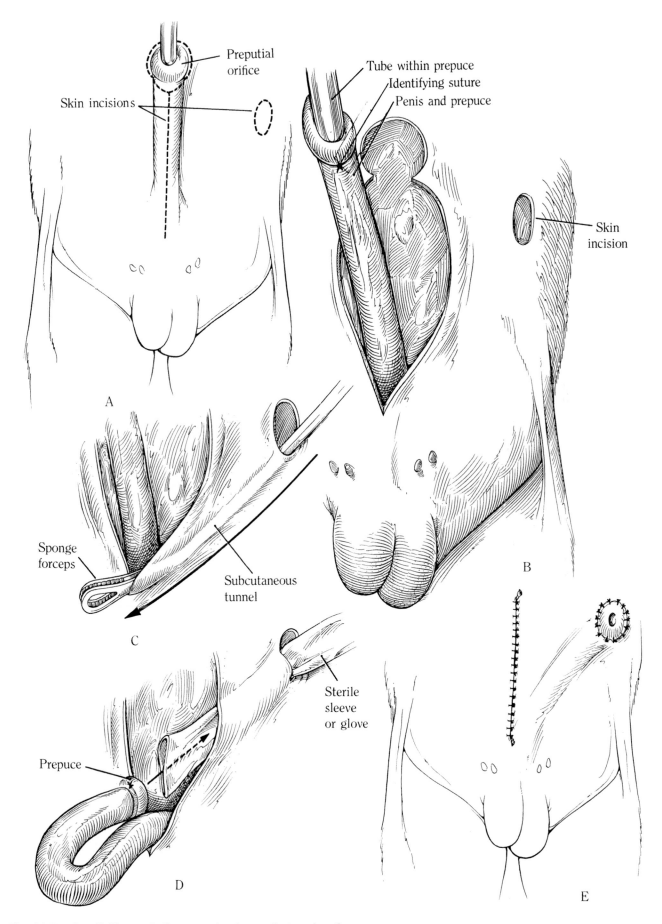

Fig. 14-5. A to E, Teaser bull preparation by penile translocation.

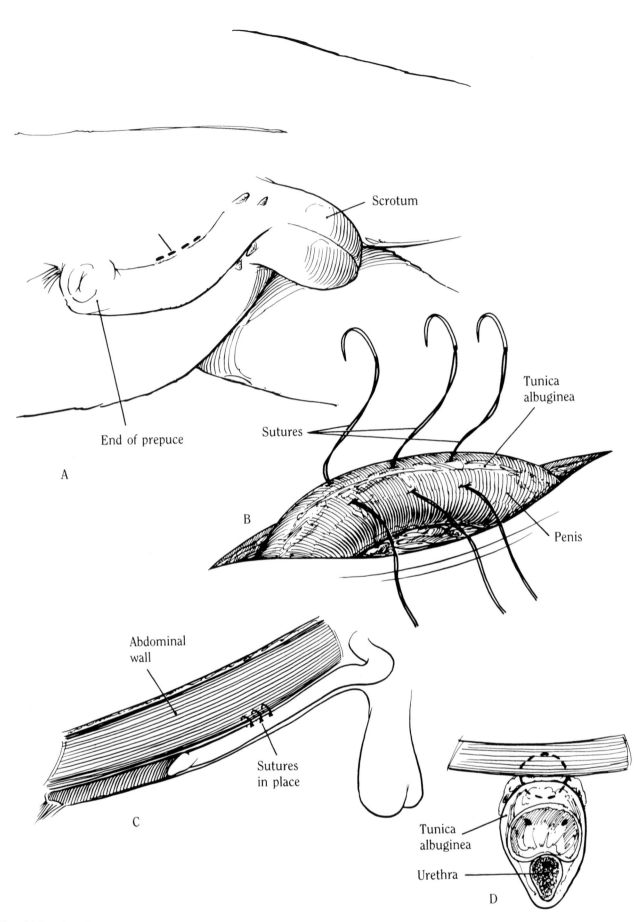

Scrotum

End of prepuce

Sutures

Tunica albuginea

Penis

A

B

Abdominal wall

Sutures in place

Tunica albuginea

Urethra

C

D

Fig. 14-6. A to D, Teaser bull preparation by penile fixation.

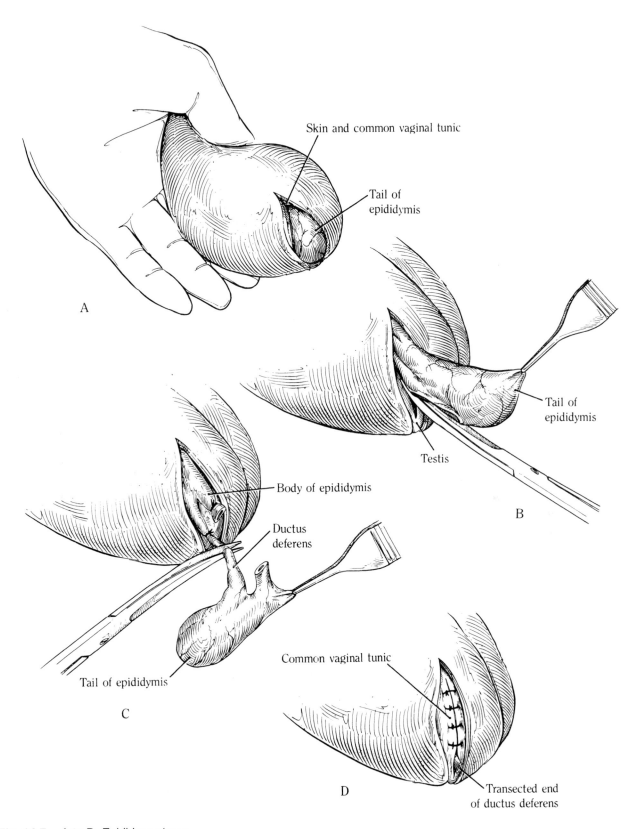

Fig. 14-7. A to D, Epididymectomy.

Skin and common vaginal tunic

Tail of
epididymis

A

Tail of
epididymis

Testis

B

Body of epididymis

Ductus
deferens

Tail of epididymis

C

Common vaginal tunic

Transected end
of ductus deferens

D

14-7C). The ductus deferens is then transected at the level of the clamp. This procedure is repeated in the body of the epididymis so that the tail of the epididymis may be removed (Figure 14-7C).

The common vaginal tunic is closed in a separate layer using simple interrupted sutures of absorbable material so that the remaining part of the epididymis is retained within the tunic, but the transected end of the ductus deferens protrudes through the suture line (Figure 14-7D). The technique is an added precaution against reanastomosis of the reproductive tract. The skin is closed with two to three interrupted sutures of nonabsorbable material. The procedure is repeated on the other testis.

Postoperative Management

If penile translocation is performed, antibiotics may be administered at the discretion of the surgeon, and the skin sutures are removed in 10 days. Sutures may be removed 2 to 3 weeks following penile fixation. The animals are not put into work for 4 to 6 weeks. Antibiotics are not administered routinely following epididymectomy. The bull may be placed in work in 3 weeks if epididymectomy is the only procedure performed. If placed in work earlier, however, the bull should be ejaculated prior to this for semen evaluation, to ensure the bull is sterile before use. Such measures are advised as liability precautions.

Complications and Prognosis

The long-term results of most techniques for teaser bull preparation have been criticized. The various charges against different techniques generally have not taken into account the probability of varying libido among bulls, however. Pariphimosis has been associated with the technique of penile translocation.[1] Successful results for penile fixation have been reported.[3] Potential complications include suture breakdown (if catgut is used), seroma formation, and insufficient retraction of the penis. Weight loss is also observed.[3] In the past, epididymectomy was commonly used as a sole procedure. It has been claimed, however, that these bulls often develop seminal vesiculitis or infections of the accessory genitalia, and they still ejaculate fluid from these glands during copulation. At present, the technique is used more often as insurance for one of the techniques that render the bull incapable of copulation.

References

1. Baird, A.N., Wolfe, D.F., and Angel, K.L.: Paraphimosis in a teaser bull with penile translocation. J. Am. Vet. Med. Assoc., 201:325, 1992.
2. Belling, T.H.: Preparation of a "teaser" bull for use in beef cattle artificial insemination program. J. Am. Vet. Med. Assoc., 138:670, 1961.
3. Hoffsis, G., and Maurer, L.M.: Evaluation of the penis tie-down method to prepare teaser bulls. Bov. Pract., 11:78, 1976.
4. Riddell, M.G.: Prevention of intromission by estrus-detector males. In Large Animal Urogenital Surgery, 2nd Ed. Edited by F.W. Dwight and H.D. Moll. Baltimore, Williams & Wilkins, 1998, pp. 335–343.
5. Walker, D.F., and Vaughan, J.T.: Bovine and Equine Urogenital Surgery. Philadelphia, Lea & Febiger, 1980.

Inguinal Herniorrhaphy in the Mature Bull

Relevant Anatomy

The inguinal canal is an opening in the caudal abdominal wall between the internal oblique muscle and the pelvic tendon of the external oblique aponeurosis.[2] In the bovine, the canal itself is considered to be nearly absent compared to other domestic species. In the normal male, the inguinal canal contains the testicular artery and vein, ductus deferens, and nerves of the spermatic cord. The vaginal tunic that encloses these structures and the testes is formed by an evagination of the peritoneum through the inguinal canal.

Indications

Inguinal herniation occurs when a loop of small intestine, occasionally omentum, or both, passes through the vaginal ring and into the canal and may be verified by rectal palpation. If the intestine and/or omentum protrudes all the way into the scrotum, it is termed a *scortal hernia*. Inguinal hernias may be further classified as *direct* and *indirect*. An indirect hernia occurs when the intestinal loops are contained within the tunica vaginalis, whereas a direct hernia occurs when the hernial sac is separate and cranial to the vaginal ring. Most hernias in the bull are indirect, but direct hernias are also seen.[1]

Inguinal hernias in the bull occur with greater frequency on the left side and are generally unilateral (Figure 14-8A shows the external appearance of a left-sided inguinal hernia). The inguinal canal of bulls in good condition is occupied by a substantial amount of adipose tissue, and this must be distinguished from an inguinal hernia.[4] A definitive diagnosis of inguinal hernia cannot be made simply by palpating the scrotum, because many bulls have external deposits of adipose tissue in this region. Sometimes, deposits of adipose tissue are seen with inguinal hernia, and the hernia itself is initiated by a protrusion of subperitoneal adipose tissue through the inguinal ring.[3] Some form of trauma may also be responsible for initiation of an inguinal hernia.[1]

Another method of repair of inguinal hernia in the bull involves a flank laparotomy.[3] The hernia is reduced by the removal of viscera from the vaginal ring, and long, sterile, nonabsorbable suture material, such as umbilical tape, is

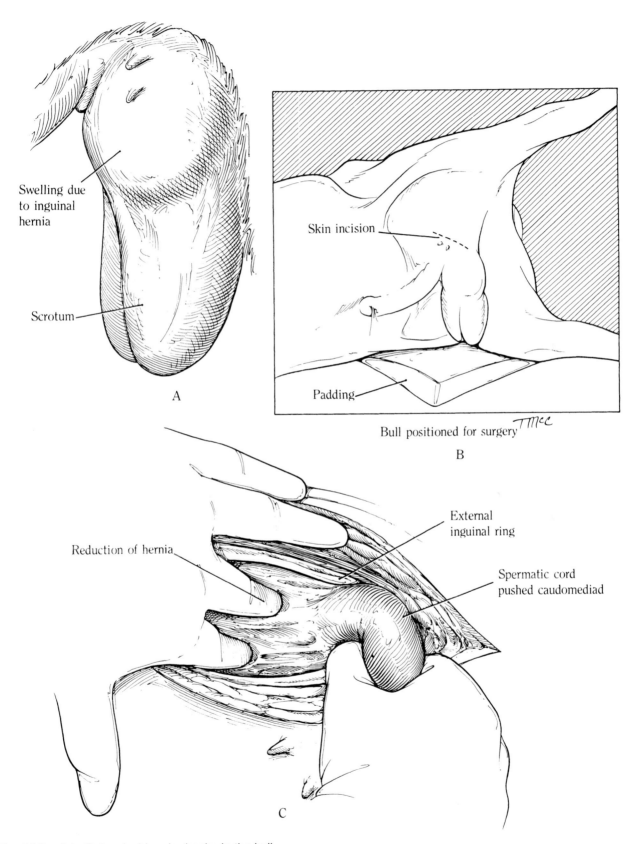

Swelling due
to inguinal
hernia

Scrotum

A

Skin incision

Padding

Bull positioned for surgery

B

Reduction of hernia

External
inguinal ring

Spermatic cord
pushed caudomediad

C

Fig. 14-8. A to G, Inguinal herniorrhaphy in the bull.

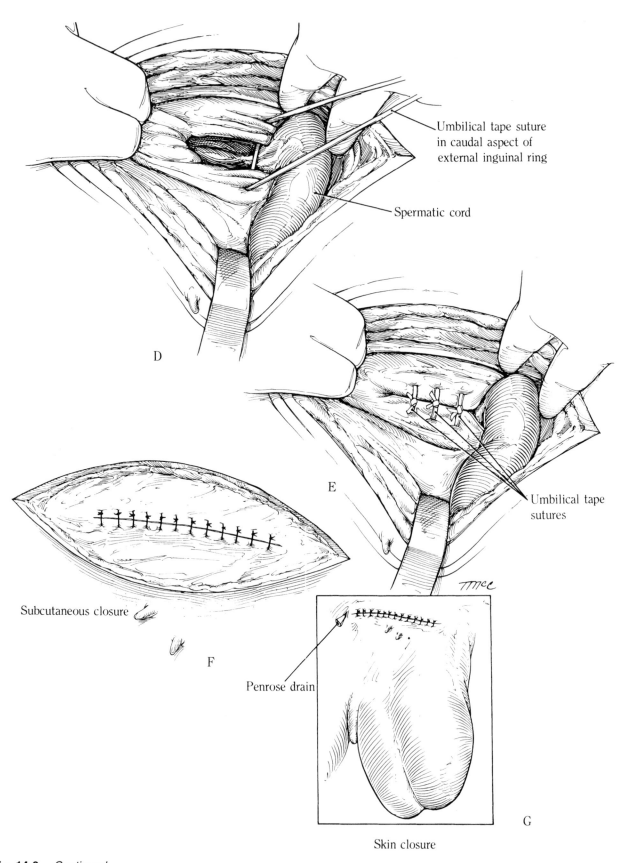

Umbilical tape suture
in caudal aspect of
external inguinal ring

Spermatic cord

D

E

Umbilical tape
sutures

Subcutaneous closure

F

Penrose drain

Skin closure

G

Fig. 14-8. *Continued.*

introduced into the abdominal cavity and is placed in the inguinal ring. Care is taken not to strangulate the spermatic cord as it passes through the vaginal ring. If adhesions are present, this method will not be successful. Moreover, placing sutures is awkward because of the constant presence of abdominal viscera at the surgical site.

Instrumentation

General surgery pack
Sterile umbilical tape, no. 2 nylon suture, or no. 2 polypropolene suture

Anesthesia and Surgical Preparation

This surgical procedure is best performed with the animal under general anesthesia and in lateral recumbency, with its hindquarters slightly elevated to aid in reduction of the hernia (Figure 14-8B). The uppermost hindlimb is secured in an upward direction and caudad, to improve exposure of the surgical area. A less-satisfactory alternative is sedation with xylazine hydrochloride supplemented with local anesthesia (see Chapter 2). The inguinal area is clipped and is prepared for aseptic surgery in a routine manner. The surgical site is draped.

Surgical Technique

A 15- to 25-cm horizontal incision is made through the skin and subcutaneous tissue over the external ring at the base of the scrotum, and hemostasis is maintained by ligation of blood vessels. A blood-free field assists progression of the surgery. Blunt dissection is performed down to the external inguinal ring to free the common vaginal tunic from the surrounding tissue. The boundaries of the ring are isolated.

If the hernia has reduced itself when the bull is positioned for surgery, it is not necessary to incise the common vaginal tunic (Figure 14-8C). If adhesions of the viscera have occurred within the scrotum, it is necessary to incise the common vaginal tunic to reduce the hernia. An incision is made through the common vaginal tunic parallel to the spermatic cord and cranial to the external cremaster muscle. The hernial contents are examined, and any adhesions are broken down. Occasionally, adhesions are so severe that circulation to intestines has been compromised and intestinal resection is required. These bulls are usually presented to the surgeon on an emergency basis for intestinal obstruction. The bowel is replaced in the abdominal cavity once the surgeon has ensured that no adhesions are present at the external inguinal ring. If the hernia is direct, located cranial to the neck of the scrotum, the subcutaneous tissue is separated, revealing the hernial contents. Adhesions are broken down to enable reduction of the hernia.

The hernial ring is repaired using no. 2 nylon or polypropolene suture or sterile double 1/8-in umbilical tape in a simple interrupted pattern. The aim of suturing is to reduce the size of the external inguinal ring so rehernation does not occur. Generally, two or three sutures in the cranial aspect of the ring are required. The sutures are tied, but are not placed under excessive tension. The spermatic cord should be positioned in the caudomedial part of the canal. The remaining ring should be of sufficient size to allow the contents of the spermatic cord to pass freely, yet prevent recurrence of the hernia. As a rule of thumb, there should be enough room for the spermatic cord and one finger. Naturally, hooking any portion of the spermatic cord with the sutures should be avoided. The first suture to be placed is the one closest to the spermatic cord, and it is generally placed about 1 cm from the spermatic cord through the medial and lateral edge of the external inguinal ring (Figure 14-8D). The sutures, which do not penetrate the peritoneum, are all preplaced by leaving the ends long and clamping the free ends with forceps. Then the sutures are tied (Figure 14-8E).

If the common vaginal tunic is entered to reduce the hernia, it is closed using fine (0 or 00) absorbable suture material in a simple continuous pattern.

Subcutaneous closure is performed using no. 0 or 1 synthetic absorbable suture (Figure 14-8F). The use of a Penrose drain is indicated because of the considerable amount of dead space. The skin is closed using a synthetic monofilament suture in a simple interrupted pattern (Figure 14-8G).

Postoperative Management

Generally, antibiotics are not indicated unless there is a break in aseptic technique or intestinal resection is performed. Considerable postoperative swelling generally occurs within 24 to 48 hours. Swelling is more severe if adhesions were present. This swelling usually responds to hydrotherapy (warm) and exercise.

The bull is confined to a clean stall for 4 weeks following surgery, and exercise should be limited for about 8 weeks. The bull should not be used for breeding for 3 to 6 months, pending the result of semen evaluation.

Complications and Prognosis

The most outstanding advantage of this method is that, if adhesions are present, they can be broken down and the affected bowel freed. A small survey of nine bulls admitted to the Colorado State University Veterinary Teaching Hospital for inguinal hernia repair showed that five of the nine had adhesions. These five bulls required incisions into their common vaginal tunics to reduce the hernias.

References

1. Aanes, W.A.: Personal communication, 1980.
2. Dyce, K.M., Sack, W.O., and Wensing, C.J.G.: Textbook of Veterinary Anatomy, 3rd Ed. Philadelphia, W.B. Saunders, 2002.
3. Frank, E.R.: Veterinary Surgery, 7th Ed. Minneapolis, Burgess, 1964.
4. Walker, D.F., and Vaughan, J.T.: Bovine and Equine Urogenital Surgery. Philadelphia, Lea & Febiger, 1980.

Cesarean Section in the Cow

Relevant Anatomy

The anatomy of the bovine uterus is very similar to that of the mares, which is described in Chapter 10. Compared to the mare, the uterus of ruminants has a relatively short body and long horns. The body appears deceptively longer because the horns travel together for approximately a third of their length before actually bifurcating externally.[6] The uterine artery, a branch of the internal iliac artery, is the main blood supply to the uterus. The uterus is also in part supplied by the ovarian artery at the tubal ends of the horns and by the vaginal artery in the caudal portion of the body. Branches of these vessels also form anastomoses with the uterine artery.

Indications

Cesarean section is indicated in various types of dystocia, including those caused by relative fetal oversize when the pelvic inlet in young heifers is too small to allow delivery, deformities of the maternal pelvis, fetal monsters, induration of the cervix, fetal malposition, hydrops amnii and allantois, uterine torsion, and emphysematous fetuses. In many cases, the choice between fetotomy or cesarean section may depend on the operator's relative experience with either technique. Case selection is also important. The cow that has suffered a long period of fetal manipulation or attempts at fetotomy and is systemically compromised is not a candidate for cesarean section.

Different approaches are indicated in various dystocia situations.[4] The left paralumbar or flank approach is the standard incision for a viable or recently expired, uncontaminated fetus and a cow capable of tolerating surgery while standing. In some situations, right-flank laparotomy is indicated if there is marked distention of the rumen or when clinical examination dictates that removal from the right side would be more convenient. For example, an oversized fetus situated in the right side of the abdominal cavity would be difficult to remove by left-flank incision. In the routine case, however, the left-flank incision is more convenient because fewer problems with encroaching bowel is encountered.

In the case of a dead and emphysematous fetus, a ventral approach should be used. A ventral paramedian incision, the most common ventral approach, requires the cow to be placed in dorsal recumbency. An alternative is the ventrolateral oblique approach, which may be performed with the animal in lateral recumbency. Both techniques reduce contamination of the peritoneum, which may occur during removal of the emphysematous, contaminated fetus and its associated debris. The ventral approaches are also indicated if the animal is recumbent and is considered incapable of standing during surgery or if the animal is so unmanageable that it is too dangerous for the operator to stand beside the patient during surgery.

Anesthesia and Surgical Preparation

Cesarean section in the cow is performed with the animal under local analgesia. If the flank approach is used, a paravertebral block, inverted L block, or a line block may be used. For the paramedian approach, a high epidural, inverted L block, or line block may be used. Casting with a rope, with or without sedation, is a supplementary restraint for cows in which a ventral approach is used. The surgical area is clipped and is prepared for aseptic surgery in a routine manner.

Instrumentation

General surgery pack

Surgical Technique

Cesarean section in the cow may be performed with the patient standing, if a chute is present, or in recumbency. Both approaches for flank laparotomy and ventral paramedian laparotomy are described in Chapter 13, "Bovine Gastrointestinal Surgery." The exact location of the incision is adapted for performing cesarean sections. For example, the incision is more ventral for the flank approach (Figure 14-9A) and farther caudad for the ventral paramedian approach. The ventral paramedian incision is made midway between the midline and the subcutaneous abdominal vein and extends from the umbilicus caudad to the mammary gland (Figure 14-9B) (as opposed to the ventral paramedian incision for abomasopexy, which extends from the umbilicus craniad to the xiphoid process). The left- and right-flank standing approaches have inherent risks, such as rumen prolapse with the left-flank approach and small intestine evisceration through the right-flank approach. The recumbent approach is preferred in many instances because it allows the uterus to be completely exteriorized, is more advantageous for extracting oversized fetuses, and is associated with a lower incidence of abdominal contamination than in the standing approach.[4] A left oblique flank approach in the standing cow has been described that may be useful for extracting large calves or for when the uterine contents are contaminated. This specific approach is described

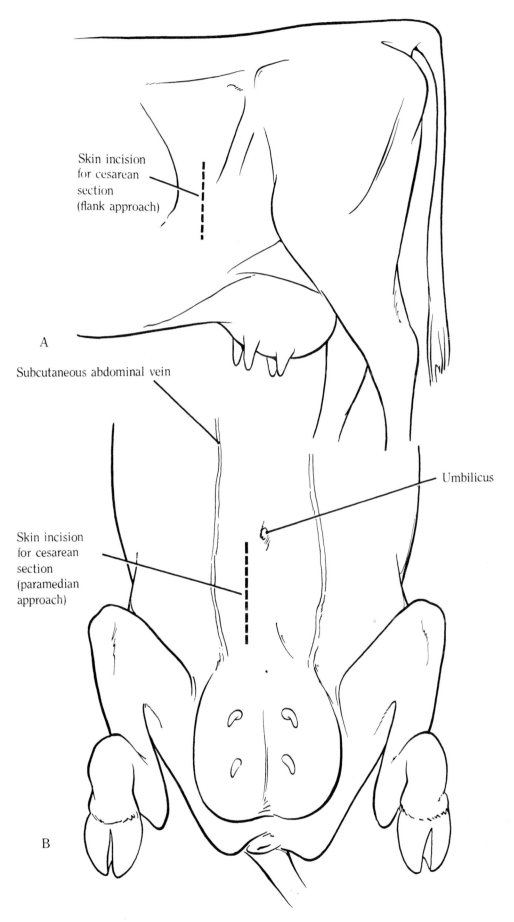

Skin incision
for cesarean
section
(flank approach)

A

Subcutaneous abdominal vein

Umbilicus

Skin incision
for cesarean
section
(paramedian
approach)

B

Fig. 14-9. A to N, Cesarean section in the cow.

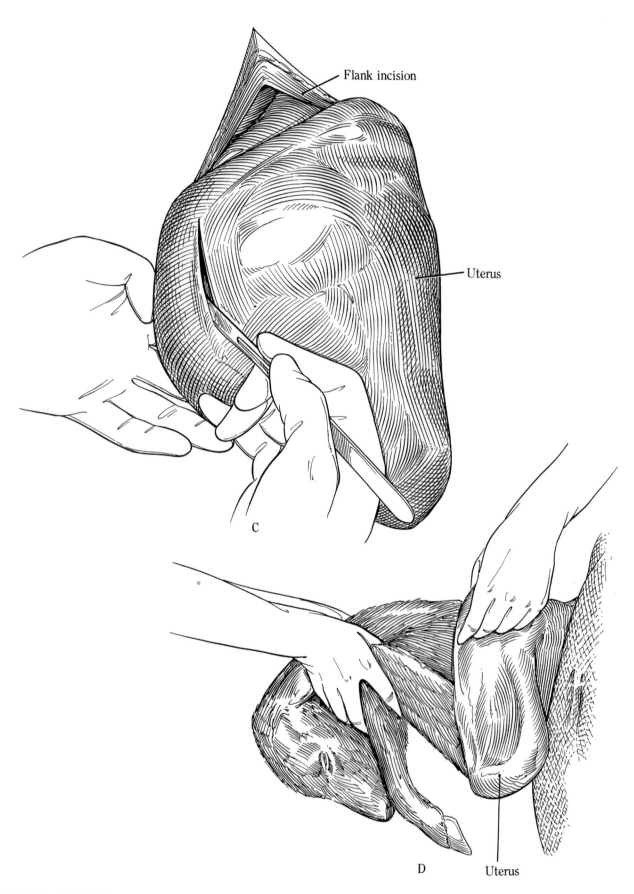

Flank incision

Uterus

C

Uterus

D

Fig. 14-9. *Continued.*

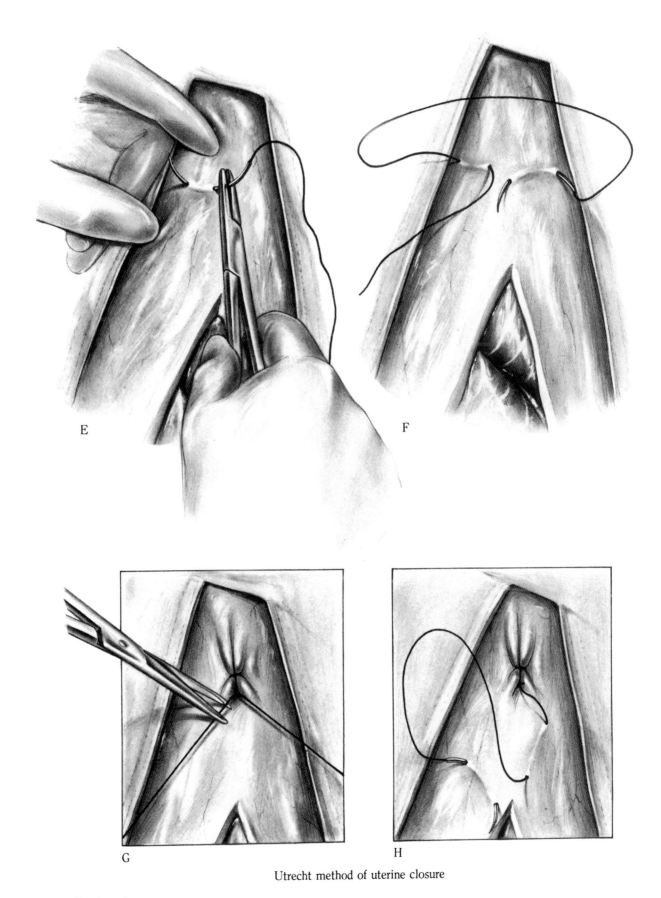

E   F

G   H

Utrecht method of uterine closure

Fig. 14-9. *Continued.*

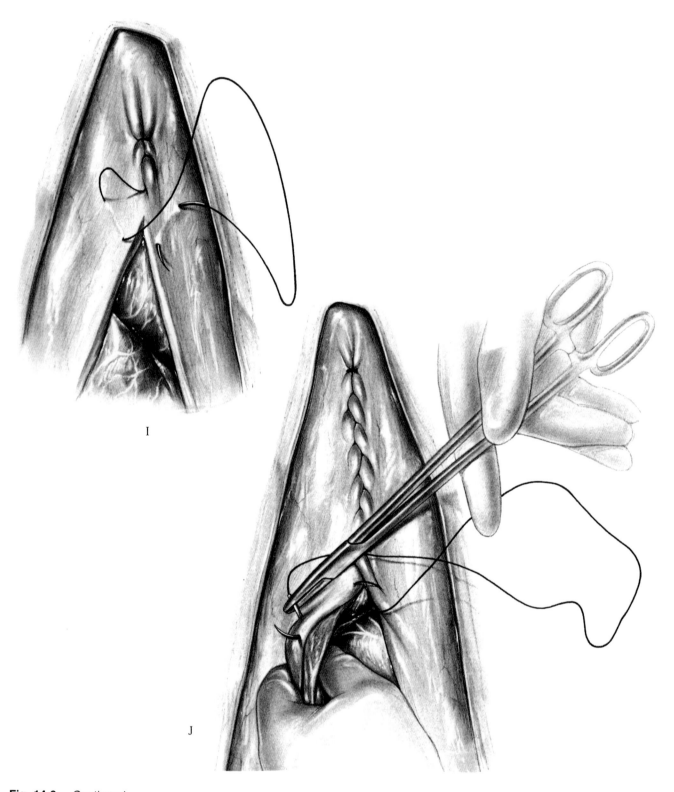

Fig. 14-9. *Continued.*

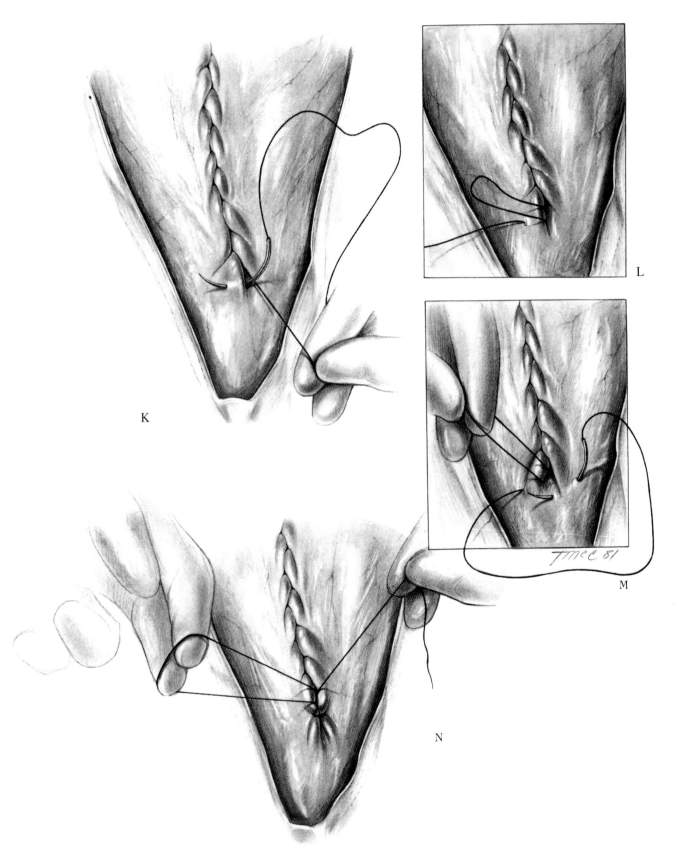

K

L

M

N

Fig. 14-9. *Continued.*

in detail elsewhere.[5] Following entrance into the peritoneal cavity, the surgeon manipulates a portion of the uterine horn containing the fetus and attempts to exteriorize an area for hysterotomy (exteriorization is often not possible). Often it is helpful to grasp a leg within the uterus and to use it as a handle to lift the uterus. The uterine incision is usually made over a limb, but in certain malpositions, the area over the head may be incised. The uterus should not be incised over a limb that is in the body of the uterus, but rather, as close to the tip of the horn as possible. This technique allows the uterine horn to be exteriorized for suturing (incisions near the body of the uterus must be sutured within the abdominal cavity).

Figure 14-9C depicts exteriorization of an appropriate part of the uterus through a flank incision. Such exteriorization would not be possible with a swollen, emphysematous fetus. In these cases, the need for a ventral approach in which the uterus can be apposed more closely to the incision is obvious. When the uterus is positioned satisfactorily, it is incised (Figure 14-9C). The incision needs to be long enough to allow removal of the fetus without further tearing or extending of the uterine incision. The incision should be made parallel to the long axis of the uterus and on its greater curvature because this area has the fewest large vessels. An attempt should also be made to avoid incising caruncles. The fetus is then removed; the surgeon attempts to retain the uterus so the fetal fluids do not fall back into the peritoneal cavity (Figure 14-9D). Although not depicted in Figure 14-9D, chains are commonly attached to the limb(s) of the calf to assist in its delivery from the uterus.

The fetal membranes should be removed only if they can be separated from the uterus without undue traction or if they are lying free within the uterus.

Antibiotic boluses are inserted into the uterus prior to its closure. The uterus is closed with a continuous inverting pattern and absorbable suture material. The Utrecht method of uterine closure is presented here and is illustrated in Figure 14-9E to N. This technique was developed at the University of Utrecht, the Netherlands, as part of a study to improve the fertility of cattle following cesarean section.[1] It was noted that adhesions often developed between the uterus and visceral organs and originated most often at the ends of the incision where exposed knots were tied; adhesions also developed along the suture line when suture patterns were exposed. Moreover, uterine healing occurred across the wound edges, rather than on the apposed peritoneal surfaces, and the inflammatory response varied with the suture material. The Utrecht method of suturing was developed as a result of these findings.

The starting knot is made using oblique bites (Figure 14-9E and F), to bury the knot within the inverted suture (Figure 14-9G). Similarly, the continuous suture pattern is inserted using oblique bites (Figure 14-9H to J), so there is minimal exposure of suture material but close

apposition of the wound edges. Figure 14-9K to N depicts the insertion and tying of the final knot so that it is not exposed. Using the Utrecht method, fertility rates improved from 75 to 92%. One surprising feature was that no. 6 nonchromic catgut produced the best results.[1] With this technique, it is important that each suture be pulled tightly following its insertion; otherwise, the wound edges may gap, and the contents of the uterus might leak. Regardless of the suture pattern used, the rapidly shrinking uterine wall will leave less tissue in each bite of the suture material and might thereby loosen the suture.

We have questioned the rationale behind the use of large-diameter plain catgut suture material because it is more reactive than chromic catgut or one of the synthetic absorbable materials. One of the reasons that adhesions may be fewer with this material is the time factor. With the abundant blood supply to the involuting uterus, the suture material is probably absorbed so quickly that adhesions have less chance to form than when suture materials remain in situ for long periods of time. Newer sutures, such as polyglytone 6211 (Caprosyn), that have rapid absorption patterns with less inflammation are even better.

The knots are the last portion of the suture line to be absorbed, probably because cellular invasion is more difficult. Therefore, burying the knots at each end of the incision should always be the goal with this suture pattern.

Once the uterus is closed, it is replaced in position. The laparotomy incision is closed as described in Chapter 13.

Postoperative Management

Antibiotics are administered, and oxytocin may be administered any time after uterine closure, to enhance uterine involution. Fluid therapy may be indicated in certain cases.

Complications and Prognosis

In dairy cattle, there is some evidence that temporary reductions in milk production may occur postoperatively.[3] Adhesions between the uterus and the surrounding tissue has been shown to occur in roughly half of all cesarean sections, regardless of whether catgut or Vicryl suture was used for closure of uterus.[2]

References

1. Ball, L.: Personal communication, 1979.
2. De Wit, F., Raymakers, R., Westerbeek, J., Mijten, P., and De Kruif, A.: A study of uterine adhesions following suturing of the uterus with catgut or vicryl in cesarean sections in cattle. Tijdschr Diergeneeskd, 118:478–479, 1993.
3. Newman, K.D., and Anderson, D.E.: Cesarean section in cows. Vet. Clin. North Am.: Food Anim. Pract. 21:73–100, 2005.

4. Noorsdy, J.L.: Selection of incision site for cesarean section in the cow. VM/SAC, 75:530, 1979.
5. Parish, S.M., Tyler, J.W., and Ginsky, J.V. Left oblique celiotomy approach for cesarean section in standing cows. J. Am. Vet. Med. Assoc., 207:751–752, 1995.
6. Wenzel, J.G.W.: Anatomy of the uterus, ovaries, and adnexa. *In* Large Animal Urogenital Surgery, 2nd Ed., Edited by D.F. Wolfe and H.D. Moll. Baltimore, Williams & Wilkins, 1998, pp. 375–380.

Retention Suturing of the Bovine Vulva (Buhner's Method)

Relevant Anatomy

The female bovine external genitalia is basically the same as described for the horse in Chapter 10.

Indications

Vaginal or cervical prolapse occurs with the greatest frequency during the last trimester of gestation in cow and ewes. The condition may also occur during early postpartum or estrus, however. Prolapses are usually classified by the duration of the condition and the extent of the prolapse. For example, first degree vaginal prolapse involves only intermittent exposure of the vaginal floor, usually occurring when the cow is lying down. Second degree vaginal prolapse infers that the vaginal floor is continuously exposed. The urinary bladder may or may not be included in the prolapsed tissue, and urination may be impeded if the urethra becomes occluded. Third degree vaginal prolapses involve a continuous exposure of the vaginal floor, the urinary bladder, and the cervix through the vulva. Third degree prolapses in *Bos indicus* and *Bos taurus* breeds have been differentiated based on the observation that third degree prolapses in *Bos indicus* are usually primary prolapses of the cervix that have not progressed from a first or second degree vaginal prolapse. The *Bos taurus* breeds, however, usually will progress from a first or second degree prolapse to a third degree prolapse. Of the prolapsed tissue, the cervical os is usually located most dorsally and an extremely edematous vaginal floor most ventrally. A fourth degree prolapse is described as either a first or second degree prolapse of a duration long enough that the prolapsed tissue has become necrotic.

The buried purse-string suture (Buhner's method) is a simple and effective way to retain vaginal or uterine prolapse in the cow.[1–3] The method consists of a deeply placed circumferential suture that effectively simulates the action of the constrictor vestibulae muscle.[2] The purse-string suture may be permanent or temporary. It is strong and does not tear out as frequently as externally placed suture patterns (lacing, Halsted, and quill).[1] These methods promote infection along the suture line, although this infection generally is of minor significance. Buhner peri-

vaginal suture tape or umbilical tape are commonly used for the purse-string suture. When the tape has been removed or has disintegrated, the fibrous connective tissue produced by the cow in response to the tape is often sufficient to prevent future prolapse. Infrequently, the scar tissue may be strong enough to result in dystocia.[2] The Buhner perivaginal tape is more expensive than umbilical tape, but is made of nylon and so lies flat and is better tolerated by tissue.[1] Umbilical tape tends to become twisted and form a string, and it is more likely to cut through the edematous tissues of the vulva. Buhner perivaginal tape can remain as a permanent suture, whereas umbilical tape may disintegrate if left in the tissues.

There are several alternative methods, described in detail elsewhere, for retention following a vaginal or cervical prolapse.[4] The Minchev technique is used to anchor the anterior dorsal vagina to the gluteal area by passing heavy suture through the anterior dorsal vaginal wall, the sacrosciatic ligament, and the skin in the gluteal area. This technique does not restrict the vaginal opening like the Buhner method but may still permit prolapse of the vaginal floor or result in necrosis of the dorsal wall in which the sutures are passed.[4]

Anesthesia and Surgical Preparation

The cow should be restrained in a chute or crush, and some cows may be recumbent during the procedure. The surgery is performed with the animal under caudal epidural analgesia (see Chapter 2). Following administration and onset of the epidural analgesic, the perianal area and prolapsed tissues are cleaned and treated with an antiseptic. Osmotic agents and massage may then be used to reduce the size of the prolapse.

Instrumentation

General surgery pack
Buhner's or Gerlach's perivaginal needle
Perivaginal suture tape or sterile, 1-cm (half-inch) umbilical tape

Surgical Technique

A typical prolapse is depicted in Figure 14-10A. The prolapse is reduced, the vagina is returned to its correct anatomic location, and the perianal area is scrubbed once again. A transverse skin incision about 1 cm long is made midway between the dorsal commissure of the vulva and the anus. Another horizontal incision is made about 3 cm below the ventral commissure of the vulva. The perivaginal needle is introduced into the ventral skin incision and is driven perivaginally through the deep subcutaneous tissues parallel to the vulva. One hand is placed in the vagina to guide the needle. The needle should be driven as deep as possible (about 5 to 8 cm) and directed out the

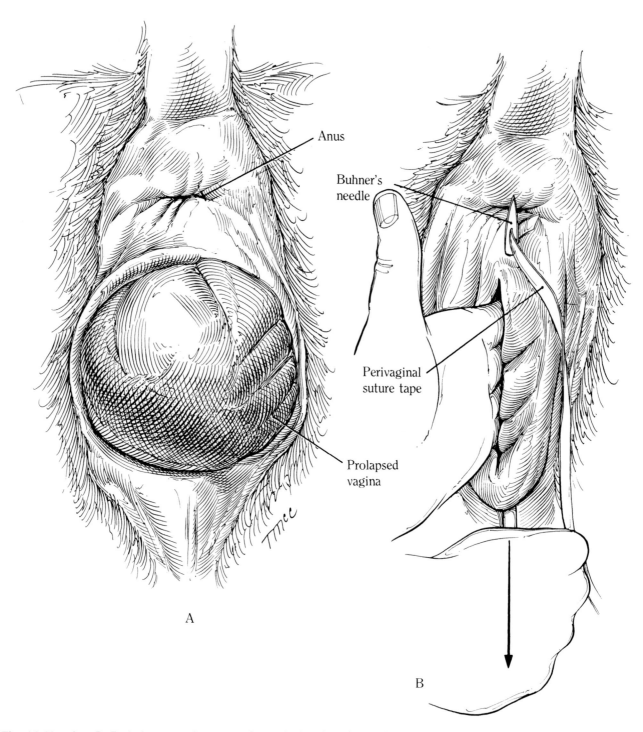

Anus

Buhner's
needle

Perivaginal
suture tape

Prolapsed
vagina

A

B

Fig. 14-10. A to D, Buried purse-string suture for vaginal and uterine prolapse.

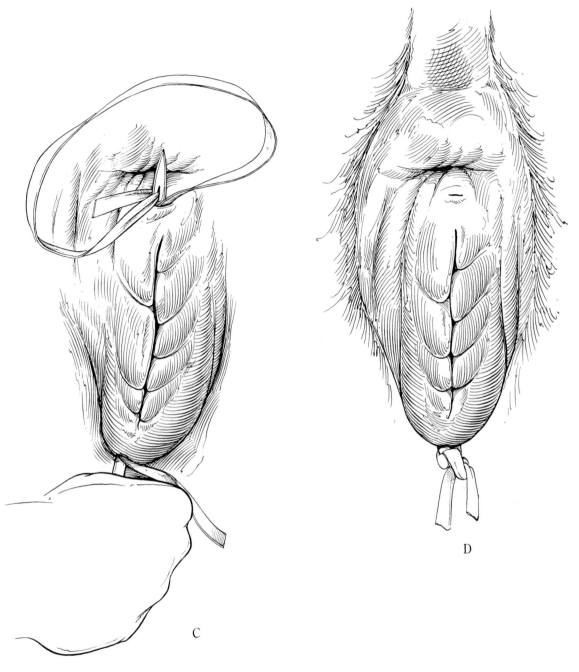

C

D

Fig. 14-10. *Continued.*

dorsal skin incision (Figure 14-10*B*). A piece of sterile perivaginal suture tape (or sterile umbilical tape) soaked in a suitable antibiotic solution, is threaded through the eye of the needle and is drawn down to emerge through the ventral skin incision (Figure 14-10*C*). At the same time, the tape is held at the dorsal incision so the end is not lost in the tissue. The tape is then removed from the needle, and the needle is threaded up the contralateral side of the vulva (about 5 to 8 cm) to emerge through the dorsal incision. The tape is threaded into the eye of the needle once again (Figure 14-10*C*), and then the needle is withdrawn ventrally, resulting in two free ends of tape emerging from the ventral skin incision.

The two free ends of the tape are tied, ensuring that the loop of tape at the dorsal incision is buried (Figure 14-10*D*). The tape is tied so the resulting suture encircling the vulva will admit two to three fingers. If a square knot is used to anchor the tape, the knot will bury itself. This minimizes the chances of contamination of the suture material and thereby avoids a wicking effect with the suture and secondary infection. The dorsal and ventral incisions may be closed with a simple interrupted suture of nonabsorbable material, to further decrease the chances of secondary infection around the umbilical tape. If the cow is close to calving, we recommend that the tape be secured in the ventral incision with a bow knot. This knot allows the suture to be removed or, at least, undone to reduce tension at the time of parturition. One of the other methods to retain the prolapse may also be used.

Postoperative Management

The cow requires close observation to time removal or loosening of the suture correctly in relationship to parturition. The knot should be untied, and the vulva should be gently dilated, to reduce tension on the suture.[2]

Complications and Prognosis

The Buhner method of repair for vaginal prolapse offers secure retention of the vagina and cervix with the convenience of quick release during calving. Calving through Buhner sutures is one of the most severe complications of this procedure and can result in severe lacerations and damage to the vulva and perineal area. Certain cattle that have a pendulous vulva may be predisposed to edema, swelling, and even necrosis of the vulva following Buhner's method of repair due to the increased tension required to retain the vagina and cervix.

References

1. Bennett, B.W.: Personal communication, 1980.
2. Hudson, R.S.: Genital surgery of the cow. In Current Therapy in Theriogenology. Vol. 2. Edited by D.A. Morrow. Philadelphia, W.B. Saunders, 1986, p. 348.
3. Sloss, V., and Duffy, J.H.: Handbook of Bovine Obstetrics. Baltimore, Williams & Wilkins, 1980.
4. Wolfe, D.F., and Carson, R.L.: In Large Animal Urogenital Surgery, 2nd Ed. Edited by D.F. Wolfe and H.D. Moll. Baltimore, Williams & Wilkins, 1998, pp. 397–412.

Cervicopexy for Vaginal Prolapse (After Winkler)

Relevant Anatomy

The external genitalia of the female bovine is basically the same as in the horse described in Chapter 10. During this procedure, the attachment of the prepubic tendon just cranial to the pelvic symphysis may be palpated through the floor of the vagina. It extends ventrad and craniad from its attachment at an angle of about 90° to the horizontal plane (Figure 14-11A).

Indications

Another method for retaining a prolapsed vagina in the cow is a technique in which the external os of the cervix is sutured to the prepubic tendon. The main advantage of the technique is that postoperative treatment is minimal.[1–3]

Anesthesia and Surgical Preparation

This procedure is performed using epidural anesthesia. Following restraint of the cow in a chute or crush, an epidural anesthetic is given, and the prolapsed tissues are cleaned, treated with the appropriate medication, and replaced.

Instrumentation

General surgery pack
8.0-cm half-circle cutting needle that has been bent into a U-shape
At least 1.2 m of nonabsorbable suture material

Surgical Technique

The prepared needle is carried into the vagina by hand. The urethra and bladder are located (preferably by inserting a urinary catheter, rather than by simple palpation), to ensure placement of the suture lateral to these structures.

The point of the needle is directed through the floor of the vagina below the vaginal end of the cervix. As originally described, the needle is directed through a triangular area toward the midline back up through the tendon and vaginal floor. This triangular area is formed by a short band of the prepubic tendon that extends caudolaterad, attaching to the iliopubic eminence of the pubis (Figure 14-11B). To decrease the possibility of breaking the needle, however, it is recommended to pass the needle down through the prepubic tendon and up through the triangular space in a medial-to-lateral direction. A bite of 1.8 cm in the prepubic tendon and 3.5 to 5.0 cm in the vaginal floor is usually adequate. The needle and suture are pulled through the prepubic tendon and vaginal wall sufficiently to continue the suture through the intravaginal part of the cervix. Tension should be applied to the suture to see whether it is adequately anchored in the prepubic tendon. A urinary catheter should be reintroduced into the bladder to ensure that the bladder and urethra have not been included in the suture. The needle is then directed across the lower half of the cervix at least 1.2 cm (half an inch) cranial to the caudal limits of the intravaginal part of the cervix. The suture ends are exteriorized, and the first throws of a surgeon's knot are performed and are then advanced craniad, tight enough to prevent caudal movement of the cervix (Figure 14-11C).

Postoperative Management

The cow should be given appropriate antibiotic therapy.

Complications and Prognosis

This procedure can be used in cows in which external retention techniques have been unsuccessful. Postoperative tenesmus has been minimal or completely absent

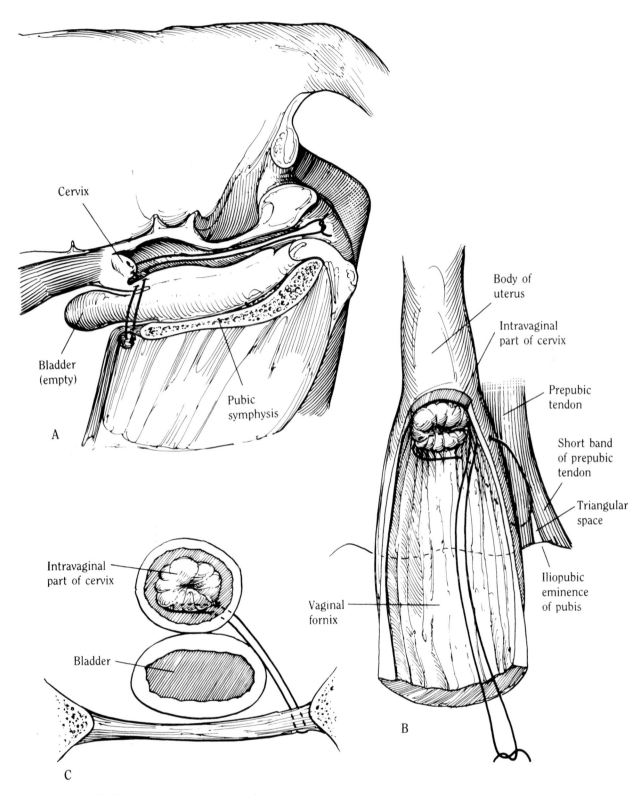

Fig. 14-11. A to C, Cervicopexy for vaginal prolapse.

with this technique. The suture has remained in position for as long as a year in some cows. In one cow, the suture was still present when the cow was slaughtered (for unrelated reasons) 7 years after repair of the prolapse.[2]

Peritonitis has been associated with this technique when umbilical tape is used, and a suture of less capillarity is recommended. Care must be taken not to deviate too far from the midline when placing the suture through the tendon; otherwise, inadvertent penetration of arteries of the pelvic cavity may result.[2]

References

1. Hudson, R.S.: Genital surgery of the cow. *In* Current Therapy in Theriogenology. Vol. 2. Edited by D.A. Morrow. Philadelphia, W.B. Saunders, 1986, p. 350.
2. Winkler, J.K.: Personal communication, 1987.
3. Winkler, J.K.: Repair of bovine vaginal prolapse by cervical fixation. J. Am. Vet. Med. Assoc., *149*:768, 1966.

Chapter 15

MISCELLANEOUS BOVINE SURGICAL TECHNIQUES

Objectives

1. Describe some surgical procedures used in treatment of common disorders in cattle, including septic arthritis and diseases of the digit, extensive neoplasia of or trauma to the eye, pericarditis, and teat lacerations.
2. Provide a technique for cosmetic dehorning.

Digit Amputation

Relevant Anatomy

In ruminants, the lateral and medial digits of each limb are connected through tough skin and interdigital ligaments until the level of the coronary band, where the distal phalanges of each digit are encased within the hoof. The distal (interdigital) collateral ligament spans the interdigital space at the level of the distal sesamoid bones and travels over the tendons of the deep digital flexor muscle to the abaxial surfaces of the middle phalanges.[4] The proximal interdigital ligament connects the axial surfaces of the proximal phalanges.[4] The distal interphalangeal joint (DIP) of each digit is formed by the articulation of two distal sesamoid bones, the distal phalanx, and the middle phalanx. There are two bursas associated with the DIP joint; the dorsal bursa lies deep to the tendon of the common digital extensor muscle, and the palmar (plantar) bursa lies deep to the tendons of the deep digital flexor and the distal sesamoid bones and associated ligaments.[4] Sepsis of the DIP joint in particular is a common pathological condition of the bovine foot and frequently necessitates surgery. Penetrations of the interdigital cleft by a foreign object, termed an *interdigital phlegmon*, and extensions of sole diseases, such as ulcers, are common causes of septic arthritis. The lateral digit bears more weight than the medial digit and is usually the larger digit in the forelimb. Unfortunately, the lateral digit is more frequently affected. In clinical studies, most cases requiring digit amputation occur in the lateral digit of the hindlimb for reasons that are not fully understood.

Indications

The following are indications for amputation of the bovine digit: severe foot rot unresponsive to antibiotics and complicated by osteomyelitis, abscess formation with osteoarthritis of the distal interphalangeal joint, tenosynovitis, or infectious arthritis and sepsis of the proximal or distal interphalangeal joints; severe phalangeal fractures; and dislocations of the phalangeal joints.[3,8]

This surgical procedure is indicated to relieve pain and to return the animal to soundness and production, as well as to prevent ascending infection of the limb. The prognosis for digit amputation is good and most cattle return to productivity rapidly; however, the survival period is not as favorable as some other techniques. Ankylosis is described elsewhere as an alternative technique to digit amputation and is successful in many cattle.[2,7] Ankylosis produces a longer survival period; however, digit amputation is still used for economical reasons and rapid recovery.[8]

The following are contraindications for digit amputation: sepsis of the fetlock joint, involvement of both digits of the same foot, and heavy bulls or cows (these animals generally break down the remaining claw). Cows with amputated digits are usually culled sooner than herdmates and have a lower market value.

The same basic technique of digit amputation is applicable to pigs and small ruminants.

Anesthesia and Surgical Preparation

The animal is usually placed in lateral recumbency by means of ropes and chemical restraint, or it is secured to a surgical table, with the affected claw uppermost. The procedure may be performed with the animal standing, but this is not generally recommended. The limb is clipped from the midmetacarpal region or midmetatarsal region distad, and the area is prepared surgically prior to administering local anesthesia. The claw and interdigital space are cleared of all fecal material and debris; a scrub brush and a hoof knife are useful for this initial preparation. Intravenous local analgesia is the preferred method of local desensitization (see Chapter 2, "Anesthesia and Fluid Therapy"), but regional nerve blocks or a ring block may also be used. Following administration of the local anesthetic, the surgical site is given a final surgical scrub. If the intravenous analgesic technique is not used, a tourniquet (rubber tubing) is applied at this stage. The limb is draped so the foot is exposed, and a sterile glove may be applied over the claw so it can be handled by the surgeon during surgery.

Instrumentation

General surgery pack
Obstetric wire saw or Gigli wire saw

Surgical Technique

The technique illustrated in Figure 15-1 uses a skin flap and attempted closure. The skin incision is made along the abaxial and axial surface of the coronary band; then vertical incisions are made cranially and caudally (Figure 15-1A). The skin and subcutaneous tissues are incised to the bone. The skin incision on the axial surface is made first so as not to obscure the surgical field with blood. The skin is then dissected free from the underlying digit, and one attempts to save as much of the skin flap as possible. Alternatively, a circumferential skin incision can be made in a similar plane to the wire cut illustrated in Figure 15-1B and C.

The amputation may be performed in two locations. A low amputation is performed when only the coffin joint and distal phalanx are diseased; this amputation is directed through the middle phalanx. We describe the technique of high amputation, which is used in cases with involvement of the coffin joint, distal phalanx, pastern joint, and middle phalanx. This amputation is directed through the junction of the middle and distal third of the proximal phalanx.

An obstetric saw is placed in the incision in the interdigital space. An assistant is needed for the sawing procedure (Figure 15-1B). The amputation is commenced with the wire saw directed parallel to the long axis of the limb until the wire is located at the distal end of the proximal phalanx. The saw is directed perpendicular to the long axis of the proximal phalanx to seat the wire in the bone, and then the position of the wire is directed so it is approximately 45° to the long axis of the proximal phalanx (Figure 15-1C). The sawing motion should not be too rapid because heat necrosis of tissues, including bone, may occur, leading to excessive sloughing during the healing period. Care should be taken to avoid invading the fetlock joint capsule. Once the digit has been removed, excess interdigital adipose tissue and all necrotic tissue,

especially that involving the tendons and tendon sheaths, should be dissected sharply from the wound. If the digital artery can be located, it should be ligated.

Some of the skin flap may be sutured down, but when the surgical site is swollen from infection and when some skin necrosis is present in the region, this is not usually possible. Complete closure is contraindicated because infection will resolve more rapidly if the skin flap is not completely sutured, to allow better ventral drainage (Figure 15-1D).[6] The value of skin flaps and of any attempt at closure has been questioned.[5] An antibiotic powder is applied to the area and is followed by sterile gauze sponges. A tight bandage is applied to prevent hemorrhage when the tourniquet is removed (Figure 15-1E), and some form of impervious covering may be indicated.

Postoperative Management

The bandage should be changed 2 to 3 days after surgery. The limb is kept bandaged until the wound has healed. The length of time the wound will need to be bandaged depends on the individual case and to what degree the wound was left open. Some cases of digit amputation may require only 10 to 14 days to heal, whereas others may require several more weeks for the wound to heal by secondary intention.

In the initial stages of healing, the animal should be housed in dry conditions where food and water are easily accessible, to avoid overuse of the remaining digit. Penicillin or another broad spectrum systemic antibiotic may be administered.

Complications and Prognosis

The most common complications of digit amputation are reductions in milk production in dairy cattle for the first 60 days postoperatively, ascending tendonitis, and development of disease on the remaining digit.[1]

In one study, a good recovery from surgery, in the authors' opinions, was achieved in 51% of cattle that underwent digit amputation. 22% were deemed a poor recovery, with the remainder of the cattle having a fair recovery.[8] The mean survival time of cattle recovering from digit amputation ranges from 68 days to 20 months.[1,8] Heavy cattle (greater than 680 kg) generally have a much poorer prognosis for digit amputation.[7]

References

1. Bicalho, R.C., Cheong, S.H., Warnick, L.D., Nydam, D.V., and Guard, C.L.: The effect of digit amputation or arthrodesis surgery on culling and milk production in holstein dairy cows. J. Dairy Sci., 89:2596–2602, 2006.
2. Desrochers, A., St. Jean, G., and Anderson, D.E.: Use of facilitated ankylosis in the treatment of septic arthritis of the distal interphalangeal joint in cattle: 12 cases (1987–1992).

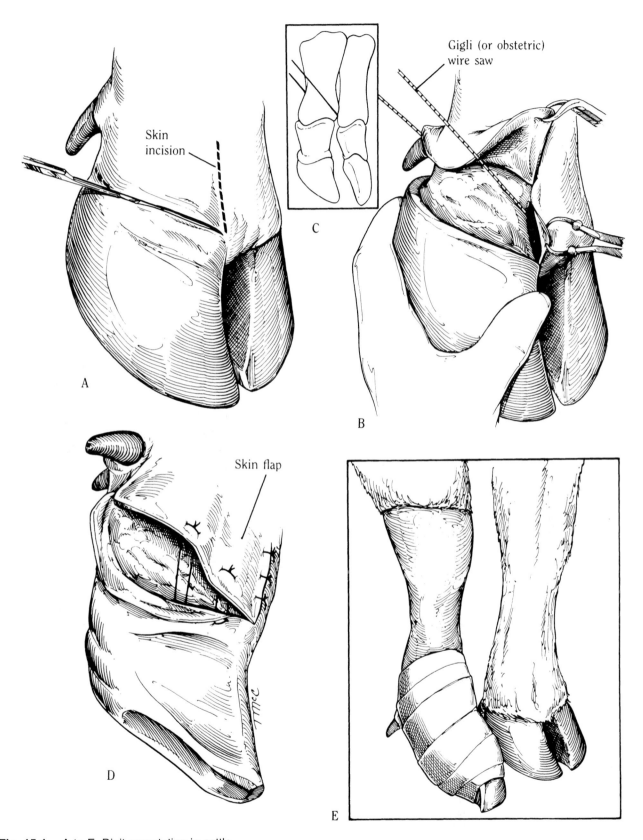

Fig. 15-1. A to E, Digit amputation in cattle.

3. Desrochers, A., and St. Jean., G.: Surgical management of digit disorders in cattle. Vet. Clin. Food Anim. Pract., 12:277–298, 1996.

4. Dyce, K.M., Sack, W.O., and Wensing, C.J.G.: Textbook of Veterinary Anatomy, 2nd Ed., Philadelphia, W.B. Saunders, 1996.

5. Greenough, P.R., MacCallum, F.J., and Weaver, A.D.: Treatment and control of digital disease. In Lameness in Cattle, 2nd Ed. Edited by A.D. Weaver. Philadelphia, J.B. Lippincott, 1981, p. 228.

6. Knight, A.P.: Personal communication, 1980.

7. Nuss, K., and Weaver, M.P.: Resection of the distal interphalangeal joint in cattle: an alternative to amputation. Vet. Rec., 128:540–543, 1991.

8. Pejsa, T.G., St. Jean, G., Hoffsis, G.F., and Musser, J.M.B.: Digit amputation in cattle: 85 cases (1971–1990). J. Am. Vet. Med. Assoc., 202:981–984, 1993.

Eye Enucleation

Relevant Anatomy

The anatomy of the eye can be divided into the structures of the eyeball (globe) and the adnexa. In the procedure described here, the adnexal structures are emphasized as the eyeball itself is removed. Structures of the adnexa include ocular muscles, orbital fasciae, the eyelids, conjunctiva, and the lacrimal apparatus. The eyelids have three basic layers: the outer skin, a fibromuscular layer, and the palpebral conjunctiva. The palpebral conjunctiva, together with the bulbar conjunctiva, comprises the conjuctival sac. The dorsal and ventral distal extremities of the sac are called *fornices*. The third eyelid attaches to a T-shaped plate of cartilage on the medial aspect of the eyeball. Between the dorsolateral wall of the orbit and the eyeball is the lacrimal apparatus.[1] Several other accessory glands of the lacrimal apparatus exist but are detailed in other anatomy texts.[1]

The muscles responsible for moving the eye are all located near the optic foramen behind the eyeball except for the ventral oblique muscle. The ventral oblique muscle originates on the ventromedial wall of the orbit and passes laterally below the eyeball. The four rectus muscles all insert anterior to the equator of the eye at a dorsal, ventral, medial, and lateral site. The retractor bulbi muscle inserts posteriorly on the eyeball and envelops the optic nerve.

The locations of the ophthalmic and maxillary nerves are also relevant to this procedure for local anesthesia of the eye. These nerves enter the orbit with the extraocular muscles through the foramen orbitorotundum, which is a combined round and orbital foramen that is unique to bovine species. This is the site of injection for anesthesia during eye extirpation.

Indications

Although the operation is called an enucleation of the eye, it is, for all practical purposes, an extirpation because everything within the orbit is generally removed; there is no demand for cosmetic repair as in other species. Enucleation involves the removal of the globe, leaving adipose tissue and muscles, whereas extirpation involves removal of everything within the orbit: globe, muscles, adipose tissue, and lacrimal gland. Extirpation in cattle is indicated for neoplasia (usually squamous cell carcinoma) of the upper and lower eyelids, third eyelid, and cornea that is too extensive to be removed by other, less radical operations, such as lid resections, H-plasties, or superficial keratectomies. Septic panophthalmitis, severe trauma beyond repair, and severe trauma with loss of globe contents are also indications for enucleation.

Anesthesia and Surgical Preparation

The animal, which is wearing a halter, should be adequately restrained in a chute and its head secured to one side. Prior to administering the retrobulbar block, the surgeon clips the hair around the animal's eyes and prepares the surgical site aseptically. Local anesthesia is administered by infiltration of the retrobulbar tissues. The four-point retrobulbar block is performed by injecting through the eyelids, both dorsally and ventrally, and at the medial and lateral canthi (Figure 15-2A). A slightly curved, 8- to 10-cm 18-gauge needle is directed to the apex of the orbit where the nerves emerge from the foramen orbitorotundum. About 40 ml of local anesthetic are injected, divided into 10 ml per site. Exophalmos, corneal anesthesia, and mydriasis indicate a satisfactory retrobulbar block.[2] Other surgeons use the Peterson retrobulbar eye block for this procedure. The four-point retrobulbar technique is quick and easier to administer.

Because this particular surgical procedure is performed for large, necrotic, ocular neoplasms or severe trauma, proper aseptic preparation of the surgical site may be impossible. Generally, draping is not performed for this procedure. If there are large amounts of necrotic, neoplastic tissue, some of it may be trimmed prior to the surgical scrub.

Instrumentation

General surgery pack
Right angled forceps

Surgical Technique

Following surgical preparation, the patient's eyelids are grasped with towel clamps and closed to minimize contamination of the surgical field. A recommended alternative is to suture the eyelids together and to leave the suture ends long. Sutures provide a better seal from necrotic debris than towel clamps. Using these methods, the instruments or ends of the sutures can be used to put traction on the eye throughout surgery. A transpalpebral

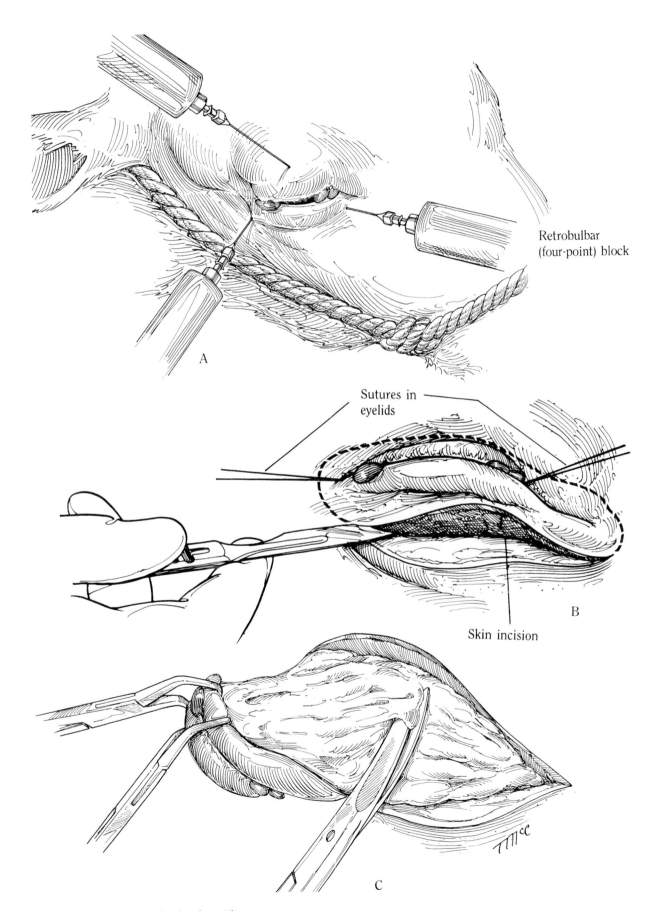

Retrobulbar (four-point) block

A

Sutures in eyelids

Skin incision

B

C

Fig. 15-2. A to E, Eye enucleation in cattle.

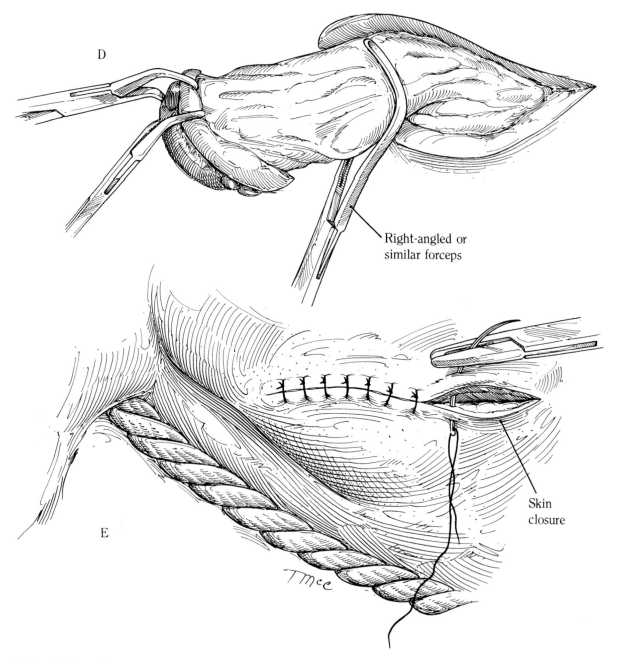

D

Right-angled or
similar forceps

Skin
closure

E

TMcc

Fig. 15-2. *Continued.*

incision is made around the orbit, leaving as much normal
tissue as possible (Figure 15-2B). The incision is generally
1 cm from the margin of the eyelid. The ventral incision
and subsequent dissection are done first. Sharp or blunt
dissection is used for 360° around the orbit continuing
down to the caudal aspect of the orbit, but avoiding
entrance through the palpebral conjunctiva (Figure
15-2C). All muscles, adipose tissue, the lacrimal gland,
and fascia are removed, along with the eyelids and eyeball.
If the indication for enucleation is neoplasia, one must
make sure that all neoplastic tissue is removed. If the eye
is enucleated for a non-neoplastic condition, such as
irreparable trauma, the surgeon can afford to leave some

of the retrobulbar tissue to reduce the amount of dead
space and intraoperative hemorrhage.

When the optic stalk and its blood supply are reached,
a pair of right-angled forceps or a similar instrument is
used to grasp the stalk, which is then severed distally
(Figure 15-2D). The optic artery may be ligated prior to
severance to minimize hemorrhage. Following removal of
the eye, considerable dead space remains and is virtually
impossible to obliterate. The cavity fills with a blood clot
that will organize during the healing period and will leave
a large depression in the orbit.

Closure consists of a layer of simple interrupted sutures,
or a simple continuous suture, in the skin using synthetic

nonabsorbable suture material (Figure 15-2E). Sutures are removed 2 to 3 weeks postoperatively. If infection is present, some of the skin sutures should be removed to permit drainage. Some surgeons prefer to pack the eye with sterile gauze to control hemorrhage and to remove the gauze a day or so after hemorrhage has stopped. Generally, this is not necessary, because a tight seal with a skin suture seems to allow pressure to build up within the orbit and to create hemostasis through a tamponade effect. Packing the orbit usually only increases the extent of postoperative management, which may be difficult in field conditions. Packing is indicated in cases of massive, uncontrollable hemorrhage.

Another variation of the enucleation technique is to pack the orbit as soon as the globe and surrounding structures have been removed and to leave the packing in place until the last skin sutures have been tied. The pack is then removed, and the closure is completed. Some surgeons prefer to use an absorbable suture in the skin, to obviate the need for suture removal; this would be useful on the range, where it may be impractical to round up the animal for suture removal.

Postoperative Management

Antibiotics are indicated if sepsis is present. If dehiscence occurs, granulation tissue will generally fill the wound satisfactorily. If healing is delayed, the surgeon may suspect a recurrence of the neoplastic process if it was the original indication for enucleation. Much hemorrhage occurs at the time of surgery, and it may alarm the inexperienced surgeon. We believe that, if the surgery progresses quickly, blood loss will be minimal. For this reason, some surgeons prefer a simple continuous pattern for closure.

Complications and Prognosis

Complications of this procedure include extensive hemorrhage from the optic artery, which may require ligation, infection, dehiscence, recurrence of disease, and convulsions due to inadvertent injection of lidocaine into the meningeal reflection of the optic nerve while performing the retrobulbar block.[3] The prognosis for this procedure is generally good but varies with the presenting disease.

References

1. Dyce, K.M., Sack, W.O., and Wensing, C.J.G.: Textbook of Veterinary Anatomy, 2nd Ed., Philadelphia, W.B. Saunders, 1996.
2. Gelatt, K.N., and Titus, R.S.: The special sense organs. *In* A Textbook of Large Animal Surgery. Edited by F.W. Oehme and J.E. Prier. Baltimore, Williams & Wilkins, 1974.
3. Welker, B.: Ocular surgery. Vet. Clin. Food Anim. Prac., *11*:149–157, 1995.

Cosmetic Dehorning

Relevant Anatomy

At the junction of horn and skin lies the corium, which consists of the cells that facilitate growth of new horn. If these cells are not removed during dehorning, regrowth will occur and a scur may form at the poll. The horn itself is attached to the porous, bony, cornual process that is covered by a papillated dermis.

Nervous supply to the dermis of the horn is primarily through the cornual nerve, which arises from the orbit and travels in the ridge of the temporal line.[1] The nerve splits and wraps around the horn beneath the frontalis muscle. Complete desensitization of the cornual nerve prior to dehorning is not always successful due to variations in branching and the location of the nerve with respect to the temporal ridge.[1] Additionally, the horn may also be innervated partially by the supraorbital or infratrochlear nerves, or nerves from the frontal sinus may extend into the cornual diverticulum.

The blood supply to the horn arises form the superficial temporal vessels, which branch and advance up the cornual process. Once severed, these branches retract and are difficult to reach with hemostats. Significant hemmorrhage can occur if the vessel is not cut close to the skull so that the artery remains embedded within soft tissue.

Indications

Dehorning is performed in cattle to reduce injuries and carcass damage caused by fighting. Cosmetic dehorning permits closure of the skin over a normal defect created by the amputation of the horn at its base. Ideally, this results in primary-intention healing, a lower incidence of frontal sinusitis, and less hemorrhage. It is generally reserved for show animals and expensive breeding livestock in which postoperative appearance of the poll is important.[2] The method is best suited for cattle under 1 year of age because there may not be enough skin to close the defect after horn removal in older animals.[4]

Anesthesia and Surgical Preparation

The animal is restrained in a squeeze chute with its head secured to one side with a halter. The hair is removed from the poll, the base of the ears, and the face as far as the eyes; the ears can be wrapped with adhesive tape and are pulled back out of the way (not illustrated). Tranquilization of the animal with intravenous xylazine or another analgesic discussed in Chapter 2 will decrease stress to the animal. The tail vein is generally the most accessible route of administration and causes the least distress in this instance.[3] If tranquilizers are used, the animal should be withheld from slaughter for the recommended period of time.

The area is then scrubbed and prepared for cornual nerve block, but it is not draped. A cornual (zygomatico-temporal) nerve block is performed using an 18-gauge, 4- to 5-cm needle. In some of the larger breeds, an 8-cm needle is more satisfactory.[4] The needle is inserted through the skin at a point midway between the lateral canthus of the eye and the base of the horn (Figure 15-3A). The needle is directed through the frontalis muscle and under the lateral aspect of the temporal portion of the frontal bone. At this point, 5 ml of local anesthetic are injected in a fanlike manner, and another 2 ml are deposited under the skin as the needle is withdrawn. Then the needle is directed subcutaneously toward the base of the horn, and an additional 2 to 3 ml of local anesthetic are deposited below the skin. The injection sites are massaged to disperse the local anesthetic. The block is repeated on the other side of the head. Generally, the head is swung around to the other side of the squeeze chute and is restrained to permit access to the sites that are to be blocked for the contralateral horn. The surgical site is given a final scrub prior to commencing surgery.

Instrumentation

General surgery pack
Obstetric wire and handle or sterilized Barnes dehorner

Surgical Technique

An incision is made from the lateral limit of the nuchal eminence (poll) in a lateral direction toward the base of the horn. The incision curves rostroventrad around the base of the horn and along the frontal crest for about 5 to 7 cm. The incision should be no more than 1 cm from the base of the horn. A second incision is begun from a point about 5 to 8 cm from the origin of the first incision, near the nuchal eminence. This incision is carried around the rostral aspect of the horn, about 1 cm from the base, to unite it with the first incision ventrally. The limits of the incisions are illustrated in Figure 15-3B. The incisions are deepened until bone is encountered, and the edges of the incision are undermined using sharp dissection. The rostral incision must be undermined in an area bounded by the ends of the incision (Figure 15-3B, shaded area). The caudal incision is undermined just enough to allow placement of the wire saw ventrally and deep to the base of the horn on the frontal crest. Care should be taken when the incisions are deepened not to divide the auricular muscles (located caudally and ventrally). Generally, bleeding is controlled by torsion of the cornual artery located rostroventral to the bony stump.

The stump is then removed using either an obstetric wire as a saw, a dehorning saw, or a Barnes dehorner, which is used like a rongeur. Many surgeons prefer the Barnes dehorner because it facilitates small, precise cuts of bone to be removed after the horn is excised to reach the desired shape. It the saw or wire is used, the rope securing the head is untied, and the head is swung around to the other side of the chute to facilitate positioning of the wire saw. The saw must seat itself in the frontal bone at an adequate distance from the base of the horn to allow removal of sufficient bone. If this is not done, the approximation of the skin edges will be under excessive tension, and closure may be impossible. If more horn must be removed, the surgeon may use a hammer and chisel or a Barnes dehorner, so the cut will be flush with the frontal bone. The remaining horn is removed in an identical manner. Once the horns and attached skin are removed, the head is repositioned in preparation for the closure of the wound.

The surgical sites are flushed with a suitable physiologic solution, such as Ringer's solution, to rinse out any bone dust. Skin closure is usually performed in one layer using a heavy, nonabsorbable material in a simple continuous pattern (Figure 15-3C). To assist in hemostasis and reduction of dead space, a roll of gauze is placed over the ventral half of the incision and is anchored by a large horizontal mattress suture in the skin (a stent bandage).

Postoperative Management

The stent bandage is removed 24 to 48 hours postoperatively, and the skin sutures are removed 2 to 3 weeks postoperatively.

Complications and Prognosis

The following are the three most common errors of the inexperienced surgeon: removal of too much skin at the base of the horn that subsequently will be removed with the horn; improper seating of the wire saw at the base of the horn, resulting in a stump of bone; and failure to undermine the skin edges adequately. These errors result in the surgeon's inability to appose the skin edges. If this happens, a varying degree of sinusitis, along with wound healing by secondary intention, is the end result. Complications are generally mild, however, and the prognosis is good.

References

1. Dyce, K.M., Sack, W.O., and Wensing, C.J.G.: Textbook of Veterinary Anatomy, 2nd Ed., Philadelphia, W.B. Saunders, 1996.
2. Greenough, P.R.: The integumentary system: skin, hoof, claw and appendages. In Textbook of Large Animal Surgery. Edited by F.W. Oehme and J.E. Prier. Baltimore, Williams & Wilkins, 1974.
3. Hoffsis, G.: Surgical (cosmetic) dehorning in cattle. Vet. Clin. Food Anim. Pract., 11:159–169, 1995.
4. Wallace, C.E.: Cosmetic dehorning. In Bovine Medicine and Surgery, 2nd Ed. Vol. II. Edited by H.E. Amstutz. Santa Barbara, CA, American Veterinary Publications, 1980, p. 1240.

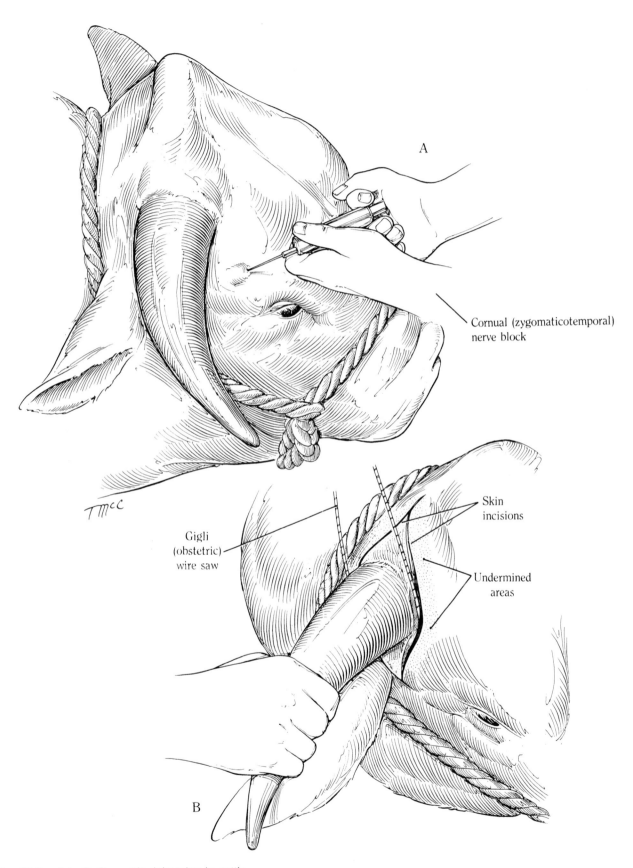

Cornual (zygomaticotemporal) nerve block

Gigli (obstetric) wire saw

Skin incisions

Undermined areas

A

B

Fig. 15-3. A to C, Cosmetic dehorning in cattle.

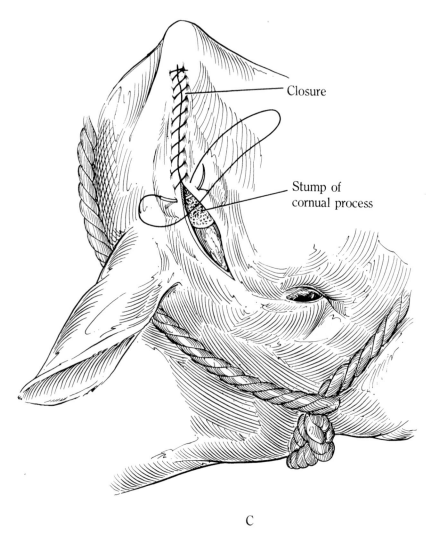

C

Fig. 15-3. *Continued.*

Rib Resection and Pericardiotomy

Relevant Anatomy

Due to the large width of the ribs and the subsequently narrower intercostal space, resection of one or more ribs may be necessary to access the thorax in the bovine.[1] The thorax is shorter than in the horse, and the diaphragm is positioned more vertically. Most of the heart lies on the left side of the thorax extending from the second intercostal space to the fifth intercostal space. The pericardium is a closed, serous sac comprised of a visceral layer that is closely adhered to the heart and a fibrous parietal layer.[1] A distance of fewer than 10 cm separates the pericardium from the reticulum, which lies caudal to the diaphragm and cranial to the rumen, occupying the space beneath the sixth to eighth rib.[5] Cattle that ingest sharp metal objects may develop traumatic reticulitis if the object is forced through the reticular wall by the normal contractions of the organ. Due to the relatively close proximity of the heart, it is also feasible that a large foreign object may be forced through the diaphragm and puncture the pericardium as well, resulting in purulent and constrictive pericarditis and chronic pericardial effusion.

Indications

Rib resection and pericardectomy in cattle are performed primarily to treat pericarditis resulting from penetration of the pericardial sac by a foreign body from the reticulum (traumatic reticulopericarditis). Generally, congestive heart failure due to pericardial and myocardial pathologic changes ensues, along with weight loss, ill thrift, and eventually, death. Drainage is indicated because the process is a closed-cavity infection, similar to an abscess, which seldom responds to antibiotic therapy alone. Drainage using a Foley catheter introduced through a large trocar may be unsuccessful because of fibrin accumulation and pocket formation in the pericardial sac.[3]

Generally, pericardiotomy is considered a salvage operation to buy time before the animal can be slaughtered. Although the aim of the surgery may be to allow time for a cow to calve, many cows with pericarditis abort from the stress of the disease process or the stress of the disease combined with surgery. When pericarditis is confirmed by clinical signs or pericardiocentesis, or when rumenotomy gives evidence of pericardial involvement, pericardiotomy is indicated.

Most animals with advanced pericarditis are in poor physical condition and have congestive heart failure, which makes them poor surgical risks. Animals under 5 years of age that can ambulate normally and are relatively normal in body function and condition can usually withstand the operation.[4] The surgery should be performed before the animal's body condition deteriorates to a point where there is no chance for survival. Advanced pregnancy and stress from other diseases hinder success.

Anesthesia and Surgical Preparation

Generally, preoperative antibiotics are indicated. *Corynebacterium pyogenes* is commonly the offending organism and is usually sensitive to common antibiotics. Mixed bacterial infections from the reticulum may be present, however, and it is preferable to culture the exudate from the pericardium and to obtain specific antibiotic sensitivities. Fluid therapy during and after surgery is beneficial in counteracting the effects of surgical and septic shock.

Because most candidates for pericardectomy are poor anesthetic risks, the surgery is generally performed with the animal under local anesthesia. Sedation may also be required. General anesthesia should be avoided if possible. The intravenous sedation techniques combined with local anesthesia are generally accompanied by struggling, but they are usually safer in an animal in poor condition.

The surgery can be performed in the standing or laterally recumbent animal. Prior to casting, a large area over the left thorax and elbow region is clipped. The surgery is performed with the animal placed in right-lateral recumbency, with the aid of casting ropes or a tilt table. If a tilt table is available, it is advantageous to operate at a 30 to 40° tilt to allow any exudate to drain from the surgical site. This position also seems less stressful than full-lateral recumbency with the animal in the horizontal position. Generally, sedation is commenced prior to placing the patient on the tilt table. Once the patient is positioned, the clipped area over the left ventral chest wall is prepared for aseptic surgery. The left thoracic limb should be pulled craniad to help expose the area over the fifth rib, and local analgesia is instituted by direct infiltration of a local analgesic agent along the incision line (line block).[4] The analgesic solution is infused initially into the subcutaneous space, into the underlying muscle, and onto the surface of the fifth rib. The operating time should be kept to an absolute minimum to reduce stress on an already compromised patient. The surgical site is given a final scrub, during which time the local anesthetic will be taking effect. Performing the surgery in the standing animal will reduce stress on the animal, but it might become recumbent during the procedure.

Instrumentation

General surgery pack
Obstetric wire saw or Gigli wire saw and handles

Surgical Technique

The skin incision extends from the costochondral junction to a point 20 cm dorsally on a line over the fifth rib (Figure 15-4A). The pericardial sac can also be approached through resection of the sixth rib. The latissimus dorsi and serratus ventralis muscles are incised to expose the rib. The periosteum is incised and is reflected from the rib (Figure 15-4B). Following exposure of 12 to 14 cm of the fifth rib, a wire saw (Gigli or obstetric) is inserted under the rib with forceps and is positioned at the dorsal commissure of the incision. The rib is transected dorsally and then is grasped and broken at the costochondral junction (Figure 15-4C). This portion of the rib is discarded. Some surgeons prefer to let the patient stand at this point in the operation before the parietal pleura is opened, to assist drainage.[2] If the animal is restrained on a tilt table, it can be positioned at a steeper angle to aid drainage of exudate. The incision is then continued through the exposed periosteum and parietal pleura for about 12 cm, using a pair of blunt-tipped scissors (Figure 15-4D).

The initial opening of the pleura should be small, because a sudden influx of air may cause respiratory distress. Usually, however, the pericardium is adherent to the parietal pleura, and pneumothorax does not occur. To avoid opening the pleural cavity, some surgeons suture the periosteum, the parietal pleura, and the pericardium together using no. 0 or 1 synthetic absorbable suture in a simple continuous pattern prior to opening the pleura. If the pericardium is not adherent to the parietal pleura, or if suturing is not performed, leakage of pus into the pleural cavity will result in contamination and pleuritis.[3]

An incision is then made between the suture lines. Once the pericardium is visible, it is opened sufficiently to allow the introduction of the surgeon's hand. A variable amount of pus will escape from the incision. Suction, if available, should be used to aid evacuation of the exudate. The pericardial sac should be explored for a foreign body. Any foreign body should be removed, but often all that is found is a firm fibrous tissue mass in the caudal aspect of the pericardial sac. As much fibrinous exudate as possible should be removed (Figure 15-4E). Adhesions should be broken down gently at this stage by passing the hand around the heart. It is unwise to proceed with a dissection that is too extensive, however, for fear

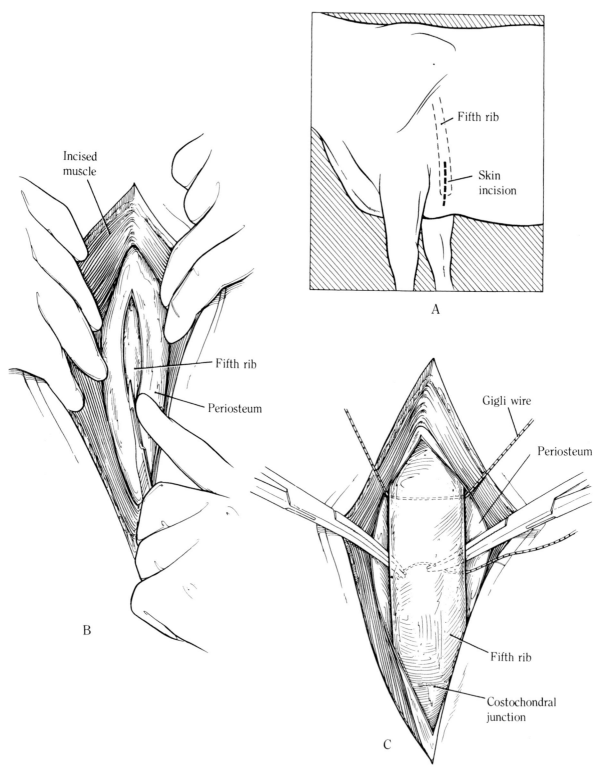

Labels in image:
A
Fifth rib
Skin incision

B
Incised muscle
Fifth rib
Periosteum

C
Gigli wire
Periosteum
Fifth rib
Costochondral junction

Fig. 15-4. A to E, Pericardiotomy.

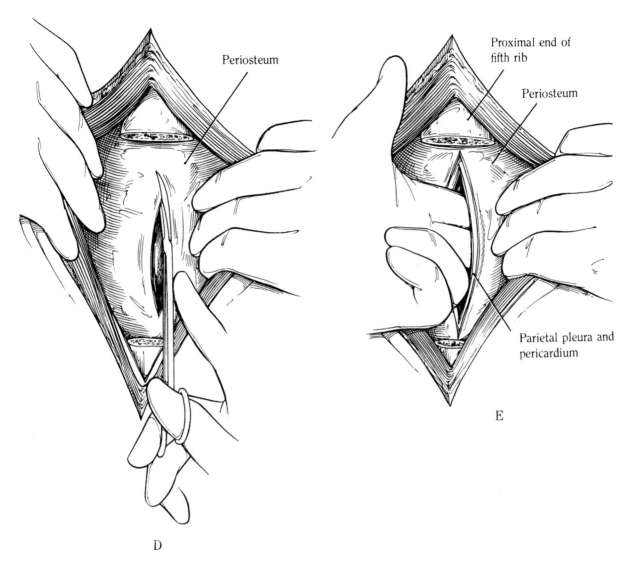

Fig. 15-4. *Continued.*

of rupturing coronary vessels.[4] Following drainage, exploration, and the removal of any foreign object, the cavity is lavaged copiously with warm isotonic electrolyte solution. The inclusion of antibiotics or antibacterial agents in the lavage solution is believed to be beneficial. Drains are sometimes indicated if postoperative flushing is to be done. The wound may be closed or left open to allow drainage.

Closure consists of simple continuous sutures of no. 0 or 1 synthetic absorbable suture. The parietal pleura, adherent pericardium, and deep periosteal layer are included in the first row. Periosteum and intercostal musculature are closed in a second row, and nonabsorbable suture material is used for the skin closure. No attempt is made to evacuate air from the pleural cavity, because normal lung function returns in about 7 to 10 days.[4] If the wound is to be left open, the combined edges of the periosteum, parietal pleura, and pericardium are everted and are sutured to the subcutaneous tissue, to create a pericardial fistula.

In some cases, a rumenotomy will be indicated if a wire foreign body is still protruding through the reticulum and was not retrieved through the pericardiotomy.

Postoperative Management

Postoperative antibiotics are administered. If drains have been placed in the wound, they are flushed daily with a mixed antibiotic-isotonic solution. These treatments are continued until it is judged either that the animal is overcoming the infectious process or that the animal should be sent to slaughter.

Complications and Prognosis

The prognosis for traumatic reticulopericarditis is poor. Long-term recovery is unusual because the resulting constrictive pericarditis is generally fatal.

References

1. Dyce, K.M., Sack, W.O., and Wensing, C.J.G.: Textbook of Veterinary Anatomy, 2nd Ed., Philadelphia, W.B. Saunders, 1996.
2. Horney, F.D.: Surgical drainage of the pericardial sac. Can. Vet. J., 1:363, 1960.
3. Mason, T.A.: Suppurative pericarditis treated by pericardiotomy in a cow. Vet. Rec., 105:350, 1979.
4. Noordsy, J.L.: The cardiovascular system. In Textbook of Large Animal Surgery. Edited by F.W. Oehme and J.E. Prier. Baltimore, Williams & Wilkins, 1974.
5. Rings, D.M.: Surgical treatment of pleuritis and pericarditis. Vet. Clin. Food Anim. Pract., 11:177–182, 1995.

Repair of Teat Lacerations

Relevant Anatomy

There are five primary layers to the lining of the teat: the innermost layers of mucosa and submucosa, a layer of highly vascularized conjunctive tissue, the muscularis, and the outermost layer of skin.[1] Proximally, the glandular cisterna collects the milk-gathering ducts. A narrowed portion of the cisterna, the annular relief, separates the glandular portion from the more distal papillary part.[1,2] The papillary part of the cisterna is comprised of longitudinal folds of mucosa that allow the cistern to expand to accommodate increases in volume. At the distal extremity of the teat, the internal opening of the papillary duct, called the *Furstenberg rosette*, probably functions to close the papillary duct between milkings and may also play an immune role in preventing infection.[1,2] The papillary duct, or teat canal, is the last portion of the mammary gland's excretory system that is held closed by a muscular sphincter.

The primary blood supply to the mammary gland of the cow is the pudendal artery, which enters the mammary gland through the inguinal canal and runs longitudinally down the teat. The artery divides into a large mammary artery that courses ventrocranially and a smaller mammary artery that runs caudally.[2] The pudendal vein drains the mammary gland and arises as a plexus from a vein encircling the sphincter and terminates at the base of the teat.[1]

Indications

Teat lacerations are common in dairy cows and can cause severe deficits in milk production. Lacerations that do not penetrate the mucosa of the teat generally heal rapidly by secondary intention with the aid of topical medication and bandaging. Teat lacerations that penetrate the mucosa of the teat require suturing to maintain normal teat function for milking and to prevent the development of teat fistulae or acute mastitis and loss of the quarter. As with any lacerations, early attention to the condition improves the success rate.

Diagnosis and treatment of teat disorders has advanced greatly since the first edition of this text. The most ideal suturing pattern for teat repair has been researched; radiography, ultrasound, and theloscopy have improved diagnostic capabilities; and surgical approaches have been refined to improve precision and reduce invasiveness. Obviously, not all this equipment is readily available to many practitioners, but the changes in technique are applicable and useful.

Anesthesia and Surgical Preparation

The methods of restraint and anesthesia are important in any teat surgery because the repair must be meticulous. A tilt table, ideal for restraint, generally is not available to most practitioners who must deal with teat lacerations in the field. Xylazine hydrochloride (Rompun) is a useful means of restraining the cow in lateral recumbency for teat surgery. Butorphanol (0.5 mg/kg) may be added for very fractious animals.[1] If the cow's disposition is good, teat surgery may be attempted with the cow in the standing position using local anesthesia, but results are more predictable if the cow is tabled or cast and is neither uneasy nor kicking. Local anesthetic injected around the base of the teat (circle or ring block) is the most common technique for anesthesia (Figure 15-5A). Epinephrine should not be used with the local anesthetic. Topical anesthetic can be infused directly into the teat canal to supplement ring block anesthesia. For topical anesthesia, 2% lidocaine (not procaine) should be used. Epidural anesthesia is an effective alternative for teat surgery (see Chapter 2).

To control hemorrhage and milk flow, a rubber tourniquet may be applied to the base of the teat. Doyen forceps clamped across the base of the teat can also be used successfully. When lacerations involve the base of the teat, suturing has to be performed without the benefit of a tourniquet.

The udder and surrounding teats should be washed thoroughly. Harsh disinfectants should be avoided because they can cause further tissue necrosis if they contact the lacerated tissue. The affected teat can be draped with a slit drape so that it protrudes from the opening in the drape. Once the borders of the laceration have been assessed carefully, a prognosis can usually be given.

Instrumentation

General surgery pack
Teat cannula (Larson's teat tube)

Surgical Technique

The wound edges should be freshened to remove any devitalized tissue and foreign material. Debridement is one of the most important procedures in repairing lacer-

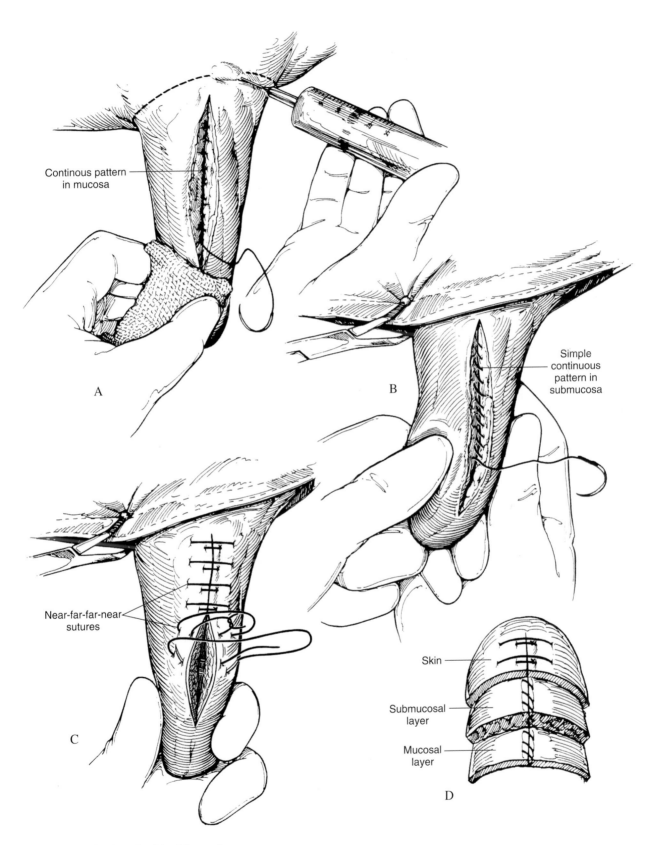

Continous pattern
in mucosa

A

B

Simple
continuous
pattern in
submucosa

Near-far-far-near
sutures

C

Skin

Submucosal
layer

Mucosal
layer

D

Fig. 15-5. A to D, Repair of teat laceration.

ated teats. Hemorrhage should be controlled because blood clots in the lumen of the teat delay healing by making milking painful and difficult for the animal.

The wound edges should be apposed under as little tension as possible. There have been many different closure techniques described in the literature for closure of teat lacerations. Evidence suggests that closure in three layers—the mucosa, muscular-submucosa, and skin—yields the most satisfactory healing.[1,3,4] The first layer closed is the mucosa. A simple continuous pattern using no. 3-0 or 4-0 synthetic, monofilament, absorbable suture material is generally preferred (Figure 15-5A).[1,3,4] When the mucosa has been closed, a teat cannula should be inserted through the teat sphincter, and the suture line should be gently probed to check its integrity. The second layer closed should be the submucosa. Again, this layer can be closed in a simple continuous pattern, using no. 3-0 or 4-0 synthetic, monofilament, absorbable suture material, and should support the delicate mucosal closure (Figure 15-5B). The remainder of the teat and the skin may be closed with a near-far-far-near or simple interrupted suture of nonabsorbable suture material, no. 0 or 2-0. This suture is placed so the deep bite is adjacent to the previously placed submucosal suture and the superficial layer is shallow (Figure 15-5C and D). The tourniquet should be removed following closure of the laceration, and, with gentle hand pressure applied to the teat, the suture line should be checked for milk leakage. Milk in the suture line will almost certainly result in a teat fistula.

Postoperative Management

Traditionally, a self-retaining teat tube, such as a Larson's teat tube, is inserted for about a week. The cap of the tube can be removed to permit the quarter to drain while the other quarters are being milked; this procedure takes advantage of the let-down phenomenon at the time of milking, or it can be left off permanently. The teat should not be hand-milked, but regular drainage is necessary to take the pressure off the suture line. If closure has been meticulous, as previously described, immediate machine-milking appears to have no adverse effects on healing.[1,4]

Intramammary antibiotics should be infused into the affected teat, and systemic antibiotics should be used as indicated. If the laceration is of some duration, mastitis will be present. This can be verified with the aid of a California Mastitis Test. Bacterial cultures and sensitivity testing are indicated in some cases.

The sutures are removed after aseptic preparation at about 8 to 10 days postoperatively to avoid inflammation and suture tract infection.[1]

Complications and Prognosis

Complications include excessive teat swelling and fibrous reaction that can impede milking. If the sutures are left in too long or the teat is handled excessively postoperatively, inflammation and infection may result.

Vertical lacerations have a better prognosis than do horizontal teat wounds because circulation to the wound edges is better. For the same reason, a V-shaped flap attached proximally has a better prognosis than a V-shaped flap attached distally. Lacerations at the distal end of the teat are considered to have a poorer prognosis because fibrosis in this area can interfere with milking. Similarly, lacerations at the base of the teat have a less favorable prognosis because they are susceptible to extensive hemorrhage due to their proximity to the pudendal venous ring.[1] Like other areas of the body, the prognosis for healing also depends greatly on the type of the injury (crushing injuries versus linear lacerations) and the degree of contamination present.

References

1. Couture, Y., and Mulon, P.Y.: Procedures and surgeries of the teat. Vet. Clin. Food Anim., 21:173–204, 2005.
2. Dyce, K.M., Sack, W.O., and Wensing, C.J.G.: Textbook of veterinary anatomy, 2nd Ed. Philadelphia, W.B. Saunders, 1996, pp. 727–736.
3. Ghamsari, S.M., Acorda, J.A., Taguchi, K., Abe, N., and Yamada, H.: Effect of different suture patterns on wound healing of the teat in dairy cattle. J. Vet. Med. Sci., 57:819–824, 1995.
4. Makady, F.M., Whitmore, H.L., Nelson, D.R., and Simon, J.: Effect of tissue adhesives and suture patterns on experimentally induced teat lacerations in lactating dairy cattle. J. Am. Vet. Med. Assoc., 11:1932–1934, 1991.

Chapter 16

SURGICAL TECHNIQUES IN SWINE

Objectives

1. Describe basic techniques for castration and inguinal herniorrhaphy in the piglet.
2. Describe a technique for cesarean section in the sow.

Castration of the Piglet

Relevant Anatomy

The testes of the boar are large in comparison to the bull, which is a direct reflection of sperm production. Located caudal to the thighs and ventral to the anus, the testes normally range from 10 to 15 cm in length and 5 to 9 cm in diameter.[5] The spermatic cord, usually 20 to 25 cm long, is comprised of the ductus deferens, testicular artery, testicular vein, lymphatics, testicular plexus of autonomic nerves, cremaster muscle, and visceral layer of the vaginal tunic. The epididymis is closely associated with the ventral aspect of the testis and terminates in the cauda epididymis at the dorsum of the testis where it becomes the ductus deferen.[5]

Indications

Generally, castration of the piglet is performed to improve the manageability of the herd; it also improves carcass quality because it removes taint. It is preferable to castrate piglets within the first 3 weeks of life. Research indicates that pain-associated behavioral responses do not differ between pigs castrated at 1, 5, 10, and 20 days. However, recorded data on pig weaning weights and weight gain appears to favor castration at 14 days rather than 1 day.[3,4] Although generally regarded as poor management, castration of larger pigs is occasionally indicated. The litter of piglets scheduled to be castrated should be clean and in good physical condition; if piglets in a litter are scouring, castration should be postponed. The area in which the castration is to be performed should be relatively clean and free of dust. If castration is to be performed in hot weather, it should be done early in the morning.

Anesthesia and Surgical Preparation

Surgical castration of piglets is a painful procedure at any age. The cutting of the spermatic cord has been identified as the most painful event. Appropriate anesthetic protocols are limited, however, due to cost effectiveness, ease and quickness of administration, and the quality of recovery. Recovery must be rapid and complete so the piglet does not develop postoperative hypothermia is not crushed by the sow.[1] For economical reasons, surgical castration of piglets younger than three weeks old is often performed without anesthesia. The herdsman restrains the piglet in a vertical position by the hindlegs by the hocks and securing the animal either against the herdsman's body or in a clean V-trough. Local analgesia is certainly indicated at this point and will help reduce stress on the animal. Intratesticular and intrafunicular administration of 2% lidocaine (4 mg/kg) were shown to be equally effective in reducing nociceptive pain responses in castrated piglets younger than 28 days old.[1] A technique for inhalational anesthesia in piglets has also been described with isoflurane, isoflurane/N_2O, and carbon dioxide.[6] It is important to note that, to date, the Food and Drug Administration has not approved an analgesic for use in meat-producing pigs in the United States. Furthermore, withdrawal times and food residues are not documented for these drugs. The practitioner is ultimately responsible for using these drugs judiciously in pigs destined for market.

Before beginning castration, the inguinal area should be carefully inspected for any evidence of inguinal hernia. Then, the inguinal and scrotal areas are scrubbed with a suitable disinfectant (Figure 16-1A).

Instrumentation

General surgery pack
No. 12 scalpel blades

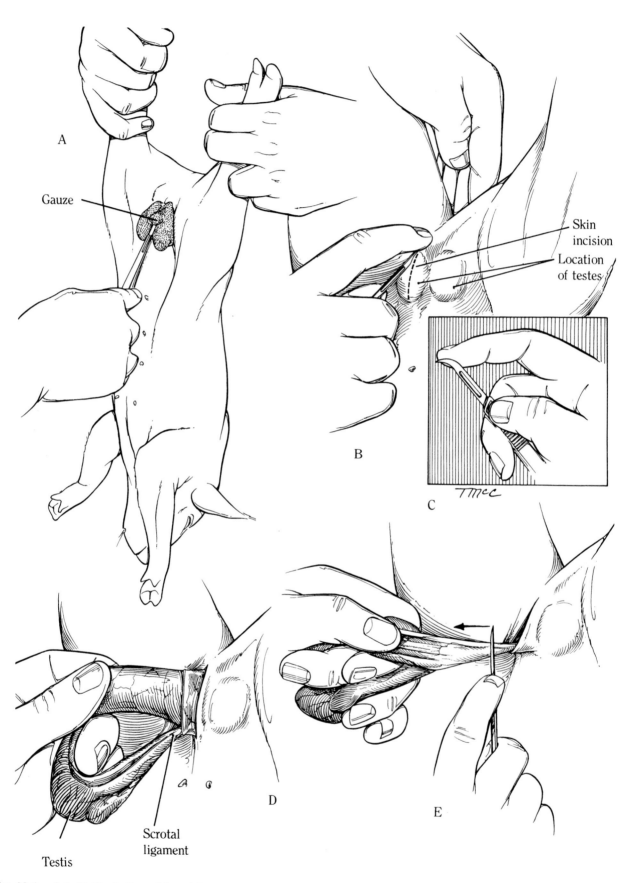

A

Gauze

B

Skin
incision

Location
of testes

C

D

Testis

Scrotal
ligament

E

Fig. 16-1. A to E, Castration of the piglet.

Surgical Technique

By pressing the fingers of the left hand into the animal's scrotum, the testes are pushed craniad into the inguinal area. A longitudinal incision through the skin, subcutaneous tissue, and fascia is made directly over each testis with a no. 12 scalpel blade (Figure 16-1B). (Figure 16-1C shows the method of holding the no. 12 scalpel blade and handle). Using blunt dissection with fingers, the surgeon grasps the testis in one hand while applying sufficient traction to break the scrotal ligament; this delivers the tunic-covered testis through the wound (Figure 16-1D). If the incision results in an open vaginal tunic, the tunic should be retrieved immediately to reduce the incidence of scirrhous cord. Traction on the testis is maintained by the left hand while a sterile scalpel blade is used to scrape and sever the tunic and cord structures. The scraping should be performed as proximal as possible on the cord, so the severed end of the cord retracts into the inguinal region. This reduces the chances of infection and scirrhous cord formation. To minimize the chances of accidentally lacerating the piglet in some other area, the scraping should be performed in a direction *away* from the animal (Figure 16-1E). This procedure is repeated on the opposite testis. The resulting incisions are located cranial to the normal position of the testes, to provide adequate ventral drainage. The left-handed operator uses the right hand to press the testis forward and holds the scalpel in his left hand.

Postoperative Management

Some surgeons prefer to dust the surgical site with an antibacterial powder; this is generally unnecessary if piglets can be turned into a clean, dry pen. The piglets should not be allowed into dirty quarters until healing is complete, usually within 5 to 7 days. If there is evidence of inguinal-scrotal hernia, the entire spermatic cord should be transfixed and ligated before it is severed (see the discussion in this chapter of inguinal herniorrhaphy in the piglet).

If intratesticular anesthesia is used to castrate boars, the testes must be disposed of carefully.

Complications and Prognosis

The prognosis for this procedure is very good. Occasionally, death may result due to intestinal prolapse from an undetected inguinal hernia. Complications most commonly associated with this procedure are abscess and behavioral side effects, including reductions in suckling time and increased lying time.[4]

References

1. Haga, H.A., and Ranheim, B.: Castration of piglets: the analgesic effects of intratesticular and intrafunicular lidocaine injection. Vet. Anaes. Analg., 32:1–9, 2005.
2. Henry, D.P.: Anesthesia of boars by intratesticular injection. Aust. Vet. J., 44:418, 1968.
3. McGlone, J.J., and Hellman, J.M.: Local and general anesthetic effects on behavior and performance of two- and seven-week-old castrated and uncastrated piglets. J. Anim. Sci., 66:3049–3058, 1988.
4. McGlone, J.J., Nicholson, R.I., Hellman, J.M., and Herzog, D.N.: The development of pain in young pigs associated with castration and attempts to prevent castration-induced behavioral changes. J. Anim. Sci., 71:1441–1446, 1993.
5. Powe, T.A.: Anatomy of the scrotum, testes, epididymis, and spermatic cord in swine. In Large Animal Urogenital Surgery. Edited by D.F. Wolfe and H.D. Moll. Baltimore, Williams & Wilkins, 1999. pp. 217.
6. Walker, B., Jaggin, N., Doherr, M., and Schatzmann, U.: Inhalational anaesthesia for castration of newborn piglets: experiences with isoflurane and isoflurane/N₂O. J. Vet. Med., 51:150–154, 2004.

Inguinal Herniorrhaphy in the Piglet

Relevant Anatomy

The inguinal canal is described as a potential space communicating between the internal and external abdominal oblique muscles.[1] The internal inguinal ring, formed by the internal oblique muscle and the inguinal ligament, leads from the canal into the abdominal cavity. An invagination of peritoneum into the scrotum, the vaginal ring, extends into the internal ring. A larger than normal vaginal ring is believed to predispose some male piglets to inguinal hernias. The superficial inguinal ring is formed by an opening in the external oblique muscle near the pecten pubis. Anatomical differences specific to swine include a larger deep (internal) ring and a relatively short inguinal canal.[1]

Indications

Frequently, inguinal hernias are discovered in piglets at the time of castration. These hernias generally do not reduce spontaneously, and when the ordinary castration procedure is used, evisceration is a frequent postcastration complication. The economics of hernia repair in the pig should be discussed with the client before surgery is undertaken.

Anesthesia and Surgical Preparation

For practical and economic reasons, no anesthetic is used routinely for small piglets; however, larger pigs require anesthesia similar to that used for castration of large pigs. The pig is restrained in a vertical position by the herdsman or by ropes in a clean V-trough, if the pig is too large. The skin of the inguinal and scrotal areas is scrubbed with a suitable antiseptic.

Instrumentation

General surgery pack

Surgical Technique

An incision approximately 7 cm long is made through the skin, subcutaneous tissues, and fascia over the external inguinal ring (Figure 16-2A). Extensive hernias may require a larger incision. The testis, spermatic cord, and surrounding fascia are isolated using blunt dissection. Steady traction is exerted on the testis, tunics, and cord, pulling them loose from their attachment in the scrotum (scrotal ligament) (Figure 16-2B). The freed vaginal tunic should not be incised. By grasping the testis, the surgeon twists the vaginal sac, to return the intestines to the abdomen. Fingers may be used to "milk" the intestines into the abdomen. A pair of Kelly forceps is used to grasp the sac while a transfixation ligature is applied on the proximal end of the cord just distal to the inguinal ring (Figure 16-2C). Generally, the ligature is of strong, absorbable suture material, such as no. 0 or 1 synthetic absorbable suture (Figure 16-2D). At this point, some operators prefer to anchor the hernia sac to the inguinal ring with the ends of the transfixation ligature. The testis and excess spermatic cord are removed (Figure 16-2E).

The skin incision may be partially closed with absorbable suture material, or it may be left completely open to allow ventral drainage. Because hernias may be hereditary, the bilateral castration of hernia-affected pigs is recommended. Hernias may be bilateral, so one should also transfix the cord of the opposite side, to prevent postoperative herniation.

Postoperative Management

The surgical site may be dusted with a suitable antibacterial powder. This is generally unnecessary if piglets can be turned into a clean, dry pen. The piglets should not be allowed in dirty quarters until healing is complete. A heat lamp is also recommended.

Complications and Prognosis

The prognosis of this procedure depends on the extent of the hernia; eviscerated inguinal hernias where the intestine has become edematous have a high rate of complications. Chronic inguinal hernias can result in intestinal incarceration and strangulation, which would necessitate resection and anastomosis. Other complications include wound infection and peritonitis.

Reference

1. Sack, W.O.: Essentials of pig anatomy. Ithaca, Veterinary Textbooks, 1982.

Cesarean Section in the Sow

Relevant Anatomy

Sows can farrow up to 25 fetuses with 12 to 13 in each horn. At the end of pregnancy, the uterine horns may occupy most of the ventral half of the abdomen. In this species, the uterine body is short but may appear longer in vivo because the uterine horns continue cranially a few centimeters before bifurcating. During a cesarean section, the surgeon should be aware of the thick layer of adipose tissue encountered before peritoneum. The neophyte surgeon may confuse the extensive subperitoneal fat for omentum with adhesions.

Indications

Cesarean section in the sow is indicated for the relief of dystocia. The following are common causes of dystocia: uterine inertia; excessive adipose tissue around the birth canal; relative fetal oversize in small, immature sows; fetal monsters; and malformation of the birth canal due to previous pelvic fractures or injuries during previous parturitions. Cesarean section is also indicated for the production of specific-pathogen-free (SPF) piglets.

The operation is successful if done early in the parturition process; however, the large animal surgeon frequently is presented with an exhausted animal subjected to numerous attempts to remove the piglets manually. Generally, tissue damage to the birth canal is considerable, and emphysematous fetuses may be present in such cases. These sows are frequently in a state of endotoxic shock and are poor risks for surgery.

Instrumentation

General surgery pack

Anesthesia and Surgical Preparation

The sow is positioned in lateral recumbency, and ropes are tied to its feet if necessary. Adequate restraint is essential, so aseptic technique is not compromised. Once the sow has been placed in either left- or right-lateral recumbency, the surgical site is prepared. Local or regional anesthesia in the form of a line block, an inverted L block, or an epidural block may be administered at this time (alternate sedative and general anesthetic techniques are presented in Chapter 2, "Anesthesia and Fluid Therapy"). Azaperone may be used for chemical restraint of the sow as well. This drug does cross the placental barrier, resulting in minor sedation of the piglet. However, respiratory depression in the piglet is usually low and the prognosis for survival is good. To avoid serious complications, the dose should be kept minimal (max dose 8 mg/kg i.m.). If additional sedation is needed, thiopental or metomidate may be administered intravenously.

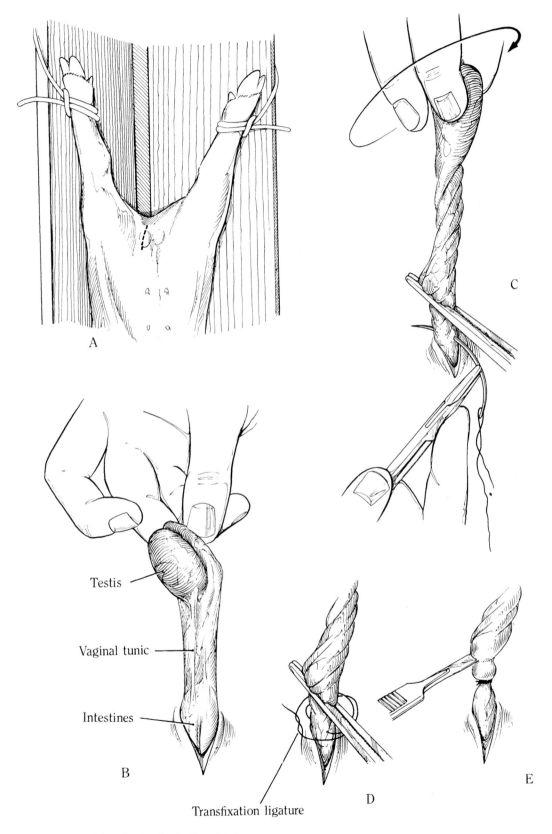

Testis

Vaginal tunic

Intestines

B

C

Transfixation ligature

D

E

A

Fig. 16-2. A to E, Inguinal herniorrhaphy in the piglet.

Three basic types of incisions are used for cesarean section in sows: the first is a vertical incision, either in the left or right paralumbar fossa and flank region; and the second is a horizontal incision in the ventral paralumbar area about 6 to 8 cm above the well-developed mammary tissue (Figure 16-3). The third, ventral midline incision, which we do not describe in this chapter, allows access to both uterine horns, but it is awkward to position the sow for this incision.

The surgical site is clipped, but shaving is generally unnecessary. Local anesthetic is administered, depending on which approach is to be used (we prefer the vertical incision). The surgical site is given an additional scrub and is prepared for aseptic surgery in a routine manner.

Surgical Technique

The following technique is for the vertical incision. The surgeon makes a 20-cm vertical skin incision that commences 6 to 8 cm ventral to the transverse processes of the lumbar vertebrae, midway between the last rib and the thigh muscles. The incision is continued through the skin, subcutaneous adipose tissue, muscles of the flank, subperitoneal adipose tissue, and peritoneum. The abdominal cavity is explored for the bifurcation of the uterus. The surgeon makes a 15- to 20-cm incision through the uterine wall, as close to the body of the uterus as possible, being careful not to cut one of the piglets. If the bifurcation can be located, the entire litter can be brought out through one incision. This leaves only one uterine incision to close and decreases surgery time. If this is not possible, an incision is made in each uterine horn close to the bifurcation, and the piglets are removed from each horn separately. If an assistant is present, piglets can be massaged down the uterine lumen toward the incision as the others are removed, but it is generally necessary for the surgeon to reach up into each uterine horn in search of more piglets while pulling the uterine walls up the surgeon's arms as one would pull on the arms of a thick woolen sweater. Great care should be exercised in exposing the ovarian end of each uterine horn. Its attachment is friable in the sow, and if one is not careful, the ovarian artery may be easily torn, possibly resulting in fatal hemorrhage. One should be sure to explore the vaginal canal for remaining piglets, and any loose placentae are removed.

Dead and emphysematous piglets usually have their corresponding placentae detached and are easily removed. Prior to closure of the uterine incisions, any intrauterine medication is administered. The uterus is closed with any of the inverting patterns described in the discussion of bovine cesarean section in Chapter 14, "Bovine Urogenital Surgery." If infection is present, a two-layer closure is recommended.[1] The uterine horns are placed in the abdominal cavity individually, making sure they are not twisted.

The combined muscle and subcutaneous layers are closed as one, using no. 0 or 1 synthetic absorbable suture material in a simple continuous pattern. The skin is closed with an interlocking pattern using polymerized caprolactam in a manner similar to closure of the bovine flank.

Postoperative Management

During closure of the uterus and body wall, an assistant should dry the piglets vigorously and should place them in warm surroundings. Once surgery is completed, the

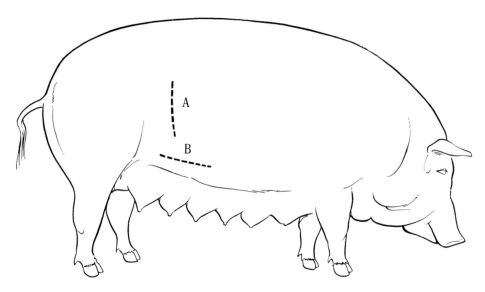

Fig. 16-3. Cesarean section in the sow.

sow is moved to a clean, dry pen, and the piglets are placed beside the sow.

Toxic patients should receive pre- and postoperative antibiotics, as well as other forms of supportive therapy for shock, such as intravenous fluids. Oxytocin can aid in contraction of the uterus and in milk let-down.

Complications and Prognosis

As mentioned previously, incorrect surgical technique or manipulation of the uterine horns may result in rupture of the ovarian artery and hemorrhage. Other potential complications include wound infection and peritonitis.

To the author's knowledge, there are no reports of survival rates for this procedure. However, assuming aseptic technique is used and little contamination occurs, the prognosis for the sow is good and most of the piglets should be successfully recovered.

Reference

1. Hokanson, J.F.: Surgery; female genital tract; experimental and miscellaneous. *In* Diseases of Swine, 4th Ed. Edited by H.W. Dunn and A.D. Leman. Ames, Iowa State University Press, 1975.

Chapter 17

MISCELLANEOUS SURGICAL TECHNIQUES

Objective

1. Describe some of the common surgical procedures in various food animals, including dehorning of the mature goat and tooth extraction in the llama.

Dehorning the Mature Goat

Relevant Anatomy

Unlike cattle, the horns of the goat are innervated by two separate cornual branches, one originating from the lacrimal nerve and the other from the infratrochlear nerve. The cornual branch of the lacrimal nerve runs superficially across the supraorbital process and may be blocked halfway between the lateral canthus of the eye and the lateral base of the horn.[3] The infratrochlear nerve may be blocked between the medial canthus of the eye and the base of the horn on the medial side.[3] The cornual artery branches, located at the ventral edge of the horns, are of particular concern for hemorrhage during this procedure.

Indications

The mature goat is dehorned if its horn(s) are broken or to reduce the danger to man and other animals. Some breed societies require dehorning to register the goat, although flock goats are generally left horned as protection from predators. Dehorning of male goats is sometimes combined with removal of the scent (horn) glands to reduce odor.[1,2] Dehorning may have profound side effects that the goat owner should be aware of: reduction in milk production, impairment of spermatogenesis, sinusitis and myiasis, and loss of social status in the herd. The surgery should be planned to minimize these effects. For prevention of myiasis, the procedure should be reserved for the cooler months.[1]

Anesthesia and Surgical Preparation

As with other ruminants, food should be withheld from the goat for 12 to 24 hours before surgery to avoid ruminal tympany, regurgitation, and possible aspiration pneumonia if general anesthesia is administered.

Goats do not tolerate pain associated with even minor surgical procedures and can die of shock if sufficient analgesia is not provided. Although the exact cause of this shock is not known, it is believed to be a reaction to intense fear or fright from a combination of restraint and pain.[1] All goats should be anesthetized or deeply sedated before dehorning; refer to Chapter 2, "Anesthesia and Fluid Therapy," for details of anesthetic techniques in goats.

Sedation needs to be supplemented with local analgesia of the horn. Once the goat is recumbent, the head region is clipped and prepared for a cornual nerve block and infratrochlear nerve block. The cornual branch of the lacrimal nerve is blocked by injecting 2 ml of local anesthetic as close as possible to the caudal ridge of the root of the supraorbital process to a depth of 1 to 1.5 cm. The cornual branch of the infratrochlear nerve is also blocked by injecting 2 ml of local anesthetic at the dorsomedial margin of the orbit. In larger goats, a ring block around the entire base of the horn may be necessary (Figure 17-1A). Lidocaine should be used judiciously in goats to avoid toxicity and the minimal dose should be used (see Chapter 2). While the anesthesia is taking effect, the area around the horn is prepared for aseptic surgery.

Instrumentation

General surgery pack
Obstetric wire saw, Gigli wire saw, or dehorning saw
Hemostats

Surgical Technique

The skin is incised 1 cm from the base of the horn. Enough skin must be removed from the caudolateral and caudomedial areas, where scars are likely to occur

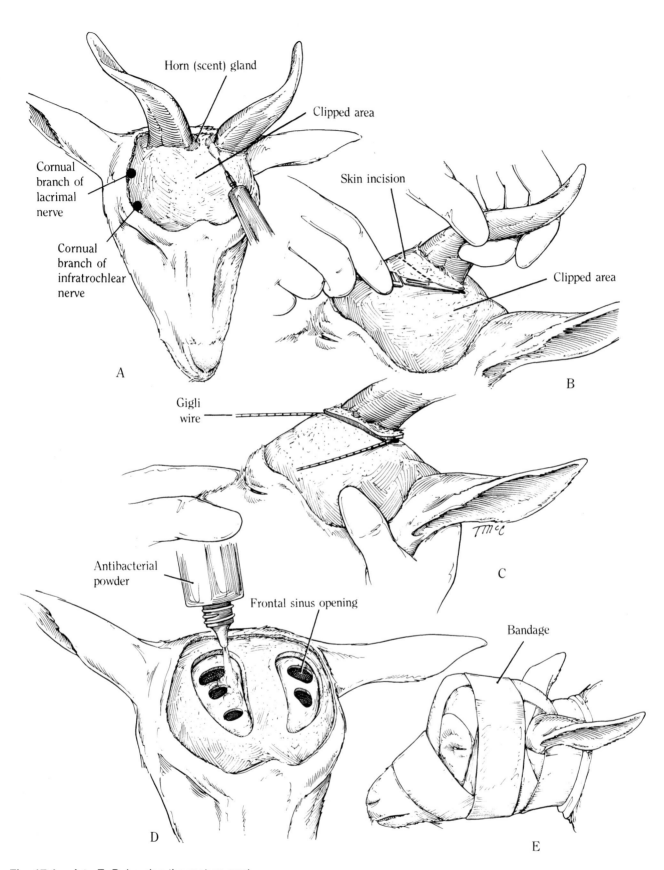

Fig. 17-1. A to E, Dehorning the mature goat.

(Figure 17-1*B*). While an assistant supports the goat's head, the surgeon seats an obstetric wire saw or Gigli wire saw in the caudomedial aspect of the incision and removes the horn by directing the saw in a craniolateral direction (Figure 17-1*C*). Some surgeons prefer a dehorning saw because it has less tendency to break and is less likely to leave a protuberance in the middle of the horn that may grow back.[1]

In male goats, the scent glands are located at the base of each horn (caudal and medial) and generally are removed during the dehorning procedure. Hemorrhage from the superficial temporal artery can be severe and should be stopped by ligating the artery or by pulling and twisting it with a hemostat.

When a goat is dehorned correctly, its frontal sinuses are exposed because of the extensive communication between the lumen of the cornual process and the frontal sinus. The head may be bandaged postoperatively to prevent both myiasis and the collection of foreign material in the sinus. Prior to bandaging, a topical antibacterial powder, such as nitrofurazone, is dusted onto the dehorning site (Figure 17-1*D* and *E*). Bandaging is not accepted by everyone. Some surgeons believe that the wound should not be covered and should be allowed to remain dry. If the wound is neglected, myiasis can develop under the bandage, and the consequences may be more serious than if the wound were left open.

Postoperative Management

Tetanus prophylaxis should be performed. If the animal's head is bandaged, the first bandage should be changed on the second postoperative day and replaced. The second bandage is left on for an additional 5 to 6 days. After this time, healing is generally sufficient, so the bandage can be removed completely.

In the summer, when flies are a problem, prevention of myiasis is important for several more weeks. The goat should be housed in an area free of dust and isolated from dirty surroundings. It is also advisable that the goat does not mix with other members of the herd until the wound has healed. Any abnormal odor, purulent nasal discharge, head shaking, or rubbing are often indications of frontal sinusitis, which necessitates removal of the bandage and treatment.

Complications and Prognosis

Dehorning can result in a reduction in milk production, impairment of spermatogenesis, sinusitis, myiasis, and loss of social status in the herd. Life-threatening complications are rare and the prognosis is good.

References

1. Bowen, J.S.: Dehorning the mature goat. J. Am. Vet. Med. Assoc., *171*:1249, 1977.
2. Guss, S.B.: Management and Diseases of Dairy Goats. Scottsdale, Arizona, Dairy Goat Journal Publishing, 1977.
3. Hull, B.L.: Dehorning the adult goat. Vet. Clin. Food Anim., *11*:183–185, 1995.

Tooth Removal in the Llama

Relevant Anatomy

The dental formula of the adult llama is I(1/3) – C(1/1) – PM (1-2/1-2) – M(3/3).[2] The shape and direction of the root of the canine teeth in llamas are important considerations to facilitate atraumatic removal of these teeth. The dentition of the llama is shown in Figure 17-2. The root of the canine follows a caudal direction, a factor important at the time of tooth removal.

Indications

As a management tool to prevent fighting, removal of canine teeth of the llama may be necessary. The other indication for removal of canine teeth is a tooth root abscess. A root abscess may occur secondary to partial removal, in which the crown has been amputated and the pulp cavity is exposed. Partial amputation is done to minimize injuries inflicted to other herd members. Infection subsequently migrates down the pulp cavity. Removal of molar teeth is usually to resolve a root abscess. The common causes of root abscesses of the molars are broken teeth. Some abscesses are caused by actinomycosis (resembling "lumpy jaw" in cattle), whereas others are spontaneous, with no apparent cause. Signs of a tooth problem include swelling of the mandible, pain, head shyness, a draining fistula, or impaired mastication. Radiographs of the affected tooth show varying degrees of bone lysis at the tooth root. Animals with chronic cases have radiographic evidence of increased bone density (sclerosis) surrounding the tooth root.

As with horses, endodontic therapy is an alternative to tooth removal that may be used in camelids as well. This technique is considered advanced, however, and is not described here.

Anesthesia and Surgical Preparation

Tooth removal in the llama is performed with the animal under general anesthesia. Xylazine, in combination with local anesthesia, has been used by some surgeons, but inhalation anesthesia (halothane) is preferred. The llama is given a guaifenesin-ketamine or guaifenesin-thiamylal combination intravenously to effect, an endotracheal tube is placed, and halothane-oxygen is administered. The llama is positioned in lateral recumbency with the affected tooth uppermost. A mouth speculum, similar to that used in dogs, is positioned to allow the surgeon free access to the incisor teeth or the ability to palpate the affected molar tooth. If a canine tooth is to be removed,

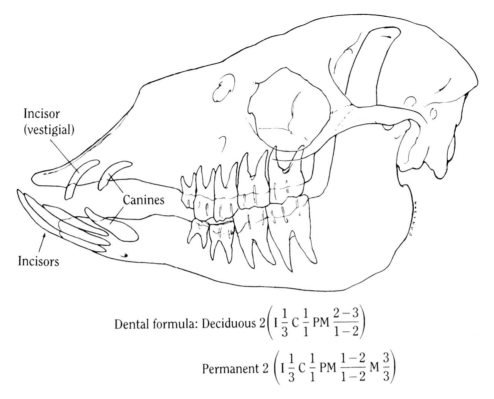

Dental formula: Deciduous $2\left(I\frac{1}{3}\ C\frac{1}{1}\ PM\frac{2-3}{1-2}\right)$

Permanent $2\left(I\frac{1}{3}\ C\frac{1}{1}\ PM\frac{1-2}{1-2}\ M\frac{3}{3}\right)$

Fig. 17-2. Dentition of the llama (*Lama glama*).

the mucosa around the tooth is surgically prepared. If a molar tooth is to be removed, the hair over the surgical site is clipped, and routine surgical preparation is performed. The exact location of the surgical site is determined by the position of the affected molar on radiographs.

Instrumentation

General surgery pack
Mouth speculum (canine mouth gag)
Small mallet
Chisel (approximately 1/4-in width)
Curette
Dental punch
Small periosteal elevator
Forceps

Surgical Technique

Removal of Canine Teeth

For removal of a canine tooth, a fusiform incision is made through the mucous membrane around the tooth and is extended down to the mandibular bone (Figure 17-3A and B). A second incision is made directly over the tooth, curving caudad, in the direction of the long axis of the tooth (Figure 17-3B). Using a periosteal elevator, the surgeon reflects the gingiva and periosteum away from the lateral surface of the mandible, in the direction of the tooth root. Similar elevation is performed on the medial side of the tooth extending about 1/8 of an inch from the gum-tooth margin. A segment of bone on the lateral side of the tooth is then removed (Figure 17-3C). Periosteum may first be reflected from this region, but this is not critical. This lateral bone is removed because this is the direction in which the tooth will be extracted. The use of a chisel on the lingual side of the tooth facilitates removal of the tooth. Knowledge of the direction of the canine tooth root is important for atraumatic removal of this tooth. As bone is removed, the tooth should be grasped periodically and moved in a side-to-side motion, to ascertain when it is ready for extraction. Eventually, the tooth can be extracted without risking fracture of the mandible. The alveolus is then curetted, to remove all diseased bone associated with the root abscess (Figure 17-3D). Debris is flushed from the site with sterile saline solution. The gingiva is then apposed over the empty socket using 2-0 synthetic, absorbable, monofilament suture (Figure 17-3E).

If the equipment is available, a Hall air drill with the appropriate bur can be used to remove the bone from the lateral surface of the canine tooth. Most important is the position of the canine tooth root within the bone. The tooth root is extensive and follows a marked caudal direction.

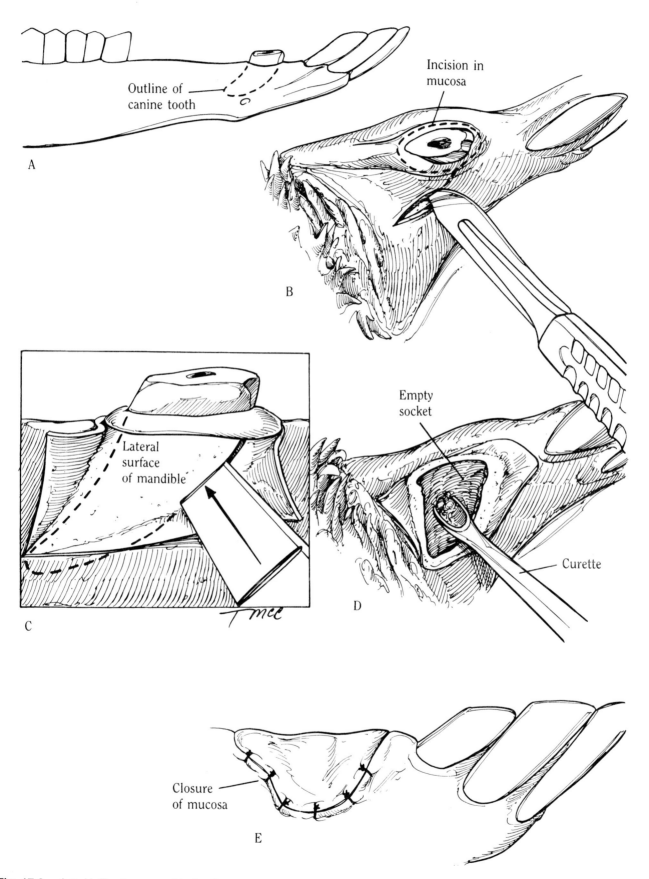

A

Outline of
canine tooth

Incision in
mucosa

B

Lateral
surface
of mandible

C

Empty
socket

Curette

D

Closure
of mucosa

E

Fig. 17-3. A to H, Tooth removal in the llama.

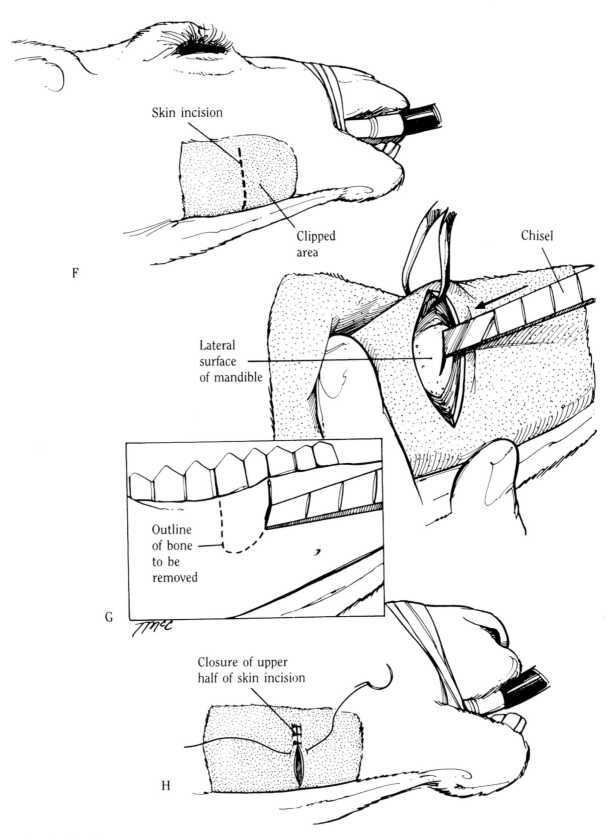

Skin incision

Clipped area

F

Lateral surface of mandible

Chisel

Outline of bone to be removed

G

Closure of upper half of skin incision

H

Fig. 17-3. *Continued.*

Removal of Molar Teeth

The exact location of the affected tooth is confirmed on the radiographs and by palpation of the crown of the tooth with the fingertips. A straight incision is made directly over the longitudinal axis of the tooth (Figure 17-3*F*). The periosteum is reflected (optional). The bone lateral to the tooth is removed, but the bone immediately ventral to the tooth is preserved (Figure 17-3*G*). The tooth should be freed of bone at its rostral and caudal surfaces using a chisel. A dental punch is placed on the tooth root, and with gentle tapping, it seats itself into the root of the tooth. The surgeon should place his fingertips over the crown of the tooth and guide the punch with the other hand. An assistant then delivers the blows to the punch. The surgeon feels the vibrations of the blows transmitted through the tooth to his fingertips. Occasionally, the punch has to be redirected. The tooth gradually loosens, and the blows of the mallet should then become less forceful. Conversely, a hole can be made over the affected roots with a trephine or hall air drill.

Following repulsion of the tooth, any small fragments of bone or teeth are removed. The alveolus is curetted and is flushed. The ventral half of the incision is left open to provide ventral drainage of the alveolus. The upper half is closed with simple interrupted sutures with nonabsorbable suture material (Figure 17-3*H*).

Postoperative Management

The llama should be placed on antibiotics preoperatively and for approximately 1 to 2 weeks following surgery. The wound where the canine tooth has been removed usually requires little postoperative care. Following molar extraction, the alveolus can be flushed daily with a mild antiseptic solution or until granulation tissue has begun to fill the defect.

Complications and Prognosis

We have seen uncomplicated healing after removal of canine and molar teeth. Daily flushing of the alveolus seems to keep food and debris from lodging in the wound in the case of molar teeth. This sort of aftercare can be performed by the owner. Reports of success and complication rates of tooth extraction in llamas are rare, but one study showed a unanimous success of surgical extraction for treatment of tooth abscesses with very few complications.[1] Medical treatment of tooth abscessation resulted in recurrence of symptoms in some animals.

References

1. Cebra, M.L., Cebra, M.K., and Garry, F.B.: Tooth root abscesses in New World camelids: 23 cases (1972–1994). J. Am. Vet. Med. Assoc., *209*:819–822, 1996.
2. Turner, A.S.: Surgical conditions in the llama. Vet. Clin. Food Anim., *5*:81–99, 1989.

Index

Page numbers in *italics* indicate figures; those followed by t indicate tables.